Ultrasonography in Urology
A Practical Approach to Clinical Problems

Second Edition

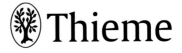

Ultrasonography in Urology
A Practical Approach to Clinical Problems

Second Edition

Edward I. Bluth, M.D., F.A.C.R.
Chairman Emeritus
Department of Radiology
Ochsner Health System
New Orleans, Louisiana

Carol B. Benson, M.D.
Professor
Department of Radiology
Harvard Medical School
Director of Ultrasound
Co-Director of High Risk Obstetrical Ultrasound
Brigham and Women's Hospital
Boston, Massachusetts

Philip W. Ralls, M.D.
Professor and Vice Chair
Department of Radiology
Keck School of Medicine
University of Southern California
Los Angeles, California

Marilyn J. Siegel, M.D.
Professor
Departments of Radiology and Pediatrics
Washington University School of Medicine
Division of Diagnostic Radiology
Mallinckrodt Institute of Radiology
Saint Louis, Missouri

Thieme
New York • Stuttgart

Thieme Medical Publishers, Inc.
333 Seventh Ave.
New York, NY 10001

Editor: Timothy Hiscock
Editorial Assistant: David Price
Vice President, Production and Electronic Publishing: Anne T. Vinnicombe
Production Editor: Print Matters, Inc.
Vice President, International Marketing: Cornelia Schulze
Chief Financial Officer: Peter van Woerden
President: Brian D. Scanlan
Compositor: Compset, Inc.
Printer: Everbest Printing Co.

Library of Congress Cataloging-in-Publication Data

Ultrasonography in urology / [edited by] Edward I. Bluth . . . [et al.]. — 2nd ed.
    p. ; cm.
    Includes bibliographical references and index.
    ISBN 978–1-58890–609-0 (alk. paper)

    1. Urology. 2. Diagnosis, Ultrasonic. I. Bluth, Edward I.
    [DNLM: 1. Urologic Diseases—ultrasonography. 2. Diagnosis, Differential. 3. Genital Diseases,
Female—ultrasonography. 4. Genital Diseases, Male—ultrasonography. 5. Pain—ultrasonography. 6.
Ultrasonography—methods. WJ 141 U47 2007]
    RC874.U35 2007
    616.6'07543—dc22   2007015101

Important note: Medical knowledge is ever-changing. As new research and clinical experience broaden
our knowledge, changes in treatment and drug therapy may be required. The authors and editors of the
material herein have consulted sources believed to be reliable in their efforts to provide information that
is complete and in accord with the standards accepted at the time of publication. However, in view of the
possibility of human error by the authors, editors, or publisher of the work herein or changes in medical
knowledge, neither the authors, editors, or publisher, nor any other party who has been involved in the
preparation of this work, warrants that the information contained herein is in every respect accurate or
complete, and they are not responsible for any errors or omissions or for the results obtained from use of
such information. Readers are encouraged to confirm the information contained herein with other
sources. For example, readers are advised to check the product information sheet included in the package
of each drug they plan to administer to be certain that the information contained in this publication is
accurate and that changes have not been made in the recommended dose or in the contraindications for
administration. This recommendation is of particular importance in connection with new or infrequently
used drugs.

Some of the product names, patents, and registered designs referred to in this book are in fact registered
trademarks or proprietary names even though specific reference to this fact is not always made in the
text. Therefore, the appearance of a name without designation as proprietary is not to be construed as a
representation by the publisher that it is in the public domain.

Printed in China

5 4 3 2 1

The Americas   ISBN 978-1-58890-609-0
Rest of the World   ISBN 978-3-13-129132-5

We dedicate this book to our families and friends, who supported us in this project:

Ed Bluth to Elissa, Rachel, Jonathan, Marjorie, Irene, and Lawry
with gratitude and love.

Carol Benson to her husband, Peter, and her children, Nicole and Benjamin.

Phil Ralls to Renee, Colin, and Whitney with love.

Marilyn Siegel to her husband, Barry.

Contents

Preface ix

Contributors x

1 Flank Pain. 1
   Lisa Lihuan Wang and Sharlene A. Teefey

2 Renal Failure. 12
   John J. Cronan

3 Hematuria. 20
   Robert L. Bree

4 Acute Abdominal Trauma. 29
   W. Dennis Foley

5 Acute Scrotal Pain: Diagnosing with Color Duplex Sonography 37
   Thomas A. Stavros and Cynthia L. Rapp

6 Erectile Dysfunction 58
   Harvey L. Nisenbaum and Steven C. Horii

7 Urinary Tract Infections in Children. 76
   Harriet J. Paltiel

8 Right Lower Quadrant Pain: Ruling Out Appendicitis 89
   Lawrence C. Chow and R. Jeffrey Brooke Jr.

9 Hypertension and Bruit 97
   Laurence Needleman

10 Elevated PSA and/or Abnormal Prostate Physical Examinations: 111
   Diagnosing Prostate Cancer
   Ulrike Hamper

11 Intraoperative Ultrasound. 123
   Robert A. Kane

12 Leg Swelling with Pain or Edema. 140
   Edward I. Bluth

13 Biopsy, Drainage, and Percutaneous Treatment of a Mass. 156
   Gerald D. Dodd III and Hayden Head

Index 165

Preface

We have been pleased by the considerable popularity achieved by the first edition of *Ultrasonography in Urology: A Practical Approach to Clinical Problems*. The second edition builds on the foundation that was originally laid at the Special Course on Ultrasound at the Meeting of the Radiological Society of North America in 1996, and then was further developed in the first edition of this text published in 2000. This new edition greatly expands and updates that previous work.

The overall aim of this textbook is to help the clinician assess and decide whether sonography or another imaging modality is the most appropriate for evaluating a clinical problem. In contrast to standard textbooks, our chapters are divided according to clinical questions rather than by organ systems. Our aim is to review the most important clinical issues faced by clinicians in their daily practice and to outline approaches for the effective use of sonography and other imaging modalities. Most chapters in the second edition have been extensively revised with new illustrations and images being added. The authors have attempted to incorporate the latest advances in ultrasound as well as to revise earlier recommendations based on advances in MRI, CT, and PET.

All of the authors are recognized authorities in the fields of ultrasound and radiology. The role of the radiologist and sonologist is changing. It is important to develop not only accurate diagnostic skills but also the appropriate consultative skills to help direct the workup of clinical problems. It is hoped that this textbook will assist radiologists, residents, medical students, and midlevel providers in developing their consultative skills regarding the use of ultrasound.

Each chapter includes practical, technical sonographic hints for studying an area or problem, basic sonographic anatomy, and the sonographic findings that can be seen in different clinical entities with the same clinical presentation. Additionally, the authors have included their recommendations regarding the use of alternative imaging modalities for solving clinical problems. The intended outcome is for the clinician to receive guidance in directing the imaging workup and in selecting the best imaging examination for a given clinical problem.

Although some of what is included in this book might be considered an opinion, our goal for the second edition of *Ultrasonography in Urology: A Practical Approach to Clinical Problems* is to provide a readable and manageable book which will offer guidance for clinicians and diagnosticians on the appropriate use of sonography to solve important clinical problems.

Acknowledgments

The authors would like to thank Drs. Peter Arger, Barbara Hertzberg, William Middleton, and Carol Stelling for their help with the conceptual origins for this project. Additionally, the authors would like to thank Dr. Peter Arger for his role as an editor of the first edition.

Contributors

Edward I. Bluth, M.D., F.A.C.R.
Chairman Emeritus
Department of Radiology
Ochsner Health System
New Orleans, Louisiana

Robert L. Bree, M.D., M.H.S.A., F.A.C.R.
Medical Director
Department of Diagnostic Imaging
Providence Everett Medical Center
Everett, Washington

R. Jeffrey Brooke Jr., M.D.
Professor
Department of Radiology
Stanford University Medical Center
Stanford, California

Lawrence C. Chow, M.D.
Associate Professor
Department of Radiology
Oregon Health and Science University
Portland, Oregon

John J. Cronan, M.D.
Professor and Chairman
Department of Diagnostic Imaging
Alpert Medical School
Brown University
Rhode Island Hospital
Providence, Rhode Island

Gerald D. Dodd III, M.D.
Professor and Chair
Department of Radiology
University of Texas Health Science Center at San Antonio
San Antonio, Texas

W. Dennis Foley, M.D.
Professor
Department of Radiology
Medical College of Wisconsin
Milwaukee, Wisconsin

Ulrike Hamper, M.D.
Professor and Director of Radiology
Department of Radiology
The Johns Hopkins University School of Medicine
Baltimore, Maryland

Hayden Head, M.D., Ph.D.
Resident
Department of Radiology
University of Texas Health and Science Center
   at San Antonio
San Antonio, Texas

Steven C. Horii, M.D.
Professor of Radiology
Department of Radiology
University of Pennsylvania School of Medicine
Philadelphia, Pennsylvania

Robert A. Kane, M.D., F.A.C.R.
Associate Chief
Department of Radiology
Director of Ultrasound
Harvard Medical School
Beth Israel Deaconess Medical Center
Boston, Massachusetts

Laurence Needleman, M.D.
Associate Professor
Department of Radiology
Jefferson Medical College
Thomas Jefferson University
Philadelphia, Pennsylvania

Harvey L. Nisenbaum, M.D.
Associate Professor of Radiology
Department of Radiology
University of Pennsylvania School of Medicine
Hospital of the University of Pennsylvania
Philadelphia, Pennsylvania

Harriet J. Paltiel, M.D., C.M.
Associate Professor
Department of Radiology
Harvard Medical School
Children's Hospital Boston
Boston, Massachusetts

Cynthia L. Rapp, B.S., R.D.M.S., R.D.C.S.
Sonographic Practitioner
Radiology Imaging Associates
Swedish Medical Center
Englewood, Colorado

Thomas A. Stavros, M.D.
Assistant Clinical Professor
Medical Director for Clinical Site Sonographer
Training Program
University of Colorado School of Medicine
Denver, Colorado

Sharlene A. Teefey, M.D.
Professor
Division of Diagnostic Radiology
Mallinckrodt Institute of Radiology
Washington University School of Medicine
Saint Louis, Missouri

Lisa Lihuan Wang, M.D.
Clinical Instructor
Mallinckrodt Institute of Radiology
Washington University School of Medicine
Saint Louis, Missouri

1 Flank Pain

Lisa Lihuan Wang and Sharlene A. Teefey

Flank pain is a common complaint and is often the primary symptom of ureteral stone disease. However, the differential diagnosis of flank pain is extensive and includes not only many renal etiologies but also nonrenal etiologies.

The approach to the patient with flank pain begins with a thorough history and physical examination followed by appropriate laboratory studies. This information will help the clinician in consultation with the radiologist to determine which radiological procedures are indicated. **Table 1–1** lists the renal and nonrenal causes of acute flank pain.[1,2] Many of the disease processes listed in this table occur commonly, including renal calculus disease, acute pyelonephritis, and fibrositis (**Table 1–2**).[1,2] Although many of the intraabdominal disease processes listed are also common, flank pain is an unusual manifestation. This chapter presents a brief summary of the important diagnostic features of these disease processes.

Differential Diagnosis

An abrupt increase in intraluminal pressure in the collecting system is the primary cause of pain from calculus disease. The severity of the pain is directly related to the rapidity with which the obstructing stone raises intraluminal pressure.[3] The pain frequently radiates from the flank

Table 1–1 Renal and Nonrenal Etiologies of Flank Pain

Retroperitoneal	Renal	Calculus disease
		Pyelonephritis/ abscess
		Xanthogranulomatous pyelonephritis
		Neoplasm/cyst
		Vascular compromise
	Nonrenal	Abdominal aortic aneurysm rupture
		Retroperitoneal fibrosis
		Retroperitoneal abscess
		Retroperitoneal adenopathy
		Retroperitoneal hemorrhage
		Retroperitoneal neoplasm
		Adrenal neoplasm with hemorrhage
Intraabdominal	Diverticulitis	
	Perforated colon carcinoma	
	Pancreatitis	
	Cholecystitis	
	Appendicitis	
	Duodenal ulcer	
	Splenic infarction/ abscess	
Musculoskeletal	Fibrositis	
	Iliac/spine osteomyelitis	
	Disk disease	
	Spinal metastases	
Miscellaneous	Münchhausen syndrome	
	Narcotic abuse	

Table 1–2 Disease Incidence[a]

Common (100)	Uncommon (5–100)	Rare (0–5)
Renal colic	Renal corticomedullary abscess	Renal cortical abscess
Acute pyelonephritis		Perinephric abscess
Fibrositis	Carcinoma of the kidney	Renal infarction
	Diverticulitis	Renal vein thrombosis
	Carcinoma of the colon with perforation	Adrenal neoplasm with hemorrhage
	Duodenal ulcer	Iliac osteomyelitis
	Acute cholecystitis	Retrocecal appendicitis
	Abdominal aortic aneurysm rupture	Splenic infarction
		Splenic abscess

[a]Incidence per 100,000 (approximate).

laterally into the abdomen and may be intermittent (renal colic) or steady. When the ureter is initially obstructed, there is an increase in the frequency of ureteral contractions causing colicky pain. Within a short time, ureteral contractions cease, and while the intraluminal pressure remains elevated, the pain takes on a more steady character.[3] Nevertheless, the patient typically paces or writhes in bed, unable to find a comfortable position. The location of pain originating from the urinary tract has been carefully mapped out by McClellan and Goodell.[3] The authors observe that if various parts of the renal pelvis and ureter are distended with small balloon catheters, the distention of the renal pelvis produces costovertebral angle pain. When the upper, middle, or lower ureter is distended, pain occurs in the flank, middle inguinal canal, or suprapubic region, respectively. Pain may also be referred from the upper or lower obstructed ureter to the ipsilateral scrotum in men or labia majora in women.[3] Symptoms of bladder irritation may occur. Because of the autonomic innervation of the kidney and stomach by the celiac ganglion, it is not unusual for patients to experience nausea, vomiting, and abdominal distention due to ileus. Diaphoresis and tachycardia may also occur in response to the pain; however, fever is not usually present unless there is a superimposed infection and pyonephrosis. Urinalysis usually reveals microscopic hematuria; however, gross hematuria occurs in 10% of patients. If ureteral obstruction is complete, then hematuria may be absent.[4]

Acute pyelonephritis is characterized by the abrupt onset of chills and fever, usually > 100°F, in association with constant, dull flank pain and/or symptoms of cystitis, which include dysuria, frequency, and urgency. In some cases, only irritative bladder symptoms are present, and differentiating pyelonephritis from cystitis is difficult.[5] The flank pain is usually less severe than that caused by stone disease and may be associated with muscle spasm and tenderness that intensify with movement. Nausea, vomiting, diarrhea, and abdominal pain may also occur. Laboratory findings show a leukocytosis with a neutrophil predominance. Urinalysis reveals numerous white blood cells and bacteria. Leukocyte casts and a specific type of cast characterized by the predominance of bacteria within the cast matrix are also frequently present in the urine.[5] Urine cultures usually grow *Escherichia coli*. When pyelonephritis occurs in the setting of stasis, calculi, pregnancy, diabetes mellitus, or a neurogenic bladder, patients are predisposed to abscess formation.[5] If renal abscess develops from a hematogenous source, then urine cultures will frequently be negative.

An uncommon infectious process of the kidney, xanthogranulomatous pyelonephritis, predominantly affects women between the fifth and seventh decades of life. Patients frequently present with nonspecific constitutional symptoms such as malaise, low-grade fever, and flank pain, which have usually been present for months to years.[6] On physical examination, there is costovertebral angle tenderness and frequently a palpable flank or abdominal mass. Laboratory findings reveal an elevated erythrocyte sedimentation rate, anemia, and leukocytosis. Urinalysis shows pyuria, proteinuria, and occasionally hematuria. *Escherichia coli* and *Proteus mirabilis* are often cultured from the urine, although urine cultures may be negative in up to one third of patients if there is complete obstruction of the kidney.[6] An interesting syndrome of reversible hepatic dysfunction has been associated with xanthogranulomatous pyelonephritis in which abnormal liver function tests with or without hepatomegaly return to normal after nephrectomy.[6]

Renal neoplasms and cysts may also cause flank pain. Fewer than 10% of patients present with the triad of flank pain, a palpable mass, and hematuria as being characteristic of renal cell carcinoma.[7] The findings of a palpable mass and flank pain are late symptoms. Usually, patients with renal cell carcinoma present with painless hematuria.[7] Large renal cysts and complications such as infection or hemorrhage into the cyst may also cause acute flank pain.

Renal vascular compromise, in particular, when acute, may cause noncolicky flank pain. Etiologies include renal artery embolus, dissection of the renal artery, rupture of a renal artery aneurysm, and renal vein thrombosis. Renal artery emboli usually originate from the left atrium or ventricle in patients with myocardial infarction, rheumatic heart disease, arrhythmias, or subacute bacterial endocarditis.[8] Atherosclerotic plaque may also embolize to the renal arteries. Sudden interruption of the renal artery blood supply causes severe, sharp, constant flank pain that may radiate to the upper or midabdomen.[9] Nausea and vomiting may also occur. Urinalysis shows microscopic hematuria and proteinuria. Renal vein thrombosis, when acute, may also cause flank pain. Etiologies are many and include malignant neoplasm, a hypercoagulable state, or an underlying renal disease such as nephrotic syndrome, membranous glomerulonephritis, systemic lupus erythematosus, and amyloidosis. Other predisposing conditions include abdominal trauma, abdominal surgery, or pregnancy (ovarian vein thrombosis with inferior vena cava extension).[10] Patients typically present with flank or upper abdominal pain, nausea and vomiting, or costovertebral angle tenderness. Laboratory findings include hematuria, proteinuria, and azotemia.[1] Other much less common conditions may compromise renal blood flow and cause flank pain such as dissection of the renal artery or rupture of a renal artery aneurysm or both.

Several nonrenal retroperitoneal processes may also cause acute flank pain, including abdominal aortic aneurysm rupture and retroperitoneal fibrosis, abscess, adenopathy, hemorrhage, or neoplasm. Patients with a ruptured abdominal aortic aneurysm most commonly present with abdominal, back, or flank pain, and syncope or loss of consciousness.[11] As seen on one study, although the classic triad of abdominal pain, back pain, and a pulsatile mass presents in only 26% of patients with a ruptured abdominal aortic aneurysm, the presence of abdominal and back pain is seen in only 42% of these patients.[12] Because an aneurysm frequently ruptures to the left of the root of the mesentery, the hematoma may extend inferiorly, causing left groin or testicular pain that may be misinterpreted as renal colic. In fact, the leading misdiagnosis of a ruptured abdominal aortic aneurysm is renal colic followed by diverticulitis and gastrointestinal hemorrhage.[12] Other retroperitoneal processes such as retroperitoneal fibrosis, abscess, adenopathy, hemorrhage, and neoplasm may also cause flank pain. Accompanying symptoms vary with the location of the process and upon which organs are encroached. Retroperitoneal fibrosis may cause colicky flank pain and tenderness due to entrapment and compression of the ureters.[13] A retroperitoneal abscess may cause abdominal or flank pain, tenderness, and fever.[14] Hemorrhage into an adrenal tumor has also been reported to cause acute flank and midback pain.[2]

There are multiple intraabdominal causes of flank pain, including diverticulitis, perforated colon carcinoma, pancreatitis, cholecystitis, appendicitis, duodenal ulcer, and splenic infarction or abscess. The pain that is felt in the back or flank region is often referred to the posterior portion of the spinal segment that innervates that organ.[15] Patients with diverticulitis frequently present with acute left lower quadrant pain that may radiate into the left lumbar and flank region. Urinary tract symptoms may occur if the inflammatory process is adjacent to the bladder.[16] Perforation of a colon carcinoma may produce an identical clinical picture.[2] Pancreatitis causes a constant, boring pain that radiates from the epigastrium into the lower abdomen, as well as the back and flanks. The pain is usually more intense in the supine position; relief is often obtained by sitting. Physical examination reveals epigastric tenderness; however, signs of peritoneal irritation are initially absent due to the retroperitoneal location of the pancreas.[17] Although acute cholecystitis classically begins with acute right upper quadrant pain and localized tenderness, less typical presentations may also occur. The pain may be pleuritic and localized to the right lower posterior chest and flank.[2] Likewise, although the classic description of the pain from appendicitis is periumbilical with a shift to the right lower quadrant, an inflamed retrocecal appendix may cause right flank pain and tenderness. Local abdominal tenderness may not be present because the appendix is posterior to the cecum and deep to the parietal peritoneum.[2,18] Midepigastric pain and localized tenderness are the most common symptoms of duodenal ulcer. However, a duodenal ulcer may also cause right lower posterolateral chest and flank pain.[2] Finally, acute left upper abdominal and flank pain and tenderness may occur from acute splenic infarction or abscess. Respiration may intensify the pain in both conditions. In the latter disease process, fever and chills are invariably present.[2]

Musculoskeletal pain from various causes such as fibrositis, iliac/spine osteomyelitis, spinal metastases, and even disk disease may produce flank pain. The pain of fibrositis is usually of a dull, aching, continuous nature and is intensified by bending or lifting.[2,15] Osteomyelitis and spinal metastases can also cause flank pain and tenderness with guarding. Cardiothoracic diseases, such as myocardial infarction and pneumonia, may also produce flank pain. Finally, it is important to remember the Münchausen syndrome and narcotic abuse patients, who present with fictitious hematuria, are well versed with the signs and symptoms of renal colic, and often give a history of contrast allergy to avoid imaging studies.[1]

Diagnostic Evaluation

Given the many different pathological processes that can produce flank pain, the clinician must obtain a thorough history and perform a careful physical examination. Important historical points include the nature, quality, and severity of the pain; associated signs and symptoms; current medications; predisposing conditions such as previous renal disease, diabetes, or recent surgery; and any underlining history of neoplasm or metabolic, cardiovascular, collagen vascular disease or family history of abdominal aortic aneurysm.[1] Findings at physical examination will assist in localizing the process to the retroperitoneum, abdominal cavity, or musculoskeletal system. Laboratory tests such as urinalysis, complete blood cell count, erythrocyte sedimentation rate, and amylase and/or lipase will further help to narrow the differential diagnosis.[1] At this point, the role of the radiologist as consultant becomes important.

The usefulness of an examination in a patient with suspected ureterolithiasis depends on its ability to confirm the diagnosis; to document stone size, burden, and location; and to assess for ancillary findings of urinary tract obstruction. The unenhanced abdominal radiograph (KUB), intravenous urogram (IVU), ultrasonography, and, more recently, unenhanced multidetector computed tomography (UECT) have all been studied for their effectiveness in confirming the diagnosis of urolithiasis. Given the lack of ionizing radiation in ultrasound, when Ellenbogen et al introduced the use of gray-scale ultrasound to exclude urinary tract obstruction nearly 3 decades ago, the potential usefulness of this particular modality sparked much interest.[19] Since that time, however, with the advent of the unenhanced helical CT, the limitations of ultrasound have come to light, especially its suboptimal detection of renal calculi less than 3 mm (~27%).[20] Ureterolithiasis is also difficult to detect, with a sensitivity of 19 to 61% and specificity of 97 to 100%.[21,22] Renal sinus fat and bowel gas limit the detection of renal calculi on ultrasound. However, when used to detect secondary ancillary signs of urinary tract obstruction (unilateral hydronephrosis, ureteral dilatation), the sensitivity of the ultrasound increases to 85%.[22] The ability of ultrasound to distinguish nonobstructive from obstructive causes of hydronephrosis is poor. Gray-scale sonography was only 65 to 69% accurate in diagnosing urinary tract obstruction.[23,24] False-positive findings are due to normal collecting system variants, high urine flow rate, postobstructive dilatation, blunted calyces (vesicoureteral reflux, papillary necrosis, or congenital megacalyces), and renal sinus structures (blood vessels and parapelvic cysts).[19,25]

In an effort to distinguish obstructive from nonobstructive dilatation, intrarenal Doppler analysis using the resistive index (RI) [(peak systolic velocity–end diastolic velocity)/peak systolic velocity] was introduced by Platt et al in 1989.[26] In their original work involving a population of patients with acute and chronic obstruction, the RI was significantly increased in obstructive pyelocalectasis in comparison with nonobstructive pyelocaliectasis. They found that an RI of 0.70 was a reasonable upper limit of normal with a sensitivity of 92%, specificity of 88%, and overall accuracy of 90%.[26] In a later study of patients with acute obstruction (< 36 h), the same authors reported an elevated RI (0.70) in 87% of kidneys.[27] However, subsequent studies have not been able to reproduce Platt's findings.[28–30] Deyoe et al reported an elevated or asymmetric RI in only 30% of patients with acute complete obstruction,[28] and Tublin et al in only 47% of patients with acute high-grade obstruction with a sensitivity of 44%,[29] although both found an elevated RI to be very specific when ureteral obstruction was suspected (**Fig. 1–1**). There are several

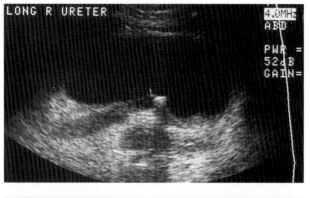

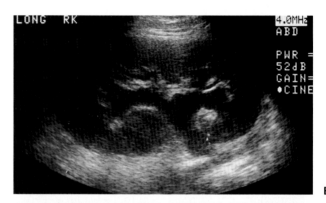

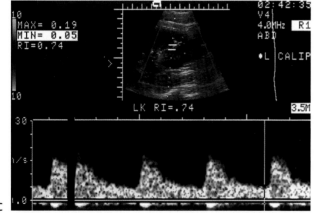

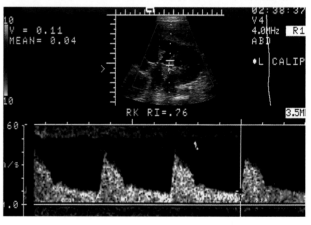

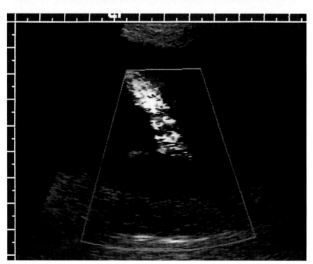

Figure 1–1 (A,B) A 61-year-old woman being treated with antibiotics for a urinary tract infection. After 5 days, fever recurred, and the patient developed acute right abdominal pain. Sonography shows moderate right hydronephrosis with a ureterovesical junction calculus. **(C,D)** Resistive indices are mildly elevated but symmetric, measuring 0.76 in the right kidney and 0.74 in the left kidney. Ureteral jet analysis shows a normal left ureteral jet, but **(E)** no right ureteral jet is visualized, indicating a high-grade ureteral obstruction.

potential reasons why the RI may be falsely negative in the setting of acute renal obstruction. If the obstruction (whether complete or not) has been present for less than 6 hours or is partial or mild, then certain mediators that cause renal vasoconstriction and increased vascular resistance may not have been released.[31] In addition, spontaneous decompression of a dilated, obstructed collecting system (i.e., forniceal rupture) may normalize an elevated RI,[27,31] and medications such as nonsteroidal antiinflammatory drugs, which may be administered in the initial management of the patient with acute flank pain, may decrease the RI.[29] On the other hand, if RI values are increased due to renal parenchymal disease, they are of little value unless the collecting system dilatation is unilateral, in which case interrenal differences may help to distinguish obstructive from nonobstructive dilatation.[31] Still other considerations include the reported normal increase in the threshold value of RI with age,[32] and the variability in RI measurements.[33] Thus, although an elevated RI is very specific for ureteral obstruction in the proper clinical setting,[26,28–31] its usefulness is limited as a diagnostic test in the patient with acute flank pain.[28–30]

Other strategies using sonography have emerged in an attempt to diagnose acute urinary tract obstruction. Mallek et al showed that the administration of furosemide before duplex sonography resulted in an accuracy rate of 95% in differentiating obstructive from nonobstructive pyelocaliectasis.[34] Laing used transvaginal sonography and detected 13 of 13 distal ureteral calculi.[35] Color and power Doppler twinkling artifact from ureteric calculi has been shown to occur frequently (83%) in a study of 36 stones by Lee et al.[36] Another technique relies on employing color Doppler sonography to search for ureteral jets. Ureteral jets are visualized with color Doppler sonography when density differences exist between bladder and ureteral urine.[37,38] Before beginning ureteral jet analysis, patient hydration may be helpful to increase jet frequency and enhance the asymmetry between the normal and abnormal sides. However, if the patient voids and refills the bladder before jet analysis, jets may not be detected due to the loss of the density difference between the bladder and ureteral urine.[37] Two other studies have shown that the absence of a ureteral jet is highly significant for complete obstruction (**Fig. 1–2**).[28,38] Deyoe et al demonstrated that the absence of

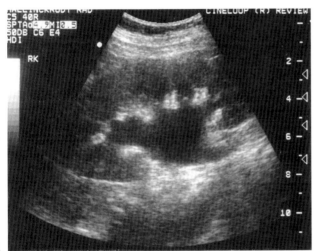

A

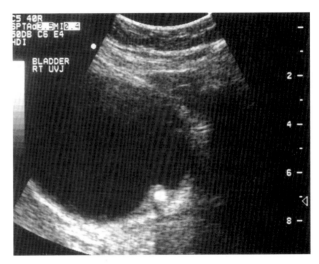

B

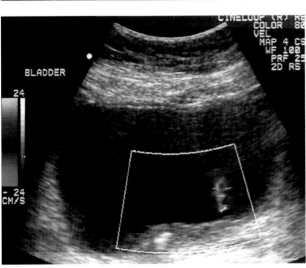

C

Figure 1–2 A 67-year-old woman with a 10-day history of right flank pain. **(A,B)** Sonography shows moderate right hydronephrosis with a ureterovesical junction calculus. Resistive indices are normal and symmetric. **(C)** Ureteral jet analysis demonstrates a normal left ureteral jet, but no right ureteral jet is visualized, indicating complete ureteral obstruction.

a ureteral jet had a sensitivity of 100% and specificity of 91% for complete ureteral obstruction.[28] Burge et al reported similar results.[38] However, ureteral jets may be normal in patients with partial or low-grade obstruction or nonobstructing stones.[38] Furthermore, it has been suggested that normal asymmetry in jet frequency may require a longer observation period to rule out obstruction than has been recommended.[39]

Haddad et al examined the combination of ultrasound with KUB and reported a sensitivity of up to 97% and specificity of 90% for diagnosing acute urinary tract obstruction when compared with the IVU.[40] In 2002, Catalano et al published a prospective study of 160 patients who underwent a combination of KUB and sonography followed by UECT. Sonography included ureteral jet analysis with color Doppler and a gray-scale exam to search for renal and ureteral calculi. When compared with CT whose sensitivity, negative predictive value (NPV), and overall accuracy were 92, 87, and 94%, respectively, the combined KUB and sonogram revealed a sensitivity of 77%, NPV of 68%, and overall accuracy of 83%.[41]

In 1995, Smith et al introduced unenhanced helical CT for urolithiasis detection.[42] In the last decade, because of its high sensitivity (95 to 100%) and high specificity (96 to 100%), UECT for urolithiasis has become the modality of choice for imaging the patient with acute flank pain.[43–49] In addition to its proven impact for diagnosing urolithiasis,[50] UECT not only offers alternative diagnoses in 9 to 29% of the cases,[43,47,49,51,52] it also expedites the treatment process without the need for patient bowel preparation and intravenous contrast administration. In patients with renal insufficiency or iodine allergy, the UECT is very useful. UECT has largely supplanted the KUB and IVU as the cornerstone in the evaluation of patients with acute renal colic. Whereas the KUB has been shown to have a sensitivity and specificity of only 45% and 77%, respectively,[48,53] the IVU has been proven to have a sensitivity and specificity of 64 to 97% and 92 to 94%, respectively,[21,48,54,55] when compared with UECT.

The primary finding in UECT is the direct visualization of the ureteral calculus within the urinary collecting system. With the exception of the indinavir stone, which may develop in patients with human immunodeficiency virus treated with this protease inhibitor,[56] virtually all other renal and ureteral stones are detectable at helical CT.[43,57] Measuring the maximal stone size is essential because stones less than or equal to 4 mm pass spontaneously 76% of the time.[58] The probability of the stone's spontaneous passage is also related to its location with respect to the urinary collecting system. The more proximal the stone, the less likely it is to pass spontaneously.[58] The stone burden itself is also much easier to assess on UECT when compared with ultrasound or KUB. Ancillary signs of acute urinary tract obstruction include a dilated collecting system (hydronephrosis and/or hydroureter), perinephric and periureteral edema, and renomegaly.[59] The presence of both ureteral dilatation and perinephric edema gives a positive predictive value of 99% and negative predictive value of 95%.[60]

The major pitfall for UECT is the presence of phleboliths, especially of the gonadal veins or pelvis. If a rim of soft tissue surrounds the calcification (the rim sign), ureterolithiasis is favored because this sign has been shown to be present in 50 to 75% of ureteric stones and in only 2 to 8% of the phleboliths.[61–64] The comet tail sign, which is a curvilinear soft tissue density that abuts a pelvic calcification, has a sensitivity of 65% and specificity of 100% for diagnosing a phlebolith.[65] The primary limitation of UECT is the dosage of the ionizing radiation. This is important not only in the pregnant and young patient but also in the high percentage of patients with recurrent ureterolithiasis who may require multiple UECTs. For follow-up of a known ureteral calculus, if the UECT scout topogram shows the calculus, the calculus will be visible on KUB.[66] If ureterolithiasis can be seen on the KUB, follow-up for the passage of the calculus can be performed with the KUB to decrease radiation. For excluding ureteral obstruction, a renal sonogram should be considered in the follow-up of known ureterolithiasis. Both the KUB and ultrasound have been shown to have a very low sensitivity for detecting stones less than 3 mm.[20,66] However, in that most of the stones 3 mm or less pass spontaneously,[58] one or a combination of these exams may be adequate for assessing ureterolithiasis and following the patient in the appropriate clinical setting. More recently, magnetic resonance urography (MRU) without and with intravenous gadopentate dimeglumine administration has been shown as an acceptable substitution in patients who do not desire radiation. However, MRU is limited in evaluating stone burden.[67]

In the pregnant patient with suspected obstruction from urolithiasis, ultrasound with gray-scale (including transvaginal), duplex, and color Doppler sonography of ureteral jets is the initial modality of choice. Few studies have examined the role of sonography in the pregnant patient with suspected urinary tract obstruction. In one study, Hertzberg et al showed that RI values are not elevated in normal pregnancy even in the presence of moderate physiological pelvicaliectasis.[68] However, the authors also stated that the effects of other pathological processes such as preeclampsia and pyelonephritis on RI values are as yet unknown and require further study.[68] A study of 65 pregnant patients by Parulkar et al showed that ultrasound had a sensitivity of 95% and specificity of 87% for the detection of urolithiasis when using the clinical scenario as the gold standard.[69]

What then is the role of sonography in the patient with acute flank pain due to suspected stone disease? The answer depends upon the question being asked. If the question is the anatomical cause rather than the physiological significance of the obstructing process, then noncontrast helical computed tomography (NECT) is the procedure of choice, especially in an older patient with new or changed

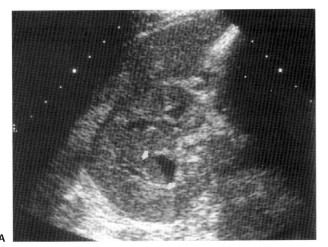

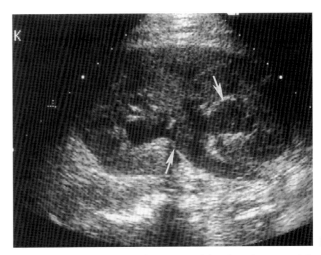

Figure 1–3 An elderly male with right nephrostomy stent placement for pyonephrosis. **(A,B)** Sonography shows urine-debris (purulent material) levels within the dilated collecting system (*arrows*). K, kidney.

symptoms of acute flank pain, because CT can also offer an alternative diagnosis. If physiological information is sought regarding the functional significance of the obstruction, then intrarenal Doppler analysis and analysis of ureteral jets may be useful. Ultrasound definitely plays a major role in the pregnant patient with suspected urinary tract obstruction.

Most patients with uncomplicated acute pyelonephritis do not require an imaging study. The diagnosis is usually established based on clinical presentation and laboratory findings. An imaging study is indicated, however, when it is important to rule out obstruction or to detect a complication such as a nephric or perinephric abscess. Patients who fail to respond to antibiotic therapy within 48 to 72 hours, or in whom the clinical diagnosis is uncertain, should be imaged, as should patients with diabetes mellitus, recur-

rent pyelonephritis, or a history of stone disease.[70] Sonography or computed tomography is frequently used to evaluate such patients. Sonography is also very specific (100%) for diagnosing pyonephrosis, a serious complication of ureteral obstruction (**Fig. 1–3**).[71] However, in this same study, Jeffrey et al reported a sensitivity of only 62% and recommended percutaneous aspiration of potentially infected urine in cases of suspected pyonephrosis.[71] Sonography is less sensitive in detecting parenchymal inflammation or small nephric or perinephric abscesses compared with CT.[72–74] In fact, most kidneys appear normal on sonography despite obvious signs of parenchymal inflammation on contrast-enhanced CT.[72] Although early sonographic reports described a variety of sonographic findings suggestive of pyelonephritis,[75–77] many of these features, such as an ill-defined hypoechoic mass (**Fig. 1–4**), are nonspecific

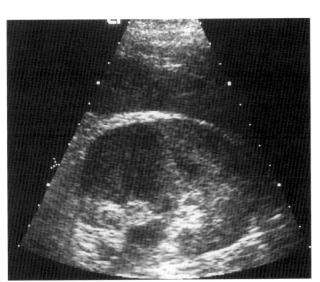

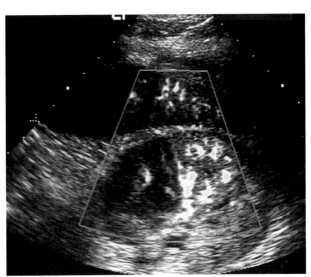

Figure 1–4 A 38-year-old woman with focal pyelonephritis. **(A)** Sonography shows a hypoechoic region in the mid–left kidney on this transverse image. **(B)** The power Doppler image shows a decrease in color flow due to intense vasoconstriction.

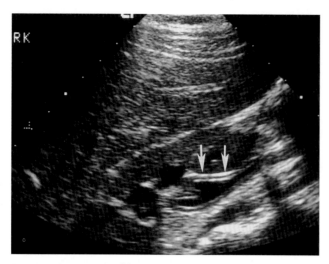

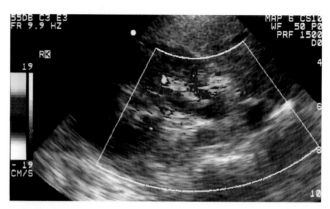

Figure 1–6 A 40-year-old woman with systemic lupus erythematosis. Sonography shows renal vein thrombosis. Collateral veins are present, indicating that the thrombosis is chronic.

Figure 1–5 A 27-year-old woman with pyelonephritis. Sonography shows urothelial thickening of the right renal pelvis (*arrows*).

and overlap with other disease processes. Thickening of the urothelium in native kidneys is a fairly reliable indication of infection in the proper clinical setting (**Fig. 1–5**) but has also been reported in patients with hydronephrosis and vesicoureteral reflux.[78,79] In addition, Morehouse et al evaluated 23 patients with pyelonephritis and found that a focal area of abnormal echogenicity had a sensitivity of only 30%, and an RI greater than 0.70, a sensitivity of only 43% for diagnosing renal infection.[80] These findings were reiterated by Keogan et al.[81] They reported that, although the mean RI in pregnant patients with pyelonephritis was significantly higher than in controls, the magnitude of the difference was too small and the overlap too great between the two groups for this index to be of clinical value.[81] Likewise, although sonography may demonstrate collecting system obstruction and a central calculus in patients with xanthogranulomatous pyelonephritis, CT will more precisely demonstrate extrarenal extension into the perirenal and pararenal spaces and soft tissues of the flank.[6]

Acute renal infarction can accurately be diagnosed in most cases with CT.[82–84] Little has been written about the role of sonography in evaluating acute native renal infarction. Absence of parenchymal flow at color Doppler sonography suggests complete occlusion of the main renal artery, whereas patchy areas of absent parenchymal flow may indicate segmental arterial occlusion in the proper clinical setting. Nevertheless, angiography or scintigraphy may be required for a definitive diagnosis. Renal vein thrombosis, on the other hand, can be confidently diagnosed with color Doppler sonography, which shows absence of flow in the main renal vein (**Fig. 1–6**). Of interest, a study by Platt et al showed that intrarenal arterial Doppler analysis (RI) was neither sensitive nor specific in diagnosing renal vein thrombosis in native kidneys due to the early development of venous collaterals and subsequent decrease in renal vascular resistance.[85] CT is capable of diagnosing renal vein thrombosis; however, optimal vi-

sualization of the renal veins is dependent on thin sections and an adequate intravenous contrast bolus with the proper scan delay. Magnetic resonance angiography (MRA) has also been shown to be a valuable technique for evaluating the renal vessels.

Although sonography may demonstrate the presence of retroperitoneal pathology, the characteristics are often nonspecific. Usually either or both biopsy and aspiration are necessary to obtain a specific diagnosis. CT and MRI are important in determining the location, size, extent, and characteristics of the retroperitoneal process, as well as its encroachment on adjacent viscera.[86,87] If the suspicion for neoplasm is high and it is visible with sonography, a sonographically guided biopsy may expedite the patient's workup.

Summary

From the preceding discussion, it is evident that, although the differential diagnosis of flank pain is extensive, the initial workup of the patient by the clinician should narrow the differential diagnosis sufficiently to allow the radiologist to recommend the appropriate imaging studies. Although the UECT has supplanted the IVU and ultrasound as the study of choice in patients with suspected urinary tract obstruction, especially for those with a severe contrast allergy or elevated creatinine, sonography remains the initial test for the pregnant patient. It may also be used to exclude obstruction or a moderate to large abscess in the setting of pyelonephritis. Duplex and color Doppler sonography is also useful in the patient with a question of renal infarction or renal vein thrombosis and in patients with abdominal aortic aneurysms. CT and MRI are superior to sonography in the diagnosis of retroperitoneal diseases, especially when the patient's symptoms are vague and nonspecific. Sonographic findings, although nonspecific, may demonstrate a retroperitoneal abnormality. Sonography is important in diagnosing many of the intraabdominal diseases that may uncommonly present with flank pain, but it is of no value in the evaluation of musculoskeletal causes of flank pain or the Münchhausen syndrome.

References

1. Hendricksen D, Eshelman B, Dill L, Frederick R. Unusual etiology for left flank pain in a 29-year-old man. Ann Emerg Med 1993;22: 1455–1462
2. Wiener SL. Acute unilateral costovertebral area and flank pain, acute bilateral costovertebral area and flank pain. In: Wiener SL, ed. Differential Diagnosis of Acute Pain by Body Region. New York: McGraw-Hill; 1993:245–257, 311–317
3. Wiker AW. Standard diagnostic considerations. In: Gillenwater JY, Grayhack JT, Howards SS, Duckett JW, eds. Adult and Pediatric Urology. 2nd ed. St. Louis: Mosby Year Book; 1991:68–69
4. Pahira JJ. Renal calculi. In: Schwartz GR, Cayten CG, Mayer TA, Mangelsen MA, Hanke BK, eds. Principles and Practice of Emergency Medicine. 3rd ed. Philadelphia: Lea & Feibiger; 1992:1664–1668
5. Schaeffer AJ. Renal infection. In: Gillenwater JY, Grayhack JT, Howards SS, Duckett JW, eds. Adult and Pediatric Urology. 2nd ed. St. Louis: Mosby Year Book; 1991:751–756
6. Hayes WS, Hartman DS, Sesterbenn IA. Archives of AFIP Xanthogranulomatous pyelonephritis. Radiographics 1991;11:485–498
7. Williams RD. Renal, perirenal, and ureteral neoplasms. In: Gillenwater JY, Grayhack JT, Howards SS, Duckett JW, eds. Adult and Pediatric Urology. 2nd ed. St. Louis: Mosby Year Book; 1991:578–580
8. Hillman BJ. Disorders of the renal arterial circulation and renal vascular hypertension. In: Pollack HM, ed. Clinical Urography. Philadelphia: WB Saunders; 1990:2140–2141
9. Badr KF, Brenner BM. Vascular injury to the kidney. In: Wilson JD, Braunwald E, Isselbacher KJ, et al, eds. Harrison's Principles of Internal Medicine. 12th ed. New York: McGraw-Hill; 1991:1192–1193
10. Mellins HZ. Renal vein obstruction. In: Pollack HM, ed. Clinical Urography. Philadelphia: WB Saunders; 1990:2119
11. Bengtsson H, Bergqvist D. Ruptured abdominal aortic aneurysm: a population based study. J Vasc Surg 1993;18:74–80
12. Marston WA, Ahlquist R, Johnson G, Meyer AA. Missed diagnosis of ruptured abdominal aortic aneurysms. J Vasc Surg 1992;16:17–22
13. Amis ES. Retroperitoneal fibrosis. AJR Am J Roentgenol 1991;157: 321–329
14. Hirschmann JV. Localized infections and abscesses. In: Wilson JD, Braunwald E, Isselbacher KJ, et al, eds. Harrison's Principles of Internal Medicine. 12th ed. New York: McGraw-Hill; 1991:517
15. Mankin HJ. Back and neck pain. In: Wilson JD, Braunwald E, Isselbacher KJ, et al, eds. Harrison's Principles of Internal Medicine. 12th ed. New York: McGraw-Hill; 1991:121
16. Naitove A, Almy TP. Diverticular disease of the colon. In: Sleisinger MH, Fordtran JS, eds. Gastrointestinal Disease, Pathophysiology Diagnosis Management. 4th ed. Philadelphia: WB Saunders; 1989:1427
17. Greenberger NJ, Toskes PP, Isselbacher JK. Acute and chronic pancreatitis. In: Wilson JD, Braunwald E, Isselbacher KJ, et al, eds. Harrison's Principles of Internal Medicine. 12th ed. New York: McGraw-Hill; 1991:1372–1375
18. Schrock TR. Acute appendicitis. In: Sleisinger MH, Fordtran JS, eds. Gastrointestinal Disease, Pathophysiology Diagnosis Management. 4th ed. Philadelphia: WB Saunders; 1989:1382–1385
19. Ellenbogen PH, Scheible FW, Talner LB, Leopold GR. Sensitivity of gray scale ultrasound in detecting urinary tract obstruction. AJR Am J Roentgenol 1978;130:731–733
20. Fowler KA, Locken JA, Duchesne JH, Williamson MR. US for detecting renal calculi with nonenhanced CT as a reference standard. Radiology 2002;222:109–113
21. Yilmaz S, Sindel T, Arslan G, et al. Renal colic: comparison of spiral CT, US, and IVU in the detection of ureteral calculi. Eur Radiol 1998;8:212–217
22. Sheafor DH, Hertzberg BS, Freed KS, et al. Nonenhanced helical CT and US in the emergency evaluation of patients with renal colic: prospective comparison. Radiology 2000;217:792–797
23. Hill MC, Rich JI, Mardiat JG, Finder CA. Sonography vs. excretory urography in acute flank pain. AJR Am J Roentgenol 1985;144: 1235–1238
24. Laing FC, Jeffrey RB, Wing VW. Ultrasound vs. excretory urography in evaluating acute flank pain. Radiology 1985;154:613–616
25. Amis ES, Cronan JJ, Pfister RC, Yoder IC. Ultrasonic inaccuracies in diagnosing renal obstruction. Urology 1982;19:101–105
26. Platt JF, Rubin JM, Ellis JH. Distinction between obstructive and nonobstructive pyelocaliectasis with duplex Doppler sonography. AJR Am J Roentgenol 1989;153:997–1000
27. Platt JF, Rubin JM, Ellis JH. Acute renal obstruction: evaluation with intrarenal duplex Doppler and conventional ultrasound. Radiology 1993;186:685–688
28. Deyoe LA, Cronan JJ, Breslaw BH, Ridlen MS. New techniques of ultrasound and color Doppler in the prospective evaluation of acute renal obstruction: do they replace the intravenous urogram? Abdom Imaging 1995;20:58–63
29. Tublin ME, Dodd GE, Verdile VP. Acute renal colic: diagnosis with duplex Doppler ultrasound. Radiology 1994;193:697–701
30. Tublin ME, Bude RO, Platt JF. The resistive index in renal Doppler sonography: where do we stand? AJR Am J Roentgenol 2003;180: 885–892
31. Platt JF. Duplex Doppler evaluation of native kidney dysfunction: obstructive and nonobstructive disease. AJR Am J Roentgenol 1992; 158:1035–1042
32. Terry JD, Rysavy JA, Frick MP. Intrarenal Doppler: characteristics of aging kidneys. J Ultrasound Med 1992;11:647–651
33. Keogan MT, Kaliewer MA, Hertzberg BS, et al. Renal resistive indexes: variability and Doppler ultrasound measurement in a healthy population. Radiology 1996;199:165–169
34. Mallek R, Bankier AA, Etele-Hainz A, Kletter K, Mostbeck GH. Distinction between obstructive and nonobstructive hydronephrosis: value of diuresis duplex Doppler sonography. AJR Am J Roentgenol 1996;166:113–117
35. Laing FC, Benson CB, DiSalvo DN, et al. Distal ureteral calculi: detection with vaginal ultrasound. Radiology 1994;192:545–548
36. Lee JY, Kim SH, Cho JY, Han D. Color and power Doppler twinkling artifacts from urinary stones: clinical observations and phantom studies. AJR Am J Roentgenol 2001;176:1441–1445
37. Baker SM, Middleton WD. Color Doppler sonography of ureteral jets in normal volunteers: importance of the relative specific gravity of urine in the ureter and bladder. AJR Am J Roentgenol 1992; 159:773–775
38. Burge HJ, Middleton WD, McClennan BL, Hildebolt CF. Ureteral jets in healthy patients and in patients with unilateral ureteral calculi: comparison with color Doppler ultrasound. Radiology 1991;180:437–442
39. Cox IH, Erickson SJ, Foley WD, Dewire DM. Ureteral jets: evaluation of normal flow dynamics with color Doppler sonography. AJR Am J Roentgenol 1992;158:1051–1055
40. Haddad MC, Sharif HS, Shahed MS, et al. Renal colic: diagnosis and outcome. Radiology 1992;184:83–88
41. Catalano O, Nunziata A, Altei F, Siani A. Suspected ureteral colic: primary helical CT versus selective helical CT after unenhanced radiography and sonography. AJR Am J Roentgenol 2002;178:379–387
42. Smith R, Rosenfield A, Choe K, et al. Acute flank pain: comparison of noncontrast enhanced CT and intravenous urography. Radiology 1995;194:789–794

43. Rucker CM, Menias CO, Bhalla S. Mimics of renal colic: alternative diagnoses at unenhanced helical CT. Radiographics 2004;24:S11–S33

44. Boulay I, Holtz P, Foley WD, White B, Begun FP. Ureteral calculi: diagnostic efficacy of helical CT and implications for treatment of patients. AJR Am J Roentgenol 1999;172:1485–1490

45. Dorio PJ, Pozniak MA, Lee FT Jr, Kuhlman JE. Non-contrast enhanced helical computed tomography for the evaluation of patients with acute flank pain. WMJ 1999;98:30–34

46. Chen MY, Zagoria RJ, Saunders HS, Dyer RB. Trends in the use of unenhanced helical CT for acute urinary colic. AJR Am J Roentgenol 1999;173:1447–1450

47. Vieweg J, The C, Freed K, et al. Unenhanced helical CT for the evaluation of patients with acute flank pain. J Urol 1998;160:679–684

48. Tamm EP, Silverman PM, Shuman WP. Evaluation of the patient with flank pain and possible ureteral calculus. Radiology 2003;___: 319–329

49. Dalrymple N, Verga M, Anderson K, et al. The value of unenhanced helical computerized tomography in the management of acute flank pain. J Urol 1998;159:735–740

50. Abramson S, Walders N, Applegate KE, Kikeson RC, Robbin MR. Impact in the emergency department of unenhanced CT on diagnostic confidence and therapeutic efficacy in patients with suspected renal colic: a prospective survey. AJR Am J Roentgenol 2000;175:1689–1695

51. Katz D, Scheer M, Lumerman J, Mellinger B, Stillman C, Lane M. Alternative or additional diagnoses on unenhanced helical computed tomography for suspected renal colic: experience with 1000 consecutive examinations. Urology 2000;56:53–57

52. Nachmann M, Harkway R, Summerton S, et al. Helical CT scanning: the primary imaging modality for acute flank pain. Am J Emerg Med 2000;18:649–652

53. Kizimenko NN, Kornienko SI, Karetin IV, Prokhorov SI, Sartakov GA. Computed tomography in x-ray-negative calculi of the ureter. Vestn Rentgenol Radiol 1996;28:44–46

54. Miller OF, Rineer SK, Reichard SR, et al. Prospective comparison of unenhanced spiral computed tomography and intravenous urogram in the evaluation of acute flank pain. Urology 1998;52:982–987

55. Niall O, Russell J, MacGregor R, Duncan H, Mullins J. A comparison of noncontrast computerized tomography with excretory urography in the assessment of acute flank pain. J Urol 1999;161:534–537

56. Blake SP, McNicholas MM, Raptopoulos V. Nonopaque crystal deposition causing ureteric obstruction in patients with HIV undergoing indinavir therapy. AJR Am J Roentgenol 1998;171:717–720

57. Federle M, McAninch J, Kaiser J, Goodman P, Roberts J, Mall J. Computed tomography of urinary calculi. AJR Am J Roentgenol 1981; 136:255–258

58. Coll DM, Varanelli MJ, Smith RC. Relationship of spontaneous passage of ureteral calculi to stone size and location as revealed by unenhanced helical CT. AJR Am J Roentgenol 2002;178:101–103

59. Katz D, Lane M, Sommer FG. Unenhanced helical CT of ureteral stones: incidence of associated urinary tract finding. AJR Am J Roentgenol 1996;166:1319–1322

60. Smith RC, Verga M, Dalrymple W, et al. Acute ureteral obstruction: value of secondary signs of helical unenhanced CT. AJR Am J Roentgenol 1996;167:1109–1113

61. Kawashima A, Sandler CM, Boridy IC, Takahashi N, Benson GS, Goldman SM. Unenhanced helical CT of ureterolithiasis: value of the tissue rim sign. AJR Am J Roentgenol 1997;168:997– 1000

62. Al-Nakshabandi NA. The soft-tissue rim sign. Radiology 2003;229: 239–240

63. Bell TV, Fenlon HM, Davison BD, Ahari HK, Hussain S. Unenhanced helical CT criteria to differentiate distal ureteral calculi from pelvic phleboliths. Radiology 1998;207:363–367

64. Heneghan JP, Dalrymple NC, Verga M, Rosenfield AT, Smith RC. Soft-tissue rim sign in the diagnosis of ureteral calculi with use of unenhanced helical CT. Radiology 1997;202:709–711

65. Boridy IC, Nikolaidis P, Kawashima A, Goldman SM, Sandler CM. Ureterolithiasis: value of the tail sign in differentiating phleboliths from ureteral calculi at nonenhanced helical CT. Radiology 1999; 211:619–621

66. Assi Z, Platt JF, Francis IR, Cohan RH, Korobkin M. Sensitivity of CT scout radiography and abdominal radiography for revealing ureteral calculi on helical CT: Implications for radiologic follow up. AJR Am J Roentgenol 2000;175:333–337

67. Sudah M, Vanninen RL, Partanen K, et al. Patients with acute flank pain: comparison of MR with unenhanced CT. Radiology 2002; 223:98–105

68. Hertzberg BS, Carroll BA, Bowie JD, et al. Doppler ultrasound assessment of maternal kidneys: analysis of intrarenal resistivity indexes in normal pregnancy and physiologic pelvicaliectasis. Radiology 1993;186:689–692

69. Parulkar BG, Hopkins TB, Wollin MR, et al. Renal colic during pregnancy: a case for conservative treatment. J Urol 1998;159:365–368

70. Renal inflammatory disease. In: Dunnick NR, McCallum RW, Sandler CM. Textbook of Uroradiology. Baltimore: Williams & Wilkins; 1991:135–146

71. Jeffrey RB, Laing FC, Wing VW, Hoddick W. Sensitivity of sonography in pyonephrosis: a reevaluation. AJR Am J Roentgenol 1985; 144:71–73

72. Talner LB, Davidson AJ, Lebowitz RL, Dalla Palma L, Goldman SM. Acute pyelonephritis: can we agree on terminology. Radiology 1994;192:297–305

73. Soulen MC, Fishman EK, Goldman SM, Gatewood OMB. Bacterial renal infection: role of CT. Radiology 1989;171:703–707

74. Hoddick W, Jeffrey RB, Goldberg HI, Federle MP, Laing FC. CT and sonography of severe renal and perirenal infections. AJR Am J Roentgenol 1983;140:517–520

75. Rigsby CM, Rosenfield AT, Glickman MG, Hodson J. Hemorrhagic focal bacterial nephritis: findings on gray scale sonography and CT. AJR Am J Roentgenol 1986;146:1173–1177

76. Lee JKT, McClennan BL, Melson GL, Stanley RJ. Acute focal bacterial nephritis: emphasis on gray scale sonography and computed tomography. AJR Am J Roentgenol 1980;135:87–92

77. Rosenfield AT, Glickman MG, Taylor KJW, Crade M, Hodson J. Acute focal bacterial nephritis (acute lobar nephronia). Radiology 1979; 132:553–561

78. Nicolet V, Carignan L, Dubuc G, et al. Thickening of the renal collecting system: a nonspecific finding at ultrasound. Radiology 1988;168:411–413

79. Babcock DS. Sonography of wall thickening of the renal collecting system: a nonspecific finding. J Ultrasound Med 1987;6:29–32

80. Morehouse H, Darwish M, Ginsberg M, Kreutzer E, Koenigsberg M. Abstract, Society of Uroradiology, Palm Beach, Florida, January 14–19, 1995

81. Keogan MT, Hertzberg BS, Kliewer MA, et al. Doppler sonography in the diagnosis of antepartum pyelonephritis: value of intrarenal resistive index measurements. J Ultrasound Med 1996;15:13–17

82. Hilton S, Bosniak MA, Raghavendra N, et al. CT findings in acute renal infarction. Urol Radiol 1984;6:158–163

83. Wong WS, Moss AA, Federle MP, Cochran ST, London SS. Renal infarction: CT diagnosis and correlation between CT findings and etiologies. Radiology 1984;150:201–205

84. Glazer GM, Francis IR, Brady TM, Teng SS. Computed tomography of renal infarction: clinical and experimental observations. AJR Am J Roentgenol 1983;140:721–727

85. Platt JF, Ellis JH, Rubin J. Intrarenal Doppler sonography in the detection of renal vein thrombosis of the native kidney. AJR Am J Roentgenol 1994;162:1367–1370

86. Patel SK. Retroperitoneal tumors and cysts. In: Pollack HM, ed. Clinical Urography. Philadelphia: WB Saunders; 1990:2413–2416

87. Lane RH, Stephens DH, Reiman HM. Primary retroperitoneal neoplasms: CT findings in 90 cases with clinical and pathologic correlation. AJR Am J Roentgenol 1989;152:83–89

2 Renal Failure

John J. Cronan

Renal failure refers to inadequate renal function with the accumulation of nitrogen waste to a toxic level that is incompatible with life. A distinction is made between renal failure and renal insufficiency. Renal insufficiency is the abnormal accumulation of nitrogen waste with preservation of sufficient renal function to sustain life. End-stage renal disease is chronic and irreversible renal failure; renal dialysis or transplantation is necessary for survival. The prevalence of renal failure is ~65 cases per million in the United States. Less than 20% of acute renal failure patients eventually require dialysis. At autopsy, ~25% of uremic patients have obstructive uropathy as either a contributory or major cause of renal insufficiency.[1]

Differential Diagnosis

Renal dysfunction, whether it be insufficiency or failure, produces the clinical state of uremia. Renal failure is the final common pathway for numerous disparate disease processes affecting the kidney. During the initial clinical evaluation, it is essential to quickly determine if renal failure is reversible. Thus determining the etiology is crucial to identify reversible causes of renal dysfunction. Diagnosis depends on evaluation and integration of the clinical history, physical exam, and laboratory data.

Maintenance of the normal internal milieu of the body depends on the ultrafiltration of blood by the kidney, followed by the secretory and resorptive functions of renal tubules. Renal function leads to the excretion of urine via the ureters, bladder, and urethra. Based on the physiology of renal function, renal failure is classified as prerenal when caused by diminished renal blood flow; intrinsic when caused by renal parenchymal damage; and postrenal when caused by blockage of urine flow (**Fig. 2–1**). For the referring clinician and radiologist, the initial step in assessing renal failure is to categorize the etiologic event as prerenal, renal, or postrenal. The ability to intervene and provide prompt improvement in defective renal function is limited to prerenal and postrenal processes. Although intrinsic renal processes may be ameliorated, the possibility of an immediate cure is unlikely.

Diagnosis of prerenal failure focuses on levels of the blood urea nitrogen (BUN) and serum creatinine. Both BUN and creatinine are filtered freely at the glomerulus. Normally, urea, but not creatinine, is reabsorbed at the tubules in peritubular capillaries. With decreased renal blood flow, capillary flow decreases and more BUN is resorbed. The resulting disproportionate elevation of blood levels of BUN compared with creatinine, can be used as a diagnostic indicator of prerenal renal dysfunction related to renal blood flow decrease.

Postrenal acute renal failure has a variable clinical presentation depending on the site and completeness of the obstruction. Urine volumes in the setting of obstruction are quite variable. Reduced urine volume and azotemia usually develop only when the obstruction is located at the level of the bladder or below. Azotemia from ureteral obstruction develops only when the obstruction is bilateral or there is a solitary kidney. Obstruction is usually reversible. When the kidney becomes obstructed, renal function changes with time. Paralleling the alteration in renal function is an alteration of the composition of urine as a result of impaired water reabsorption and electrolyte transport.

Intrinsic disorders affecting the renal parenchyma cause decreased glomerular filtration rate (GFR) and resultant elevation of the BUN and creatinine. There is a difference between hospital-acquired and non-hospital-acquired intrinsic (acute) renal failure. Most hospital-ac-

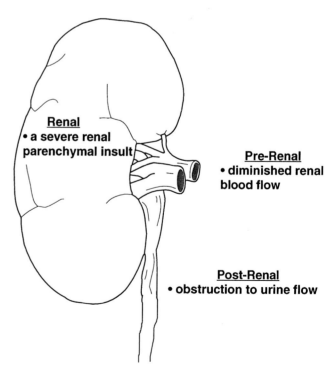

Figure 2–1 The three main types of renal failure are based on an etiologic classification.

quired acute renal failure is caused by acute tubular necrosis (ATN). Intrinsic acute renal failure acquired outside the hospital is usually caused by acute glomerular, interstitial, or vascular disease. When prerenal and postrenal acute renal failure are excluded, the cause of acute renal failure must be an acute renal parenchymal insult.

Diagnostic Evaluation

Nonimaging Evaluation

The clinical difficulty in diagnosing the cause of acute renal failure arises from the plethora of potential etiologies and the difficulty distinguishing among them. It is often difficult or impossible to determine if the cause is prerenal, intrinsic, or postrenal. Compounding the diagnostic confusion is the possibility that several different causes of renal dysfunction may interact to produce acute renal failure.

Prerenal acute renal failure should be considered if there is a history of congestive heart failure or hypotension. Changes in the patient's weight can indicate fluid shifts caused by hypoperfusion, either from dehydration or "third spacing" of fluid. Physical examination to assess skin turgor, edema, blood pressure, and pulse is helpful. The referring clinician will usually be able to diagnose or exclude prerenal acute renal failure without imaging assistance.

Postrenal acute renal failure due to obstruction is easily corrected if promptly diagnosed. For this reason, it is important to consider the possibility of obstruction as a cause of renal failure in every patient. Sonography can usually diagnose obstruction quickly and simply. It is important to evaluate the clinical history because the presence of a single kidney or preexisting renal disease will alter the presentation. A history of stone disease or malignancy suggests possible causes of obstruction.

Urine volume is a nonspecific test for acute renal failure. Anuria, defined as a 24-hour volume of 100 mL or less, may occur with prerenal, obstructive, and intrinsic renal disease. The urine-specific gravity or osmolality is measured to assess the concentration of solute in the urine. With hypovolemia, water is reabsorbed, and the urine becomes concentrated. With urine osmolalities below 350 mOsm, intrinsic renal disease is most likely. With osmolalities above 500 mOsm, the likely etiology is prerenal acute renal failure. There is great overlap, however, between the range of 350 and 500 mOsm. The normal specific gravity of urine is 1.002 to 1.028.

Creatinine is formed from the breakdown of muscle creatinine phosphate. Daily production is proportional to muscle mass. With acute renal failure, creatinine can rise 1 to 2 mg per dL per day. The normal range of creatinine in females is ~0.6 to 1 mg/dL and in males 0.8 to 1.3 mg/dL. Plasma levels of urea may also be used to assess renal function. Blood urea levels, unlike serum creatinine values, are commonly influenced by external factors; for example, an increased dietary load of protein or intestinal bleeding increases the plasma urea levels. Normal BUN is 7 to 18 mg/dL and may rise 10 to 25 mg/dL per day in acute renal failure.

Renal biopsies should be performed in only a small subset of patients with intrinsic renal disease. In most situations, the diagnosis and likely etiology of intrinsic renal disease is sufficiently certain with clinical history, urinalysis, and physical exam that appropriate treatment can be instituted. Less than 20% of patients with intrinsic renal disease require a kidney biopsy to establish the cause of acute renal failure.

Imaging other than Ultrasound

Plain Film

A plain film of the abdomen can be useful in assessing renal size and shape and identifying radiopaque stones and renal calcification (**Fig. 2–2**). Normal renal size is 3.7 ± 0.37 × the height of the second lumbar vertebral body. Approximately 90% of renal stones are radiopaque. Thus, potentially obstructing stones can often be identified on plain radiographs. Renal osteodystrophy, a complication of

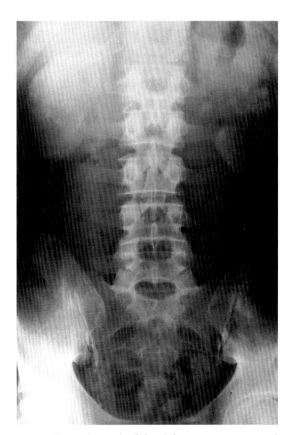

Figure 2–2 Plain radiograph of the abdomen in a patient with ARF demonstrates diffuse bilateral cortical nephrocalcinosis.

chronic renal failure, or metastatic bone disease, may also be identified on the plain film.

Excretory Urography

Excretory urography is usually not performed in patients with acute renal failure because of the risks that contrast material may exacerbate renal failure or cause a hypersensitivity reaction. The utility of renal sonography has also contributed to decreased demand for excretory urography. When renal function is normal, 25 mg of iodine per kg body weight is appropriate for the excretory urogram. With acute renal failure, 40 to 60 mg of iodine per kg is necessary to achieve opacification of the collecting system. The urogram can provide information regarding the size and shape of the kidneys. With severe azotemia, tomography is necessary to assess the renal contour (**Fig. 2–3**). Small kidneys with smooth or scarred contours indicate chronic renal failure. Bilaterally normal or large kidneys are suggestive of ATN, obstruction, renal vein thrombosis, or infiltrative disease. When renal obstruction is present, contrast excretion and collecting system opacification are delayed, which often permits determination of the site and etiology of obstruction.

Retrograde Pyelography

The retrograde pyelogram is rarely employed in acute renal failure because of the reliability of excretory urography and renal sonography. Retrograde pyelography can opacify the ureter directly, showing excellent radiographic detail. The ureteral access also provides the urologist a means to

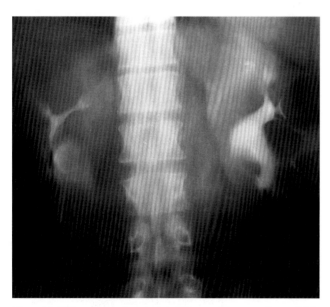

Figure 2–3 Excretory urogram in a 24-year-old man with renal failure. Kidneys are large bilaterally, with masses caused by polycystic disease of the kidneys.

pass a stent. Hence, the retrograde pyelogram is employed when there is a high probability of ureteral obstruction requiring stent placement.

Renal Scintigraphy

Intravenous injection of a radioisotope permits assessment of renal blood flow, filtration, and urinary excretion. A major limitation of renal scintigraphy is poor delineation of the anatomy. This makes it difficult to assess the etiology of acute renal failure with renal scintigraphy.

Computed Tomography

Computed tomography (CT) is rarely used as the primary imaging technique in renal failure. CT should be considered, however, when sonography is inconclusive. Even without intravenous contrast material, CT permits evaluation of the presence of the kidneys, their size, and their location. Renal stones are readily visualized. A dilated collecting system can easily be recognized and the ureters can be followed from the kidneys to the bladder or to the point of obstruction.[2]

Aortography

Placement of a pigtail catheter into the aortic lumen followed by the injection of contrast material provides excellent opacification of the renal arteries and is most useful when there is concern regarding the integrity of renal blood flow. Visualization of the renal arteries eliminates arterial occlusion as a cause of prerenal failure. Similarly, delayed filming following aortic injection will often permit visualization of the renal veins. On occasion, however, direct selective injection of the renal veins is necessary to properly establish venous patency.

Magnetic Resonance Imaging

The role of magnetic resonance imaging (MRI) in evaluating acute renal failure has increased significantly in the past decade. The absence of radiation and iodinated contrast has elevated its use in renal failure evaluation. In assessing renal blood flow, MRI with magnetic resonance angiography (MRA) is replacing angiography and nuclear medicine in evaluation of renal arteries.[3] Magnetic resonance urography is competing successfully against the excretory urogram.[4] However, with heavily T2-weighted fast imaging techniques, MR urograms can be produced that visualize the ureters.[4,5] The MR urogram is particularly helpful in assessing postrenal processes (**Fig. 2–4**). Similarly, MR angiography can assess the presence and patency of the renal arteries. MRI will probably become more important in the assessment of renal failure as faster imaging sequences evolve.

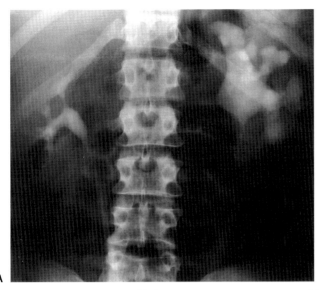

A

B

Figure 2–4 Comparison of **(A)** 5-minute excretory urogram with **(B)** maximum intensity pixel image of magnetic resonance urogram using three-dimensional fast-spin echo technique. The patient had undergone a left pyeloplasty. (Case courtesy of Martin E. O'Malley, MD, Department of Radiology, Boston University Medical Center, Boston, MA)

Ultrasound Imaging

Postrenal causes of acute renal failure are likely to be reversible. Sonography is the optimal imaging technique in renal failure patients because it is a quick and simple tool to diagnose or exclude obstruction. Sonography rapidly provides useful information about the kidney, both noninvasively and independent of renal function. Sonography can establish the presence of the kidneys and their size and shape. If the kidneys are small, renal failure is chronic (**Fig. 2–5**). If the kidney size is normal or enlarged, acute renal failure is likely.[6] Although prerenal acute renal failure is likely to be diagnosed by the clinician, renal blood flow can be evaluated with color Doppler or spectral Doppler, assessing the patency of renal arteries bilaterally (**Fig. 2–6**). Renal veins can also be evaluated with Doppler sonography.

Normal renal size is quite variable. Using ultrasound measurements, two standard deviations above and below the mean yields a normal renal length of 8.4 to 13.1 cm. It is very important to assess the amount of renal parenchyma, which can best be determined by noting the thickness of the renal cortex (**Fig. 2–7**). A thin renal cortex provides an excellent indication of renal tissue loss. Nor-

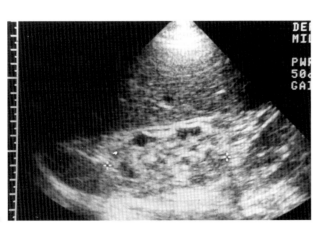

A

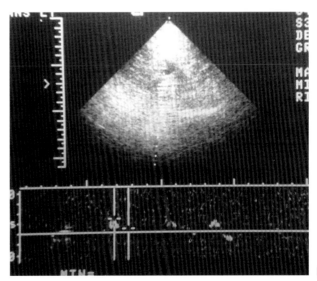

B

Figure 2–5 Chronic renal failure. **(A)** Sagittal view demonstrates a small dense kidney (8 cm). **(B)** Pulsed Doppler of left kidney demonstrates an elevated resistive index (RI) of 90%, comparative with intrinsic renal disease.

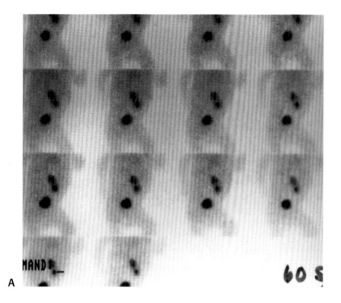

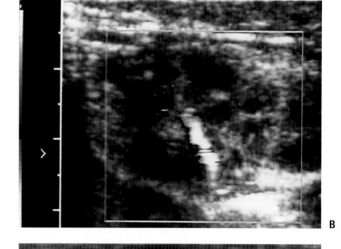

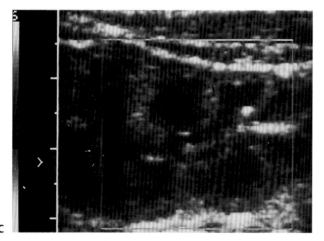

Figure 2–6 Acute renal failure developed in a neonate after placement of an intraaortic line. **(A)** Nuclear medicine scan obtained with diethylenetriamine-pentacetic acid injection shows no flow or function of the left kidney. **(B)** Color Doppler of the right kidney shows normal flow. **(C)** Color Doppler of left kidney demonstrates no flow. **(D)** Ultrasound image of the aorta shows a catheter (*arrow*) in the distal aorta with a clot extending into the left renal artery.

mal renal parenchyma, as measured from the outer margin of the renal pyramids, is greater than 1 cm thick. The normal kidney surface is smooth. Indentations between the calyces (renal pyramids) are usually due to fetal lobulation or scarring from vascular occlusion, often caused by analgesic nephropathy. Renal size is usually normal with lobulation. Scarring of any etiology is usually accompanied by some reduction in size. It is important to note that in assessing renal tissue loss, renal length is often preserved, even when there is a reduction of overall weight or volume of the kidney, because lost parenchyma is replaced with renal sinus fat—so-called replacement lipomatosis.[7] The

telltale indicator of tissue loss is the decreased parenchymal thickness.

Increased echogenicity of the renal cortex indicates intrinsic acute renal failure. Normal echogenicity of the kidney is less than or equal to that of the liver.[8] Renal echogenicity greater than that of the liver or spleen suggests intrinsic renal disease. Similarly, the resistive index, a measure of the systolic and diastolic variability of the arterial signal, can be measured to suggest the presence of intrinsic renal disease. Because of slight variation in flow, several measurements of the RI should be taken and averaged.[9] In the absence of hydronephrosis, an elevated RI

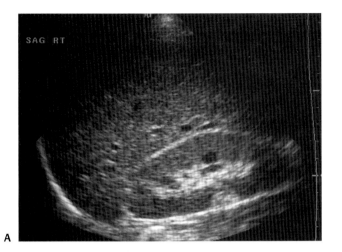

A

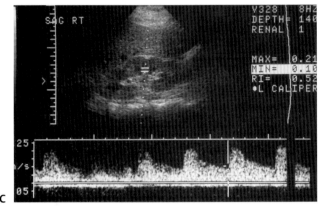

C

B

Figure 2–7 Images of a kidney from a 20-year-old female patient with a history of analgesic abuse and early nephrotic syndrome. Kidneys are scarred because of persistent analgesic abuse. **(A)** Initial scan demonstrates smooth renal parenchyma. **(B)** Two years later, the kidney is diffusely scarred; **(C)** Note the lobulated renal contour. The resistive index remains normal at 52%.

(greater than 0.70) suggestive of intrinsic renal disease.[10] Elevation of the RI in the setting of renal disease is unpredictable. For example, the RI is more likely to become elevated with tubular interstitial processes and is less likely to rise when isolated glomerular disease is present. A normal RI does not exclude intrinsic renal disease. There is evidence that an elevated RI in the setting of renal failure argues against reversibility of the renal failure.[11]

Sonography's sensitivity in detecting postrenal acute renal failure in the azotemic patient is 94%. False-negatives occur in some patients with stone disease or when minimal dilatation of the collecting system is ignored.[12] When assessing obstruction in a general population, sonography has a reported sensitivity of 98%.[13] However, the false-positive rate of sonography is 10 to 26%. False-positive images are due to pseudohydronephrosis, which may be caused by blood vessels or a parapelvic renal sinus cyst mimicking the appearance of hydronephrosis.[14] Sonography of the kidneys with diuresis has been proposed to distinguish mechanical obstruction of the renal excretory system from renal sinus cysts.[15] Another problem is that hydronephrosis can occur in the absence of obstruction. It is essential, therefore, to determine if hydronephrosis is obstructive or nonobstructive in nature. Nonobstructive hydronephrosis can be related to a prior episode of obstruction or damage from reflux. The resistive index

has been advocated as a technique to distinguish obstructive versus nonobstructive hydronephrosis.[14,16,17] If the RI is greater than 0.70, then this suggests an obstructive etiology for the hydronephrosis. Unfortunately, the reliability of the RI in diagnosing obstruction is suspect.[18,19] Of note is the fact that sonographically observed hydronephrosis is more likely to be caused by obstruction when clinical evaluation suggests the presence of obstruction.[15,16]

As peristalsis expels urine from the ureter into the bladder, it creates a "jet." This ureteral jet may be detected with color Doppler. The presence of a ureteral jet indicates patency of that ureter (**Fig. 2–8**).[22] Color Doppler visualization of a ureteral jet requires a difference in specific gravity between the urine in the bladder and the urine passing into the bladder from the ureter. If there is no difference in specific gravity between the ureteral urine and urine in the bladder, no jet will be seen with color Doppler. Thus, bilateral absence of jets has no significance. Unilateral absence of a ureteral jet is highly significant and indicates total obstruction on the affected side. If a jet is seen on one side only after 10 minutes of observation, obstruction of the ureter on the side with the absent jet is almost certain. Unfortunately, a ureteral jet can be present with partial obstruction, although it is usually diminished in magnitude compared with the normal side. In addition to scanning the bladder searching for ureteral jets, signs of

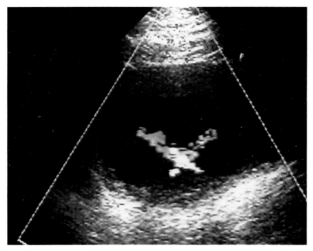

Figure 2–8 Transverse color Doppler image of bladder demonstrates bilaterally patent ureters indicated by the ureteral jets.

bladder outlet obstruction (**Fig. 2–9**) should be sought. Outlet obstruction is suggested when the bladder wall is thickened and trabeculated and the bladder is distended. Tumors such as transitional cell carcinoma or prostate carcinoma may obstruct the bladder and can often be visualized sonographically.

Summary

In summary, sonography should be the initial imaging tool used to evaluate the kidney in patients with acute renal failure. If all ultrasound techniques are employed, including color and pulsed Doppler, the radiologist should be able to assist in excluding pre- and postrenal obstruction. On occasion, the presence of echogenic small kidneys will indicate chronic intrinsic renal disease—end-stage renal disease. It is important that the radiologist not limit

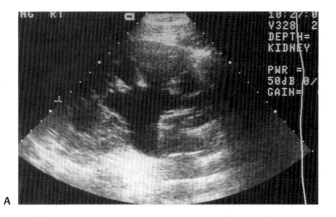

A

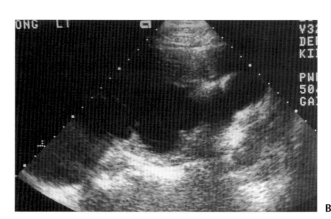

B

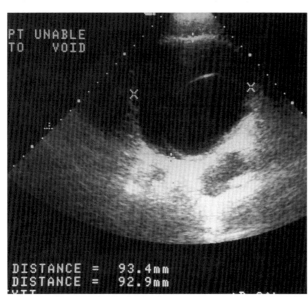

C

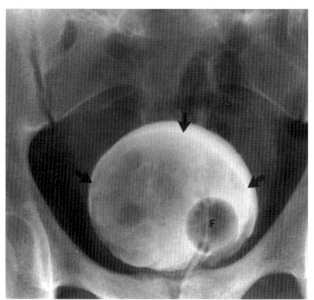

D

Figure 2–9 A 19-year-old male presented with a recent history of hypertension and acute onset of anuria. A ureterocele was causing bladder outlet obstruction. **(A,B)** Renal ultrasound demonstrates bilateral hydronephrosis. **(C)** Bladder ultrasound shows a 9 cm cys-

tic mass that proved to be a ureterocele. **(D)** Contrast-enhanced cystogram reveals Foley (F) and mass (*arrows*) that represents the ureterocele.

the use of sonography to ruling out obstruction. If other etiologies of renal failure are sought, a diagnosis can be achieved in most patients. The American College of Radiology Appropriateness Criteria (UR-10.1, Renal Failure–Acute)[23] suggests sonography as the primary imaging technique in acute renal failure. All other techniques, for example, CT or scintigraphy, play a distinctly secondary role. Their use depends upon the experience and preferences of individual institutions.

A diagnosis of chronic renal failure implies that the process is not reversible. Acute obstructive processes causing acute renal failure must be diagnosed quickly and corrected if renal function is to be preserved. Prerenal processes are readily evident clinically and the patient will not likely be sent for imaging. Intrinsic renal disease is more difficult to diagnose but it may be suggested by excluding postrenal acute renal failure or diagnosing echogenic kidneys with an increased RI.

References

1. Klahr S, Buerkert J, Pakerson ML. The kidney in obstructive uropathy. Contrib Nephrol 1977;7:220–249
2. Webb JA, Reznek RH, White FE, et al. Can ultrasound and computed tomography replace high dose urography in patients with impaired renal function? Q J Med 1984;211:411–425
3. Woolfson RG. Renal failure in artherosclerotic renovascular disease: pathogenesis, diagnosis, and intervention. Postgrad Med J 2001;77:68–74
4. Blandino A, Gaeta M, Minutoli F, et al. MR urography of the ureter. AJR Am J Roentgenol 2002;179:1307–1314
5. Regan F, Bohlman M, Khazan R, Rodriguez R, Schultz-Haakh H. MR urography using HASTE imaging in the assessment of ureteric obstruction. AJR Am J Roentgenol 1996;167:1115–1120
6. Sustic A, Mauric Z, Fuckar Z, et al. Kidney length in postoperative acute renal failure. J Clin Ultrasound 1998;26:251–255
7. Simon AL. Normal renal size: an absolute criterion. AJR Am J Roentgenol 1964;92:270–272
8. Platt JF, Rubin JM, Bowerman R, Marn CS. The inability to detect kidney disease on the basis of echogenicity. AJR Am J Roentgenol 1988;151:317–319
9. Keogan MT, Kliewer MA, Hertzberg BS, et al. Renal resistive indexes: variability in Doppler US measurement in a healthy population. Radiology 1996;199:165–169
10. Platt JF, Rubin JM, Ellis JH. Acute renal failure: possible role of duplex Doppler US in distinction between acute prerenal failure and acute tubular necrosis. Radiology 1991;179:419–423
11. Splendiani G, Parolini C, Fortunato L, Sturniolo A, Costanzi S. Resistive index in chronic nephropathies: predictive value of renal outcome. Clin Nephrol 2002;57:45–50
12. Talner LB, Scheible W, Ellenbogen PH, Beck CH Jr, Gosink BB. How accurate is ultrasonography in detecting hydronephrosis in azotemic patients? Urol Radiol 1981;3:1–6
13. Ellenbogen PH, Scheible FW, Talner LB, Leopold GR. Sensitivity of gray scale ultrasound in detecting urinary tract obstruction. AJR Am J Roentgenol 1978;130:731–733
14. Scola FH, Cronan JJ, Schepps B. Grade I hydronephrosis: pulsed Doppler evaluation. Radiology 1989;171:519–520
15. Nicolau C, Vilana R, Del Amo M, et al. Accuracy of sonography with a hydration test in differentiating between excretory renal obstruction and renal sinus cysts. J Clin Ultrasound 2002;30:532–536
16. Platt JF, Rubin JM, Ellis JH, DiPietro MA. Duplex Doppler US of the kidney: differentiation of obstructive from nonobstructive dilatation. Radiology 1989;171:515–517
17. Platt JF, Rubin JM, Ellis JH. Acute renal obstruction: evaluation with intrarenal duplex Doppler and conventional US. Radiology 1993;186:685–688
18. Lee HJ, Kim SH, Jeong YK, Yeun KM. Doppler sonographic resistive index in obstructed kidney. J Ultrasound Med 1996;15:613–618
19. Rawashdeh YF, Djurhuus JC, Mortensen J, Hørlyck A, Frokiaer J. The intrarenal resistive index as a pathophysiological marker of obstructive uropathy. J Urol 2001;165:1397–1404
20. Kamholtz RG, Cronan JJ, Dorfman GS. Obstruction and the minimally dilated renal collecting system: US evaluation. Radiology 1989;170:51–53
21. Curatola G, Mazzitelli R, Monzani G, Cozzupoli P, Maggiore Q. The value of ultrasound as a screening procedure for urological disorders in renal failure. J Urol 1983;130:8–10
22. Burge HJ, Middleton WD, McClennan BL, Hildebolt CF. Ureteral jets in healthy subjects and in patients with unilateral ureteral calculi: comparison with color Doppler US. Radiology 1991;180:437–442
23. American College of Radiology Appropriateness Criteria. 2001; UR-10.1.

3 Hematuria

Robert L. Bree

Hematuria is a very common clinical problem that challenges both primary care and specialty physicians. Hematuria may be defined as gross or microscopic and symptomatic or asymptomatic. Asymptomatic hematuria occurs in ~13% of men over 35 and women over 55.[1] Asymptomatic hematuria is defined as microscopic hematuria [three to five or more red blood cells (RBCs) per high-power field] seen on two of three urinalyses; one episode of 100 RBCs per high-power field; or gross hematuria.[2] One or two RBCs per high-power field are found in ~15% of asymptomatic persons.[1] Unfortunately, the degree of hematuria does not necessarily correlate with its significance. All hematuria requires evaluation. This discussion includes both gross and microscopic hematuria. This chapter does not discuss patients suspected of having a renal or ureteral calculus, who present with flank pain and hematuria.

cola-colored urine, renal insufficiency, red-cell casts, dysmorphic red cells, and proteinuria. Methods to assess red cell morphology have not been widely accepted in medical practice.[8,9]

Older patients and patients with frankly bloody urine are at higher risk for a significant lesion. Sixty percent of patients with painless gross hematuria will have a diagnosis made by a combination of imaging and cystoscopy. The majority of these diagnoses are not life threatening. Conversely, 40% of patients with gross hematuria have no diagnosis made.[5,7] The vast majority of patients over the age of 50 who present with hematuria will have significant diseases. Because urological cancer is more common in males, those men over 50 who present with hematuria should have a complete and thorough evaluation of the urinary tract (**Fig. 3–1**).[5,10]

Differential Diagnosis

Only ~20% of patients with microscopic hematuria have a significant abnormality as the cause and only 4% have life-threatening lesions (**Table 3–1**).[1,3–6] When gross hematuria occurs, almost 60% have significant abnormalities and 20% have life-threatening disorders.[7] When lower abdominal symptoms are associated with hematuria, the cause is commonly in the lower urinary tract D a significant percentage will have treatable pathology.[2,3] **Table 3–1** lists the more common diseases, stratified by severity, that are associated with hematuria. It is not always clear that the associated diagnosis is the cause of the hematuria. In fact, only about half of the patients investigated for hematuria have a related diagnosis discovered in the initial evaluation. When the remaining, undiagnosed patients with persistent hematuria are followed, a small percentage will have a cause for hematuria detected within 3 years of the discovery of hematuria. These diseases include glomerulonephritis, calculi, and, rarely, bladder or prostate cancer.[6]

Because transient hematuria is common, the insistence on multiple positive tests is important when trying to separate disease from no disease. It can be useful to try to separate glomerular from nonglomerular hematuria. Findings that favor a glomerular source include

Table 3–1 Common Causes of Hematuria

Life-Threatening and Significant Diseases

Bladder cancer

Renal cell carcinoma

Transitional cell carcinoma of ureter or kidney

Ureteral calculus

Abdominal aortic aneurysm

Prostate cancer

Generalized renal parenchymal disease

Moderately significant diseases

Pyelonephritis

Cystitis

Hydronephrosis

Bladder calculus

Bladder diverticulum

Urethral stricture

Neurogenic bladder

Prostatitis

Insignificant Diseases

Renal cyst

Benign prostatic hyperplasia

Urethritis

Bladder diverticulum

Caliceal diverticulum

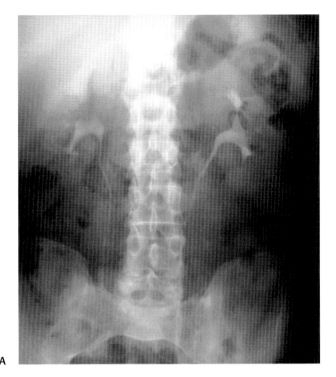

A

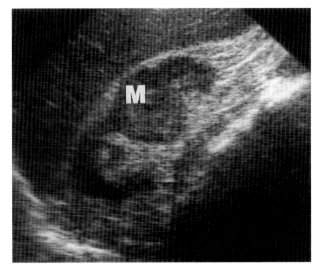

B

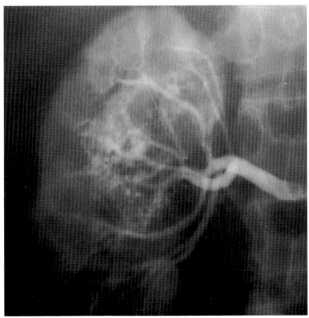

C

Figure 3–1 Central renal cell carcinoma in a 60-year-old man. **(A)** Intravenous pyelogram shows very subtle dilatation of upper pole collecting system on the right. Tomograms did not suggest a mass. **(B)** Right renal ultrasound shows a large solid mass (M) in the midportion of the kidney. **(C)** Arteriogram confirms typical findings of renal cell carcinoma.

Diagnostic Evaluation

Nonimaging Evaluation

In addition to imaging evaluations, common testing performed in patients with hematuria include (1) search for proteinuria (seen in glomerulopathies); (2) urine cytology; (3) urine culture; (4) renal function tests; and (5) endoscopic evaluations, including evaluation of the bladder, ureter, and renal collecting system.[11] Appropriate sequenc-

ing of these procedures is important. The frequency with which invasive and more expensive procedures (e.g., ureteroscopy or retrograde pyelography) are used depends on the quality and reliability of the less invasive studies, particularly the imaging studies. Risk–benefit choices must be made when deciding whether to administer iodinated intravenous contrast media to a patient of a certain age or sex. This evaluation is made relative to the extent of hematuria and the chances of finding a significant or life-threatening abnormality. In general, meta-analyses and clinical decision-making models suggest that

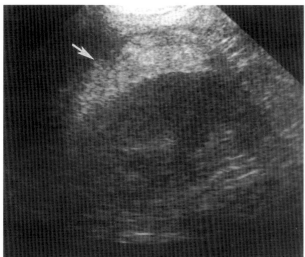

A

Figure 3–2 Infiltrative transitional cell carcinoma. **(A)** Ultrasound of the right kidney in a patient with gross hematuria. Normal renal architecture is absent and there is increased echogenicity in the perirenal space (*arrow*). **(B)** Computed tomogram demonstrates in-

B

filtrative neoplasm with perirenal hemorrhage. The kidney was surgically removed and contained extensive transitional cell carcinoma with spontaneous perirenal hemorrhage.

patients with hematuria who harbor a urological malignancy are over 90% curable, whereas the risk of adverse events from the evaluation is ~1%. Therefore, evaluation is always warranted except in women under 40, where the yield of pathology is less than the risk of adverse events.[5,11–14]

Imaging Other than Ultrasound

Imaging tests for hematuria range from noninvasive to invasive. The intravenous pyelogram (IVP) has been the standard examination for many years. Other examinations that are capable of making a diagnosis in more difficult or enigmatic cases are retrograde pyelography computed tomography (CT) (**Fig. 3–2**), magnetic resonance imaging (MRI), renal scintigraphy, renal arteriography, renal venography, and antegrade pyelography. CT of the entire urinary tract can be augmented by images of the contrast-opacified collecting systems, ureters, and bladder (24); the combined exam is known as CT urography.

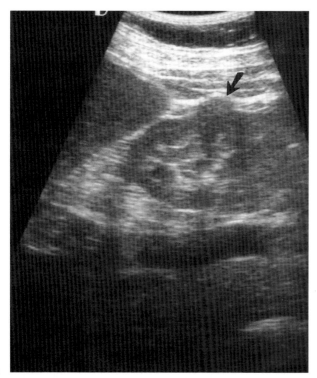

A

Figure 3–3 Small renal cell carcinoma. **(A)** A 55-year-old woman was initially investigated with ultrasound and a small solid mass (*arrow*) was discovered on the lateral cortex of the left kidney.

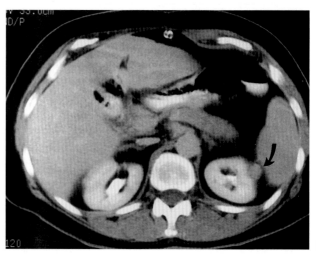

B

(B) Computed tomogram confirms the solid nature of the mass (*arrow*) and suggests a neoplasm. A small renal cell carcinoma was removed surgically.

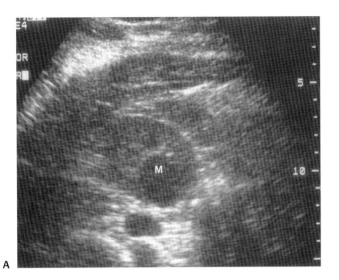

A

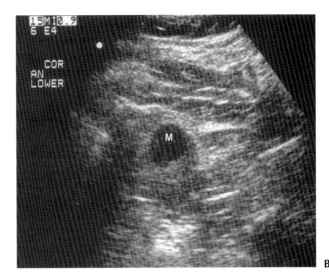

B

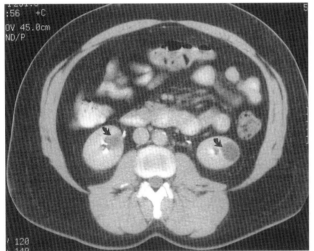

C

Figure 3–4 Bilateral focal pyelonephritis. A 45-year-old man presented with hematuria and fever. **(A)** Ultrasound of the right and **(B)** left kidneys reveals bilateral hypoechoic masses with internal echoes (M). **(C)** Computed tomogram performed at the same admission shows similar bilateral masses (*arrows*), which are nonspecific. In view of the suspected infection and lack of strong evidence of abscess, treatment with antibiotics commenced, and the symptoms resolved. Follow-up ultrasound was normal.

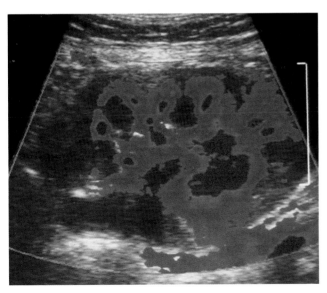

Figure 3–5 Renal arteriovenous fistula with power Doppler. A patient who underwent a biopsy of a renal transplant and who subsequently developed hematuria was examined with ultrasound. Gray-scale imaging was not revealing. Power Doppler examination shows turbulent flow in the renal hilus, proven to represent an arteriovenous fistula.

The IVP-like portions of the exam may be obtained when contrast administered for the CT has opacified the bladder and collecting systems. Images may alternatively be produced by reformatting delayed CT images to show this anatomy. The pyelogram portion of this exam is comparable to a standard IVP exam, and the CT is more accurate than ultrasound or nephrotomography for small focal renal parenchymal abnormalities. For conditions such as infiltrative tumors, small carcinomas (**Fig. 3–3**), or pyelonephritis (**Fig. 3–4**), contrast-enhanced CT or MRI may be necessary to make the diagnosis.[15–17] DMSA renal scintigraphy can define renal masses when an IVP cannot be performed.[18] Renal arteriography may be the best technique capable of identifying vascular causes for hematuria, such as arteriovenous malformations or hemangiomas, although newer ultrasound techniques such as power Doppler can rival conventional or MR angiography. Vascular lesions such as this are most commonly found in young patients with gross hematuria (**Fig. 3–5**). Renal venography may be necessary to diagnose venous abnormalities, primarily renal vein varices. Finally in the patient with a nonfunctioning or obstructed kidney, antegrade pyelography may be the best choice, particularly when urothelial cancer is suspected.[2,11]

Ultrasound

The role of ultrasound in the evaluation of hematuria is controversial and has not been studied extensively.[19,20] Because the IVP and CT remain standard and reliable examinations, ultrasound has not received much attention. There are, however, many advantages to ultrasound in this patient population. Ultrasound requires no preparation and does not use intravenous contrast material. That eliminates the possibility of an adverse event, particularly in a population at low risk for significant disease. The

actual cost of ultrasound is lower than IVP and CT. Even in an asymptomatic patient who is suspected of having a ureteral calculus, ultrasound can identify the obstructed collecting system and, occasionally, identify the stone in the distal ureter (**Fig. 3–6**).[21]

Mokulis et al,[22] in a study of 101 patients who had ultrasound after a normal IVP, found that 20% of patients had an abnormal ultrasound study. All of these proved to be false-positive ultrasounds when subsequent evaluation was done. Therefore, they conclude that ultrasound is unnecessary in patients with a normal IVP and microscopic hematuria. On the other hand, IVP can miss anterior and posterior renal masses that can be seen with ultrasound.[17] In a more extensive review of 193 patients with microhematuria, Aslaksen et al[21] demonstrated a clear advantage for ultrasound in detecting significant abnormalities,

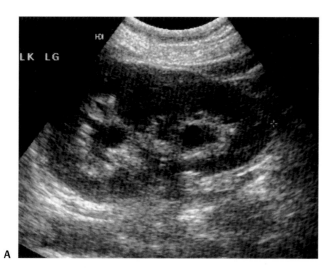

A

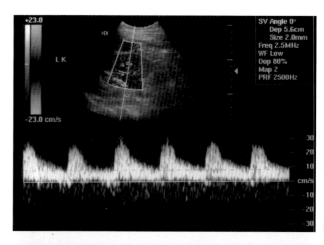

B

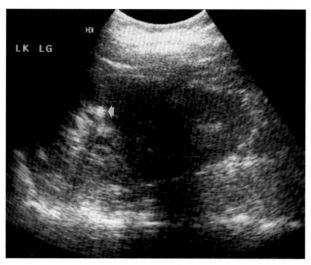

C

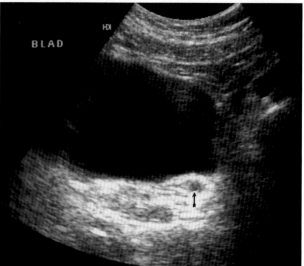

D

Figure 3–6 Obstructing distal ureteral calculus. A young woman presented to her physician after recovering from an episode of left flank pain and hematuria, but no stone was passed. An ultrasound was requested. The right kidney ultrasound was normal. **(A)** Hydronephrosis is demonstrated on the left. **(B)** Left renal Doppler indicates an elevated resistive index (0.74) indicating obstruction. **(C)** A calculus with shadowing (*arrow*) is seen in the upper pole of the left kidney. **(D)** Ultrasound of the bladder shows dilated left distal ureter (*arrow*). (*Continued*)

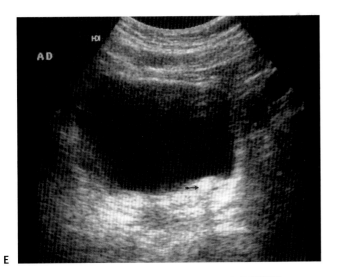

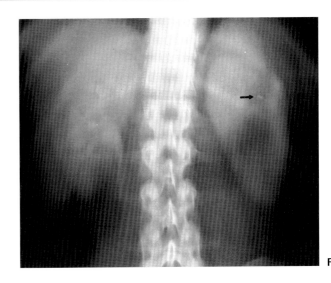

E

F

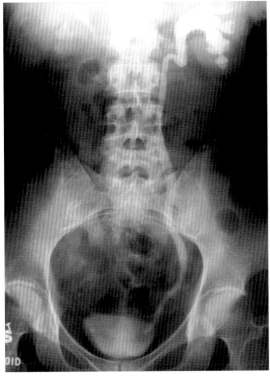

G

Figure 3–6 (*Continued*) **(E)** A few millimeters caudal to **(D)** a stone (*arrow*) is demonstrated at the ureterovesical junction (IVJ) in the intramural portion. **(F)** Early tomogram from intravenous pyelogram (IVP) shows delay in excretion on the left and an upper pole calculus (*arrow*). **(G)** Delayed film from IVP after voiding demonstrates obstructing calculus at the UVJ.

especially renal masses. Unfortunately, some stones were missed by both modalities (**Fig. 3–7**).

An additional advantage of ultrasound is the evaluation of the bladder. In the current practice standard, the bladder is included in the examination of the retroperitoneum when the urinary tract is suspected of being abnormal. Bladder tumors, hemorrhagic cystitis, calculi, and diverticula can be found with ultrasound but are sometimes not seen well with IVP (**Fig. 3–8**).[21–23]

In the patient with known or suspected renal parenchymal disease, the most common cause of gross or microscopic hematuria is the renal disease itself. When a glomerulopathy is evident because of proteinuria, red cell casts, and red cell dysmorphism, hematuria can be attributed to

the underlying disease. In these patients, IVP may be contraindicated because of the risk of provoking renal failure. Ultrasound is warranted to confirm the findings of generalized renal disease, as well as to exclude other superimposed pathology (**Fig. 3–9**).[2,4,9,11]

In the patient who is known to have an acute hemorrhagic cystitis, imaging is typically not warranted unless there is failure of therapy. In this circumstance, an underlying additional cause must be investigated, particularly in men and women over 40 years of age. In younger women, because hemorrhagic cystitis is very common, imaging is only necessary in a very severe or refractory case.[2,10]

In some patients with hematuria, economic savings result when ultrasound is used instead of CT or IVP. In

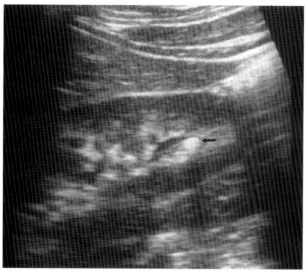

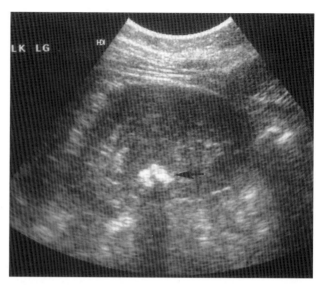

Figure 3–7 Nephrolithiasis without obstruction. **(A)** Sagittal scan of the right kidney in a patient with hematuria demonstrates a small nonobstructing calculus (*arrow*) in a lower pole calyx. This stone was not identified on an intravenous pyelogram. **(B)** Large left renal calculus (*arrow*) in the midportion of the kidney that was identified on a plain abdominal radiograph.

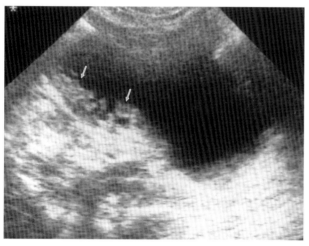

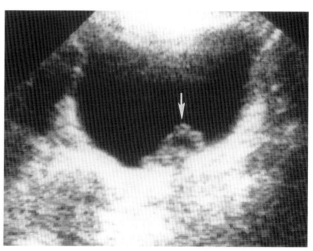

Figure 3–8 Bladder pathology. **(A)** Bullous cystitis. Focal mucosal thickening with cystic change (*arrows*) in a woman with chronic bullous cystitis and hematuria. **(B)** Bladder cancer. Focal polypoid mass (*arrow*) discovered in a patient being evaluated with ultrasound for hematuria. The bladder should be included in all scans directed to the retroperitoneum for suspected urinary tract abnormalities.

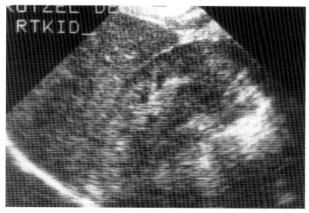

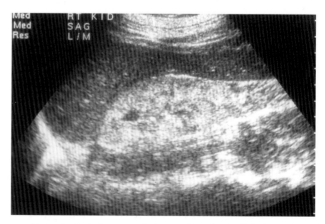

Figure 3–9 Two patients with renal parenchymal disease. **(A)** Acute glomerulonephritis. Ultrasound of the right kidney showing normal size but increased echogenicity compatible with the clinical and biopsy diagnosis of glomerulonephritis. The patient had hematuria and other urinalysis features of glomerulonephritis. **(B)** Chronic renal failure. Patient with hematuria and renal failure. The kidney is small and echogenic and has a thin cortex. No other reasons for hematuria were found, and further evaluation was not deemed necessary.

Corwin and Silverstein's series,[12] the expense of finding one renal cell carcinoma with ultrasound was half the cost of finding a renal cell carcinoma using IVP. Even if additional IVPs must be performed in patients with caliectasis and stones seen with ultrasound, significant cost savings resulted if patients were screened with ultrasound.[21]

The most significant limitations of ultrasound are the inability to evaluate the ureters and, in some instances, the inability to define urothelial lesions. The sensitivity of ultrasound can be enhanced, particularly when blood is found coming from an individual ureter at the time of cystoscopy, by adding CT urography or retrograde pyelography.[3,12,21]

Recommendations for Imaging

Although there is scant literature on the role of ultrasound in hematuria, the American College of Radiology Task Force on Appropriateness Criteria for hematuria[25] suggests ultrasound, CT, and IVP as the first-line imaging tests. When imaging is indicated, the choice of IVP, CT, or ultrasound may depend upon factors such as age, extent of hematuria, and result of urinary cytology, which, if positive, would suggest CT or IVP. Risk factors for contrast administration and radiation dose also enter into the decision algorithm. Both IVP or ultrasound can, on occasion, miss significant disease and further evaluation with CT may be warranted. The American College of Radiology Task Force on Appropriateness Criteria recommendations following here are meant to guide the initial evaluation of hematuria and may not apply to difficult or complex patient problems.

Hematuria in patients other than young women with cystitis or patients with generalized renal parenchymal disease
IVP: Indicated
CT urography: Indicated
Urological ultrasound: Probably indicated
Retrograde pyelography: Probably not indicated
Other imaging examinations: Not indicated

Hematuria in patients with generalized renal parenchymal disease
Urological ultrasound: Indicated
Other urological imaging exams: Not indicated

Hemorrhagic cystitis in woman under 40 that clears with treatment
All imaging tests: Not indicated

References

1. Mohr DN, Offord KP, Owen RA, Melton LJ. Asymptomatic microhematuria and urologic disease: a population-based study. JAMA 1986;256:224–229
2. Grossfeld GD, Wolf JS Jr, Litwin MS, et al. Asymptomatic microscopic hematuria in adults: summary of the AUA best practice policy recommendations. Am Fam Physician 2001;63:1145–1154
3. Bryden AAG, Paul AB, Kyriakides C. Investigation of haematuria. Br J Hosp Med 1995;54:455–458
4. Golin AL, Howard RS. Asymptomatic microscopic hematuria. Urology 1980;124:389–391
5. Mariani AJ, Mariani MC, Macchoini C, et al. The significance of adult hematuria: 1,000 hematuria evaluations including a risk-benefit and cost-effectiveness analysis. Urology 1989;141:350–355
6. Murakami S, Igarashi T, Hara S, Shimazaki J. Strategies for asymptomatic microscopic hematuria: a prospective study of 1,034 patients. J Urol 1990;144:99–101
7. Barkin M, Lopatin W, Herschorn S, Comisarow R. Unexplained hematuria. Can J Surg 1983;26:501–503
8. Ahmed Z, Lee J. Asymptomatic urinary abnormalities; hematuria and proteinuria. Med Clin North Am 1977;81:641–650
9. Webb JAW. Imaging in haematuria [editorial]. Clin Radiol 1997;52:167–171
10. Froom P, Ribak J, Benbassat J. Significance of microhaematuria in young adults. Br Med J 1984;288:20–22
11. Sutton JM. Evaluation of hematuria in adults. JAMA 1990;263:2475–2480
12. Corwin HL, Silverstein MD. The diagnosis of neoplasia in patients with asymptomatic microscopic hematuria: a decision analysis. J Urol 1988;139:1002–1006
13. Green LF, O'Shaughnessey EJ Jr, Hendricks ED. A study of five hundred patients with asymptomatic microhematuria. JAMA 1956;161:610–613
14. Thompson IM. The evaluation of microscopic hematuria: a population-based study. J Urol 1987;138:1189–1190
15. Caoili EM, Cohan RH, Korobkin M, et al. Urinary tract abnormalities: initial experience with multi-detector row CT urography. Radiology 2002;222:353–360
16. Bree RL, Schultz SR, Hayes R. Large infiltrating renal transitional cell carcinomas: CT and ultrasound features. J Computer Assist Tomogr 1990;14:381–385
17. Glen DA, Gilbert FJ, Bayliss AP. Renal carcinomas missed by urography. Br J Urol 1989;63:457–459
18. Chisholm RA, Millet B, Sherwood T, Wraight EP, Doyle PT. The investigation of painless haematuria: a comparison of intravenous urography and DMSA scintigraphy. Clin Radiol 1988;39:494–495
19. Spencer J, Lindsell D, Mastorakou I. Ultrasonography compared with intravenous urography in the investigation of adults with haematuria. Br Med J 1990;301:1074–1076
20. Stonelake PS, Wallace DMA. Investigation of adults with haematuria. BMJ 1990;301:1396–1397
21. Aslaksen A, Gadeholt G, Göthlin JH. Ultrasonography versus intravenous urography in the evaluation of patients with microscopic haematuria. Br J Urology 1990;66:144–147
22. Mokulis JA, Arndt WF, Downey JR, Caballero RL, Thomason IM. Should renal ultrasound be performed in the patient with microscopic hematuria and a normal excretory urogram? J Urol 1995;154:1300–1301
23. Bree RL, Silver TM. Sonography of bladder and perivesical abnormalities. AJR 1981;136:1101–1104
24. Brun B, Gammelgaard J, Christoffersen J. Transabdominal dynamic ultrasonography in the detection of bladder tumors. J Urol 1984;132:19–20
25. American College of Radiology Task Force on Appropriateness Criteria. American College of Radiology: Appropriateness Criteria for Imaging and Treatment Decisions. 2005:UR5.1–UR5.6

Suggested Readings

Abuelo JG. Evaluation of hematuria. Urology 1983;21:215–225

Benson GS, Brewer ED. Hematuria: algorithms for diagnosis, II: Hematuria in the adult and hematuria secondary to trauma. JAMA 1981; 246:993–995

Copley JB. Review: isolated asymptomatic hematuria in the adult. Am J Med Sc 1986;291:101–111

Fairley KF. Clinical evaluation of the kidney. Urinalysis 359–390

Lowe FC, Brendler CB. Evaluation of the urologic patient: history, physical examination, and urinalysis. 307–331

Messing EM, Young TB, Hunt BV, Emoto SE, Wehbie JM. The significance of asymptomatic microhematuria in men 50 or more years old: findings of a home screening study using urinary dipsticks. J Urology 1987;137:919–922

4 Acute Abdominal Trauma

W. Dennis Foley

The most common cause of morbidity and mortality in the second, third, and fourth decades of life is trauma. The leading cause is automobile accidents, with penetrating injury, battery, and sports-related injury also important factors. The prevalence of trauma and cost to society are increasing. The spectrum of major trauma encompasses neurological, thoracic, abdominal, and musculoskeletal injuries. Life-threatening consequences may result from injury to any body region. Blunt abdominal injury poses a particular problem because there may be minimal physical findings, particularly if the patient's state of consciousness is impaired. In addition, blunt abdominal injury may coexist with other significant trauma, including intracranial hemorrhage, ruptured thoracic aorta and pneumothorax, and musculoskeletal injury (e.g., major spinal, pelvic, and long-bone fractures). An accurate evaluation of abdominal injury is required to select the patient's management.

With the advent of sequential computed tomographic (CT) scanning for blunt abdominal injury in the late 1970s and early 1980s, surgeons began to refine their indications for exploratory laparotomy based on an evolving understanding of the natural history of blunt abdominal injury.[1,2] In a hemodynamically stable patient, both major and minor lacerations of the liver, spleen, and kidneys will usually resolve with conservative management and no sequelae. Hepatic and splenic lacerations with intraperitoneal blood are not primary indications for laparotomy. Intervention, either angiographic or surgical, is usually reserved for lacerations associated with active bleeding, manifest as vascular contrast extravasation at the time of emergency CT scanning.[3] Other CT findings in a hemodynamically stable patient that may prompt immediate laparotomy include intestinal rupture, central renal pedicle injury, pancreatic transection, and intraperitoneal bladder rupture. The major indication for laparotomy in a hemodynamically unstable patient is hemoperitoneum (without obvious extraabdominal blood loss) and hypotension unresponsive to intravenous fluid resuscitation. In the past, clinical evaluation and diagnostic peritoneal lavage determined the need for laparotomy.[4] Sonography has largely supplanted diagnostic peritoneal lavage for detecting hemoperitoneum.[5-8]

CT is the preferred technique for evaluating normotensive patients with documented abdominal injury.[9] It provides accurate global diagnostic information about abdominal and pelvic injury. However, the relatively high rate of negative abdominal and pelvic CT scans following blunt trauma, particularly in patients who are neurologically impaired, has prompted the use of sonography as a more cost-effective and efficient screening study.[5-8] Hemodynamically stable patients with documented intraperitoneal fluid on sonography should proceed to CT evaluation. An abdominal sonogram that is negative for intraperitoneal fluid has been assumed to be sufficient to exclude significant blunt abdominal trauma in a patient without hematuria and with no clinical evidence of occult injury following 6 hours of observation.[10]

This chapter discusses the role of abdominal sonography and CT scanning in evaluating patients with suspected blunt abdominal injury. Both hemodynamically unstable and hemodynamically stable patients are discussed. The goal of sonographic imaging in trauma is to provide a cost-effective triage with high sensitivity and negative predictive value that leads to appropriate patient management and outcome.

Differential Diagnosis

Intraperitoneal Fluid

Intraperitoneal fluid may be blood, bile, urine, pancreatic juice, lymph, intestinal content, or preexistent ascites. Intraperitoneal fluid following blunt trauma is most often intraperitoneal blood resulting from hepatic, splenic, or mesenteric laceration. A periportal liver laceration or gallbladder rupture may cause leakage of bile into the peritoneal cavity. In acutely injured patients, bile is usually not the predominant component of intraperitoneal fluid. Other types of intraperitoneal fluid in the patient with blunt trauma are unusual. Urinary ascites usually results from intraperitoneal rupture of the bladder. The dome of the bladder is the most common site of rupture. Pancreatic ascites may result when there is pancreatic transection associated with disruption of the posterior parietal peritoneum. Pancreatic ascites is usually caused by delayed intraperitoneal rupture of a pancreatic pseudocyst. Chylous ascites is very uncommon. It results from transection of the cisterna chyli or proximal thoracic duct. Patients with underlying liver disease with portal hypertension and hypoproteinemia may have preexisting ascites.

Hepatic and Splenic Injury

Injuries to the liver and spleen result from compression or shearing force.[11] The resultant lacerations may be localized or multifocal and may or may not be associated with a capsular tear. Grading schemes, such as CT injury severity scores, have been used to classify the extent of solid organ injury.[12] However, there is no direct correlation between the injury severity score and the likelihood of delayed bleeding.[12]

Parenchymal and capsular tears usually result in a localized perihepatic or perisplenic hematoma, such as a sentinel clot,[13] as well as intraperitoneal bleeding in the perihepatic or perisplenic spaces, paracolic gutters, or pelvis. This common pattern of hemoperitoneum distribution means that a rapid four-quadrant sonographic assessment will usually detect intraperitoneal fluid associated with hepatic or splenic injury.

Mesenteric and Bowel Injury

Injuries to the mesentery or bowel are more problematic. Hematoma may be confined to the bowel wall or mesentery without lateral or inferior distribution into the dependent intraperitoneal spaces.[14] Because there may be no hemoperitoneum, an emergency sonogram may not detect these injuries.

Extraperitoneal Organ Injury

Extraperitoneal organ injury does not usually result in intraperitoneal bleeding. Injuries to the kidneys, pancreas, and duodenum, and disruption of the aortoiliac arterial system (caused by seat belt injury or pelvic fracture) are in this category. Thus, a negative sonogram for intraperitoneal fluid in patients with a central abdominal compression injury or hematuria does not exclude the possibility of significant injury.[15] Patients with hematuria and those with lumbar spine or pelvic fractures should have an abdominal pelvic CT scan to exclude injuries even when sonography is negative.[15] In addition, care must be taken to avoid missing traumatic pneumothorax, which has a relatively high association with blunt abdominal injury.[16]

Diagnostic Evaluation

Nonimaging Evaluation

Patients with abdominal injury are assessed for hemodynamic stability and the presence of associated injuries, including neurological, thoracic, and orthopedic injuries. Patients should be triaged into a hemodynamically unstable or hemodynamically stable category to guide further evaluation.

If patients are unresponsive, either due to neurological injury or alcoholism, then external signs of abdominal trauma, including body wall contusion, should be assessed on a clinical examination. For patients who are conscious and responsive, clinical evaluation for focal guarding and rebound tenderness is vital.

Plasma expanders are usually infused via intravenous lines. Bladder catheterization is used to evaluate for hematuria and to measure urine output. Tube thoracostomy is performed if any significant hemopneumothorax is present. Endotracheal intubation may be required for neurologically impaired patients or those in respiratory difficulty following aspiration or tube thoracostomy. The early triage diagnostic evaluation by sonography is usually performed concurrent with these diagnostic or resuscitative procedures.

The Hemodynamically Unstable Patient

The hemodynamically unstable patient with suspected abdominal injury requires urgent evaluation for possible hemoperitoneum. Diagnostic peritoneal lavage can fulfill this role with very high reported sensitivity and specificity.[4] Limitations of diagnostic peritoneal lavage include its inability to detect contained intracapsular hemorrhage in the liver or spleen, and relative insensitivity to bowel perforation and mesenteric hemorrhage. Diagnostic peritoneal lavage is insensitive to retroperitoneal injury, including pancreatic, duodenal, and renal injuries. A false-positive diagnostic peritoneal lavage may result from a traumatic peritoneal tap.

Sonography can be performed as an alternative test to diagnostic peritoneal lavage.[5,8] In general, sonography and diagnostic peritoneal lavage share the same limitations: suboptimal detection of solid organ injury, mesenteric hemorrhage, bowel perforation, and retroperitoneal injury.[17]

A positive diagnostic peritoneal lavage or positive sonogram in the hemodynamically unstable patient should result in urgent laparotomy. It may be appropriate to delay laparotomy in some patients with multiorgan injuries. Severe associated neurological injury may require early evaluation by neurological CT. Thoracic injury may require portable chest radiography, tube thoracostomy, or a vascular phase multidetector CT examination to evaluate for possible thoracic aortic rupture. A negative diagnostic peritoneal lavage or negative sonogram in a hemodynamically unstable patient should lead to urgent evaluation of the thorax, abdominal retroperitoneum, pelvis, or extremities as sources of continuing blood loss.

The Hemodynamically Stable Patient

The hemodynamically stable patient may be assessed by sonography. Detection of intraperitoneal fluid or sentinel clot should be an indication for an abdominal pelvic CT study. A negative emergency abdominal sonogram, in the

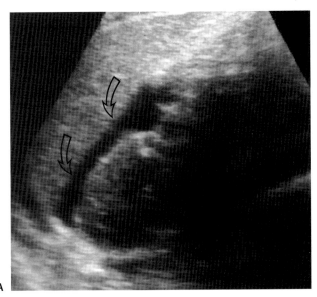

A

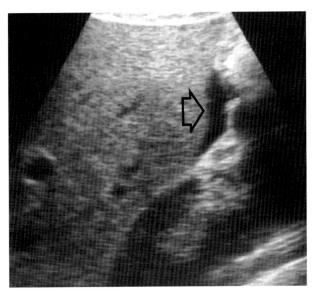

B

Figure 4–1 Hemoperitoneum in the hepatorenal space following blunt injury. **(A)** Fluid (*curved arrows*) is present in the posterior right subhepatic space and extends to the diaphragm.

(B) Longitudinal sonogram in a more medial plane demonstrates contiguous fluid in the anterior right subhepatic space (*arrow*) between the right colon and the inferior surface of the liver.

hemodynamically stable patient, does not exclude the possibility of contained intrahepatic or intrasplenic hematoma, mesenteric or bowel wall injury, or retroperitoneal injury.[15] Sirlin et al indicate the clinical findings that mandate additional testing despite negative screening ultrasound study to include persistent pain, decreased hematocrit levels, abdominal wall echomyoses, hemodynamic instability, and sepsis.[18] Additionally, hematuria and fractures of the lower ribs, lumbar spine, and pelvis would warrant additional testing. At institutions where a period of observation following a negative ultrasound study is not routine practice, a negative ultrasound scan may not be adequate to exclude occult injury. In these circumstances, CT should be considered as the primary study.

Ultrasound Imaging

Small-footprint, 3 to 5 MHz sector transducers, either linear phased array or curved array, are the most appropriate choice for an abdominal trauma sonographic study. As with all sonographic studies, attention to appropriate depth and width of field, gain, and time gain compensation (TGC) curve, and focal zones is important for image quality.

A four-quadrant rapid survey sonographic technique is recommended. This involves evaluation of the perihepatic and perisplenic spaces, the paracolic gutters, and posterior deep pelvis. The right and left pleural spaces are evaluated concurrent with imaging of the perihepatic and perisplenic spaces. Operator speed and expertise are essential. Examination time to assess for fluid in the four abdominal quadrants, right and left pleural space, and, in selected instances, the pericardial space, should be limited to less than 5 minutes. Although examination speed is critical,

adequate documentation of findings is also important. This includes annotated hard-copy recordings obtained online at the time of examination, or images transferred from an ultrasound unit to a departmental electronic archive and viewed at a workstation.

In the right upper quadrant, the hepatorenal space and subphrenic spaces should be evaluated. Parasagittal and coronal imaging planes, using intercostal and subcostal access, are used to evaluate this region (**Fig. 4–1**). A similar approach is used in the left upper quadrant to define the left anterior subphrenic and perisplenic spaces (**Fig. 4–2, Fig. 4–3**). The lesser sac is frequently obscured by gas and

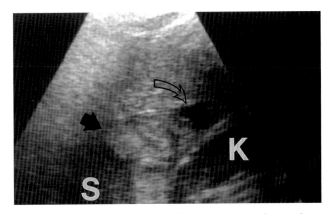

Figure 4–2 Splenic laceration with intrasplenic and perisplenic blood clot. Oblique coronal image of left upper quadrant. There is echogenic blood clot (*arrow*) extending from the region of the splenic hilum anterior to the upper pole of the left kidney (splenorenal recess) and toward the diaphragm. This is a perisplenic "sentinel clot." An adjacent, more inferior hypoechoic defect (*curved open arrow*) represents an adjacent intrasplenic laceration containing unclotted blood. S, spleen; K, left kidney.

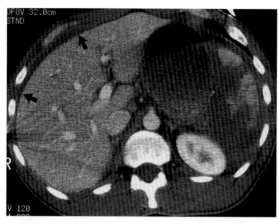

A

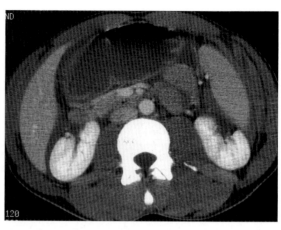

B

Figure 4–3 Dynamic helical computed tomographic scan of patient illustrated in **Fig. 4–2** with splenic laceration and hemoperitoneum. **(A)** Scan at a more cephalad level demonstrates splenic laceration with a perisplenic fluid collection containing relatively high attenua-

tion coagulum and relatively low attenuation presumed unclotted blood. Perihepatic hemoperitoneum (*arrows*), lower in attenuation than the perisplenic blood clot, is noted. **(B)** A more inferior-level scan demonstrates subhepatic and perisplenic hemoperitoneum.

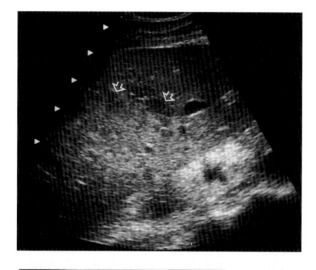

A

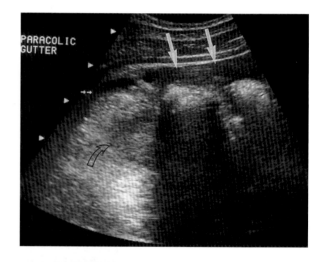

B

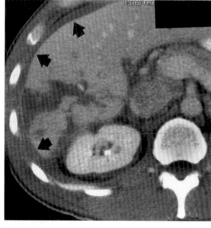

C

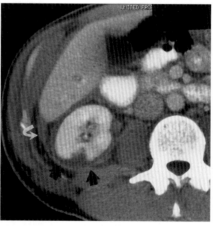

D

Figure 4–4 Hepatic lacerations following blunt trauma. **(A)** Coronal plane right upper quadrant sonogram demonstrates linear hypoechoic defects in the hepatic parenchyma (*arrows*). **(B)** Coronal scan at a more inferior and posterior level demonstrates fluid in the paracolic gutter between the abdominal wall and right colon (*arrows*). Note the inferior tip of the liver (*straight arrows*) and the upper pole of the right kidney (*curved arrow*). **(C)** Contrast-enhanced computed tomo-

graphic (CT) scan documents multiple transverse lacerations in the right hepatic lobe extending to the capsule with perihepatic hematoma (*arrows*). **(D)** More caudal level CT scan through the inferior right hepatic lobe demonstrates hemoperitoneum (*curved arrow*) and perinephric hematoma (*arrowheads*) related to a small posterior margin renal laceration. The renal injury was not detected by abdominal sonogram.

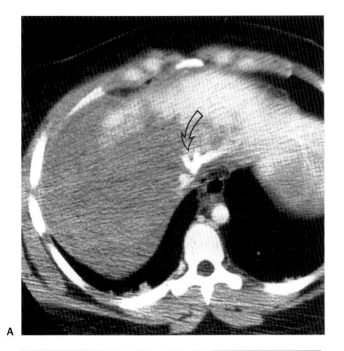

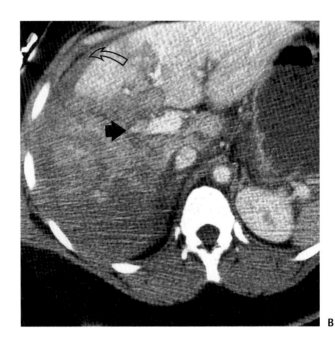

A

B

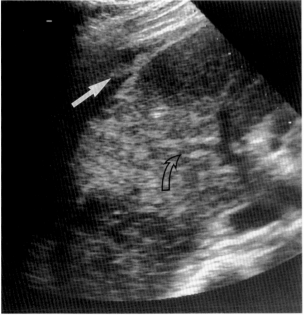

C

Figure 4–5 Right hepatic lobe laceration with interruption of the right hepatic vein and right portal vein. **(A)** Computed tomographic (CT) scan at a cephalic level demonstrates a patent conjoint left and middle hepatic vein (*arrow*) and absent right hepatic vein at the hepatic vein/inferior vena cava confluence. Laceration margin is adjacent to the major fissure. No enhancement of the right hepatic lobe is seen at this level. **(B)** CT scan at the level of the hepatic hilum shows an amputated right portal vein (*arrow*) and relatively high attenuation coagulum in the anterior right hepatic lobe extending to the capsule. There is a high attenuation perihepatic hemoperitoneum—"sentinel clot" (*curved arrow*). The more posterior right hepatic lobe is hypoattenuating, reflecting infarction. **(C)** Sonogram of the right upper quadrant using an oblique transverse plane. Echogenic intrahepatic coagulum is identified in the anterior right hepatic lobe, and the heterogeneous hypoechoic posterior right hepatic lobe corresponds to infarction. Perihepatic hematoma and coagulum are identified (*arrow*). The right portal vein (*curved arrow*) was amputated.

ingested material in the stomach. Hepatic and splenic lacerations can be recognized as linear or branching hypoechoic defects in the parenchyma (**Fig. 4–4**). Subcapsular and perihepatic and perisplenic hematomas—"sentinel clots"—may be relatively echogenic because of the aggregated red cells and blood products in the coagulum (**Fig. 4–5**).

The spectrum of renal injuries following blunt trauma includes laceration, fracture, vascular pedicle disruption (laceration and/or thrombosis), infarction, and pyelocalyceal/ureteric disruption. Sonography is less sensitive in detecting renal injury than hepatic or splenic injury, probably because acoustic access is more difficult in a supine

patient in the trauma setting. The distinction of perirenal hematoma from perirenal urinoma cannot be obtained by sonography, but may be evident on a delayed image sequence obtained in an intravenous contrast-enhanced CT examination.

The pleural spaces and diaphragm are evaluated by cephalad tilt of the transducer probe in both the parasagittal and coronal imaging plane. Pleural space fluid is anechoic and demarcated by the diaphragm inferiorly, the costal pleural surface and chest wall peripherally, and the lower lobe of the lung superiorly (**Fig. 4–6**). Frequently, compression atelectasis of the lower lobes can be seen within the pleural fluid, moving during inspiration and expiration.

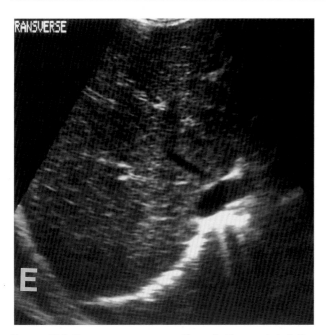

Figure 4–6 Transverse sonogram through the cephalad liver demonstrates a small right pleural effusion (E). The diaphragm was intact and moved appropriately with respiration.

Sonography cannot be relied on to exclude diaphragm rupture because it is insensitive in the detection of diaphragmatic defects. Direct ultrasonic findings of rupture of the diaphragm include focal diaphragmatic disruption, and herniation of liver, spleen, or bowel loops through the diaphragmatic defect. A "floating diaphragm," the appearance

of the free edge of a disrupted diaphragm outlined by pleural and peritoneal fluid, may be noted. In the hemodynamically stable patient, diagnosing rupture of the diaphragm is not urgent. It can be diagnosed in a more elective setting using reformatted coronal or sagittal images from helical CT data or by direct coronal MRI. On the left side, gastric and colonic herniation can be recognized by radiography.

Intraperitoneal fluid in the lower abdomen will usually collect in the posterior deep pelvis (retrovesical or retrouterine space) (**Fig. 4–7**). In the acute setting, in which the patient is examined without bladder distension, sonography may not be able to image this compartment of the peritoneal cavity.[19] The lower-quadrant examination evaluates the inferior aspect of the paracolic gutters and the perivesical spaces (**Fig. 4–8**).

Midline compression injuries may result in myocardial contusion or pericardial tamponade. A posttrauma echocardiogram limited to evaluation of the pericardium can be performed utilizing a subxyphoid approach, with parasagittal and coronal imaging planes directed to the cardiac apex.

Evaluation of Sonographic Imaging in Blunt Abdominal Trauma

Publications in the surgical and emergency medicine literature attest to the interest and potential utility of emergency abdominal sonography in the blunt trauma patient.[20,21] The use of sonography as a replacement for diagnostic peritoneal lavage in the hemodynamically unstable patient following blunt injury appears well supported.[5,8] Sonography can be performed more expeditiously and avoids potential false-positive results from

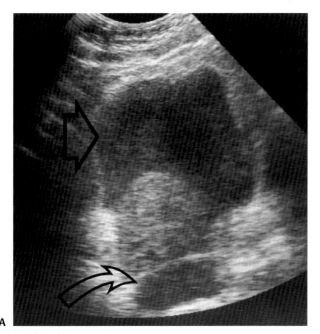

A

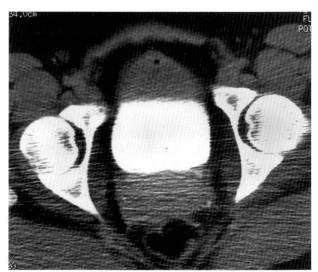

B

Figure 4–7 Hemoperitoneum in the posterior deep pelvis. **(A)** Transverse sonogram through the bladder (*straight open arrow*) demonstrates a fluid collection with low-level internal echoes in the rectouterine space (*curved arrow*). Patient was examined after bladder catheterization allowing acoustic access through a relatively distended bladder. **(B)** Computed tomographic scan through the distended bladder confirms relatively high-attenuation hemoperitoneum in the posterior deep pelvis. Contrast layers in the urinary bladder. A small anterior gas bubble was related to bladder catheterization.

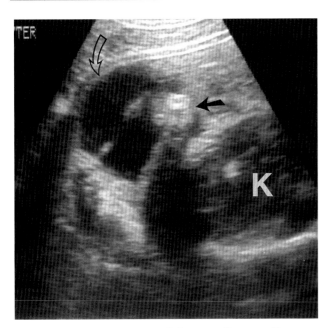

Figure 4–8 Transverse imaging of the paracolic gutter. Transverse imaging of the right paracolic gutter at the level of the inferior right kidney (K) demonstrates paracolic gutter fluid (*curved arrow*) lateral and posterior to the collapsed right colon (*straight arrow*). The quadratus muscle is posterior to the paracolic gutter.

traumatic peritoneal taps. A false-negative abdominal sonogram is unusual in the hypotensive patient, with a sensitivity of 97% for surgical injuries quoted in the literature.[22] Both techniques are insensitive to contained intracapsular hepatic or splenic injury, localized mesenteric hematoma or bowel wall injury, and injury to extraperitoneal structures, including pancreas, duodenum, and kidneys. If the hemodynamically unstable patient has no free intraperitoneal fluid, then attention should be directed to possible bleeding in the extraperitoneal spaces or bleeding associated with thoracic, pelvic, or long-bone injury. This appraisal may require combinations of radiography (portable chest, spine and pelvis, long bones), thoracoabdominal and pelvic CT, and tube thoracostomy.

Sonography as a screening test in the hemodynamically stable patient is a more controversial issue. A positive sonogram with documented intraperitoneal fluid is valuable information and should lead to an abdominal pelvic CT study. CT studies should be performed on patients with negative abdominal sonograms who have hematuria, spinal or pelvic fractures, or suspicion of midline compression injury that could result in trauma to the duodenum, pancreas, central renal vascular pedicle, or aortoiliac vessels.[18] In other circumstances, the value of a negative sonographic study is more problematic. Studies comparing emergency abdominal sonography to diagnostic peritoneal lavage, CT, and surgery have demonstrated sensitivity of sonography in detecting free intraperitoneal fluid to vary between 63 and 80%.[5,8] Similar findings have been

noted in sonographic evaluation of blunt trauma in pregnant patients and children.[23,24] The most common cause for false-negative sonographic studies has been free fluid in the pelvis, detectable on CT but not on sonography, owing to a collapsed bladder.[19] In addition, in Chiu et al's large series, in which 7% of blunt trauma victims had abdominal injury, one third of those with documented abdominal injury had no hemoperitoneum by CT study or emergency abdominal sonography.[15] All these patients had contained intrasplenic or intrahepatic hematomas detected only on CT study and were at risk for delayed bleeding. Some of these patients with contained intracapsular hematomas and lacerations and negative abdominal sonograms underwent laparotomy.

Reported patient studies utilizing emergency abdominal sonography have high accuracy rates and high negative predictive values. However, the vast majority of patients had negative studies with good outcomes. Only a small proportion of blunt trauma victims have abdominal injury with intraperitoneal bleeding, or are found to have contained intraparenchymal hematomas on CT study. Sensitivity values for blunt abdominal injury varying between 63 and 80% are relatively poor—critical diagnostic information will not be obtained in up to one third of patients with blunt abdominal injury. Thus, claims that sonography is a sensitive tool in the evaluation of blunt trauma may be suspect because the overwhelmingly negative patient population masks a significant false-negative rate.

There are two possible approaches in hemodynamically stable patients. Triage CT could be performed instead of triage sonography in all patients. This would require either or both lower-cost CT and refining the indications for CT in contast to the almost universal application of sonography to trauma patients in the emergency room. The second option is the continued liberal use of sonography with close clinical observation of those patients with negative sonograms and without hematuria. Even under the circumstances of a 6- to 12-hour postsonographic clinical observation in the emergency room, a small proportion of patients are likely to re-present with delayed internal bleeding. There has been no reported mortality in such patients.

Summary

The role of abdominal trauma ultrasound is to document the presence or absence of intraperitoneal fluid—a parameter that is critical in patient management decisions. In the hemodynamically unstable abdominal trauma patient, intraperitoneal fluid is an indication for exploratory laparotomy. In the hemodynamically stable abdominal trauma patient, intraperitoneal fluid is an indication for abdominal pelvic CT scan to document the site and extent of solid and hollow viscus injury. Used in this fashion, sonography replaces diagnostic peritoneal lavage. Sonography provides equivalent sensitivity and specificity for the detection of intraperitoneal fluid. Abdominal sonography can be performed expeditiously and the study may detect fluid in the pleural spaces and pericardium.

A negative sonogram does not exclude the possibility of contained intracapsular hemorrhage in the liver or spleen, mesenteric or bowel injury, or injury to the extraperitoneal structures—the pancreas, duodenum, and kidneys. Patients with suspicious clinical findings, hematuria, and spinal or pelvic fractures should have abdominal pelvic CT scans. Patients with negative sonography can be observed for a period of 6 to 12 hours and, if clinically stable, discharged. A few of these patients may re-present with delayed internal bleeding.

Effective use of sonography in abdominal trauma requires 24-hour coverage on site by experienced sonologists or sonographers competent in abdominal scanning techniques. Experienced sonologists and sonographers can rapidly adapt scanning parameters to different patients to provide the requisite diagnostic information.

References

1. Knudson MM, Lin RC, Oakes DD, Jeffrey RB. Nonoperative management of blunt liver injuries in adults: the need for continued surveillance. J Trauma 1990;30:1494–1500
2. Foley WD, Cates JD, Kellmann GN, et al. Treatment of blunt hepatic injuries: role of CT. Radiology 1987;164:635–638
3. Federle MP, Courcoulas AP, Powell M, Ferris JV, Peitzman AB. Blunt splenic injury in adults: clinical and CT criteria for management with emphasis on active extravasation. Radiology 1998;206:137–142
4. Gomez GA, Alvarez R, Poasencia G, et al. Diagnostic peritoneal lavage in the management of blunt abdominal trauma: a reassessment. J Trauma 1987;27:1–5
5. McKenney M, Lentz K, Nunez D, et al. Can ultrasound replace diagnostic peritoneal lavage in the assessment of blunt trauma? J Trauma 1994;37:439–441
6. McKenney MG, Martin L, Lentz K, et al. One thousand consecutive ultrasounds for blunt abdominal trauma. J Trauma 1996;40:607–610
7. Boulanger BR, McLellan BA, Brenneman FD, et al. Emergent abdominal sonography as a screening test in a new diagnostic algorithm for blunt trauma. J Trauma 1996;40:867–874
8. Lentz KA, McKenney MG, Nunez DB Jr, Martin L. Evaluating blunt abdominal trauma: role for ultrasonography. J Ultrasound Med 1996;15:447–451
9. Foley WD. Abdominal trauma. In: Bradley N, Stevenson, GW, eds. Margulis and Burhenne's Alimentary Tract: Radiology. 5th ed. Philadelphia: Mosby; 1994:2120–2142
10. McKenney KL, Nunez DB, McKenney MG, et al. Sonography is the primary screening technique for blunt abdominal trauma: experience with 899 patients. AJR Am J Roentgenol 1998;170:979–985
11. Anderson CB, Ballinger WF. Abdominal injuries. In: Zuidema GD, Rutherford RB, Ballinger WF, eds. The Management of Trauma. 4th ed. Philadelphia: WB Saunders; 1985:449–504
12. Mirvis SE, Whitley NO, Gens DR. Blunt splenic trauma in adults: CT based classification and correlation with prognosis and treatment. Radiology 1989;171:33–39
13. Orwig D, Federle MP. Localized clotted blood as evidence of visceral trauma on CT: the sentinel clot sign. AJR Am J Roentgenol 1989;153:747–749
14. Levine CD, Gonzales RN, Wachsberg RH, Ghanekar D. CT findings of bowel and mesenteric injury. J Comput Assist Tomogr 1997;21:974–979
15. Chiu WC, Cushing BM, Rodriguez A, et al. Abdominal injuries without hemoperitoneum: a potential limitation of focused abdominal sonography for trauma (FAST). J Trauma 1997;42:617–623
16. Miller JA, Ghanekar D. Pneumothoraces secondary to blunt abdominal trauma: aids to plain film radiographic diagnosis and relationship to solid organ injury. Am Surg 1996;62:416–420
17. Richards JR, McGahan JP, Simpson JL, Tabar P. Bowel and mesenteric injury: evaluation with emergency US. Radiology 1999;211:399–403
18. Sirlin CB, Brown MA, Andrede-Barrego OA, et al. Blunt abdominal trauma: clinical value of negative screening US scans. Radiology 2004;230:661–668
19. McGahan JP, Rose J, Coates TL, Wisner DH, Newberry P. Use of ultrasonography in the patient with acute abdominal trauma. J Ultrasound Med 1997;16:653–662
20. Rozycki GS, Ochsnner MG, Jawfin JH, Champion HR. Prospective evaluation of surgeons use of ultrasound in the evaluation of trauma patients. J Trauma 1993;34:516–526
21. Bode PJ, Niezen RA, van Vugt AB, Schipper J. Abdominal ultrasound as a reliable indicator for conclusive laparotomy in blunt abdominal trauma. J Trauma 1993;34:27–31
22. Farahmand N, Sirlin CB, Brown MA, et al. Hypotensive patients with blunt abdominal trauma: performance of screening US. Radiology 2005;235:436–443
23. Richards JR, Bormsby EL, Romo MV, Gillen MA, McGahan JP. Blunt abdominal injury in the pregnant patient: detection with US. Radiology 2004;233:463–470
24. Richards JR, Knopf NA, Wang L, McGahan JP. Blunt abdominal trauma in children: evaluation with emergency US. Radiology 2002;222:749–754

5 Acute Scrotal Pain: Diagnosing with Color Duplex Sonography

Thomas A. Stavros and Cynthia L. Rapp

Differential Diagnosis

The differential diagnosis for acute scrotal pain includes testicular torsion (spermatic cord torsion), infection (epididymitis, orchitis, epididymo-orchitis), torsion of the appendix testis, trauma, incarcerated or strangulated inguinal hernia, hemorrhage into or necrosis of a testicular tumor, vasculitis, spermatic cord thrombosis or compression (during inguinal hernia surgery), and complications of vasectomy. The most common causes vary with age, but in all age groups, spermatic cord torsion and infection are the leading causes of acute scrotal pain. In adults, infection is more common than torsion, but in children (including neonates), torsion is more common. Torsion of the appendix testis or appendix epididymis is also relatively common in children. The remaining causes of acute scrotal pain are less common in all age groups (**Table 5–1**).

Diagnostic Evaluation

Differentiations Torsion from Infection

Differentiating torsion from infection is an urgent problem. Torsion can lead to infarction of the testis within a few hours, so rapid reduction of the torsion is necessary. The mechanism of infarction is initially venous and lymphatic obstruction, later followed by arterial obstruction. The soft lymphatic and venous structures are prone to obstruction at lower degrees of torsion than are the thicker-walled testicular arteries. The rapidity with which torsion causes infarction varies with the degree of torsion. Infarction may not occur for days if there is only 90 degrees of torsion. On the other hand, 720 degrees of torsion may cause infarction within 2 hours. Intermediate degrees of torsion can lead to infarction in intermediate lengths of time.

An underlying anatomical abnormality, the "bell-clapper deformity," predisposes the patient to torsion in most cases. In the bellclapper deformity, the normal, "low, broad attachment" of the tunica vaginalis to the posterior surface of the testis is absent. Instead, the tunica vaginalis attaches in an abnormally high position to the spermatic cord, and the mesorchium is abnormally long. The lack of attachment of the testis to the tunica vaginalis predisposes the testis to torsion around the high point of attachment to the spermatic cord. Thus, testicular torsion should more properly be termed spermatic cord torsion. The bell-clapper deformity is usually bilateral, predisposing both sides to torsion.

The urgent reduction of torsion can be performed surgically or nonsurgically under local anesthetic. Regardless of whether reduction of torsion is surgical or nonsurgical, orchiopexy is required to prevent repeat torsion at a later date. Orchiopexy is almost always performed bilaterally because the bell-clapper deformity, which is the underlying predisposition to torsion, is usually present bilaterally.

The patient's clinical history can be helpful, but is sometimes quite atypical. The precipitating factor is thought to be an unusually strong contraction of the cremasteric muscle, which can be caused by trauma, strenuous exercise, or sexual activity. However, in many patients the onset of pain occurs during sleep, without any apparent cause for forceful contraction of the cremasteric muscle. The onset of pain in spermatic cord torsion is usually acute. Gradual onset of pain is more typical of infection, but up to 25% of torsion patients also have gradual onset of pain. Spontaneous detorsion does occur, and careful questioning sometimes reveals a past history of repeated episodes of scrotal pain due to intermittent spontaneously resolving episodes of torsion. Urinary symptoms such as dysuria are relatively rare in torsion in comparison with epididymitis.

Table 5–1   Differential Diagnosis of Acute Scrotal Pain

Children
Torsion
Infection
Appendage torsion
Tumor
Trauma
Hernia
Spermatic versus occlusion
Vasculitis
Adults
Infection
Torsion
Appendage torsion
Tumor
Trauma
Hernia
Spermatic versus occlusion
Vasculitis

Like the clinical history, the patient's physical examination may not reveal the classical signs of torsion. The torsed testis is usually swollen, painful, and tender, but may be nontender. Swelling of the testes and scrotal skin is usually present in both torsion and infection. The torsed testis is usually in an abnormally high, transverse position, with the epididymis rotated anteriorly, but in some cases it is not. The high, transverse testicular position is related to the degree of torsion. It is said that the pain from infection improves if the testis is elevated and supported, but the pain due to torsion does not. However, this is not always the case. The physical examination can be limited and difficult because of pain and tenderness, but injection of the spermatic cord in the inguinal canal with lidocaine may facilitate both a more thorough and accurate physical examination and nonsurgical external reduction of the torsion.

In patients in whom the history and physical examination are not classical for torsion, ultrasound with Doppler can be used to help differentiate torsion from infection. Our ability to demonstrate specific gray-scale patterns of edema within the testes, epididymis, and spermatic cord has improved. The sensitivity of color duplex sonography and power Doppler sonography for demonstrating the relatively slow and sparse flow within the testes has also improved markedly over the years. The combination of improved gray-scale imaging and Doppler capabilities now make ultrasound and Doppler the imaging procedures of choice for evaluation of acute scrotal pain.

Ultrasound Imaging

Ultrasound Equipment and Machine Setup

Scrotal sonography requires both high-frequency, high-resolution, near-field, real-time, gray-scale imaging and superb color and/or power Doppler sensitivity. These are best accomplished with high-frequency electronically focused transducers in the 10 to 12 MHz range. In children, frequencies as high as 17 MHz can be used. Lower frequency transducers, such as 5 MHz linear array transducers, are designed for peripheral vascular Doppler, not small parts imaging, and will less frequently show normal intratesticular flow than will higher-frequency transducers. Failure to show normal flow on the contralateral asymptomatic side reduces the value of Doppler in assessment of acute scrotal pain caused by torsion. In addition to Doppler sensitivity limitations, most 5 MHz transducers also have short-axis fixed focal lengths that are too deep for optimal scanning of the scrotal contents, especially in children. However, in patients with large hydroceles or hematoceles, severe testicular enlargement, a large testicular mass, or severe skin swelling, the greater focal length of the 5 MHz linear probe may be an advantage.

Power Doppler imaging is more sensitive than color Doppler flow imaging for showing relatively slow flow in small vessels, such as those within the substance of the normal testes. This is especially true in young boys and very old men, who tend to have less flow within the testes. Power Doppler is also less angle dependent than color Doppler, showing small vessels that course near 90 degrees to the Doppler beam better than does color Doppler. Being able to demonstrate flow within the normal contralateral asymptomatic testis is critical to the diagnosis of torsion because failure to do so makes lack of demonstrable flow in the symptomatic testis meaningless, and in a few cases power Doppler can show normal flow better than color Doppler does.

Some ultrasound equipment enables the user to downshift the Doppler frequency to a lower frequency than is normally used for imaging (i.e., the Doppler frequency on a 10 MHz linear transducer might be 7 MHz rather than 10 MHz). This downshift allows better penetration for peripheral vascular applications and also allows a greater degree of beam steering to optimize angles of incidence in peripheral vessels, such as the carotid and femoral arteries. However, downshifted Doppler frequencies and beam steering both reduce Doppler sensitivity and generally should not be used for evaluating intratesticular blood flow except in rare cases where large masses or marked scrotal enlargement makes penetration with higher frequencies suboptimal. If the vessels of interest within the scrotum are coursing at an obtuse angle of incidence, it is easy to move the probe along the surface of the scrotum to a position in which the angle of incidence is more acute. Angles as close to 0 degrees as possible should be sought and are usually possible. Sliding the transducer parallel to its long axis to a different location on the surface of the scrotum is a better way to improve angles of incidence than is beam steering.

Doppler sensitivity settings should be maximized. This is especially important in young children and old men, who have less flow and slower flow than young adult and middle-aged men. Full color and pulsed Doppler power, low-velocity scales, low wall filters, and high gray-scale-write-priorities maximize sensitivity. Many units, due to U.S. Food and Drug Administration requirements, boot up at low-power settings for safety purposes. These low-power settings can adversely affect Doppler sensitivity for the detection of normal intratesticular blood flow, especially in children and elderly men. The risk:benefit ratio of Doppler imaging in these patients demands full power, if flow within the asymptomatic testis cannot be demonstrated at the default low-power setting. Low-velocity scales (pulse-repetition frequency) and low wall-filter settings also maximize our chances of demonstrating flow. The ultrasound unit can usually only write either color or gray scale to each pixel, but not both. The write-priority tells the unit how white a gray-scale pixel can be overwritten with color. Peripheral vascular applications, with large lucent vessels, require low write-priority settings (that is, toward the black end of the gray scale). In such cases, high write-priorities (toward the white end of the gray-scale spectrum) would result in too much artifactual color being written into echogenic tissues outside of the vessels. In contrast to large peripheral vessels, the testes and epididymis are relatively echogenic. Many of the vessels within them that are being interrogated are too small to resolve on the B-mode image. Therefore, color flow must be displayed on a relatively white background by using a high write-priority. If the B-write-priority settings are too low (like those used for peripheral vascular imaging), color may not be written onto the image of the testis, even when the unit has correctly detected it. Some ultrasound units do not have a separate control for write-priority and have combined control of this parameter with other parameters (i.e., threshold control).

In most cases, color Doppler or power Doppler imaging alone is sufficient to distinguish between infection and torsion by showing markedly increased or decreased flow within either or both the symptomatic testis and epididymis. However, occasionally, obvious color or power Doppler asymmetry may not be demonstrable. In such cases, pulsed Doppler spectral analysis can be helpful. As is the case for color and power Doppler imaging, electronic beam steering reduces the sensitivity of pulsed Doppler spectral analysis and should not be used. In our experience, it is possible to maneuver the transducer on the surface of the scrotal skin to create an angle of incidence of the pulsed Doppler beam that is near 0 degrees without steering in virtually all cases. We have also found that using a wider sample volume improves the quality of the spectral tracing when the vessel being interrogated is small and the angle of incidence is near 0 degrees.

Occasionally, the testis is too long to measure with a standard 38 mm long 10 or 12 MHz linear array transducer. Five centimeter long transducers, trapezoidal beam shapes, extended field of view, or 5 MHz curved linear array transducers all offer workarounds to this problem.

Sonographic and Duplex Technique

Ultrasound examination of the scrotum in patients with acute scrotal pain should always include Doppler studies in addition to gray-scale imaging. On the other hand, Doppler evaluation is usually not necessary when the patient has a nonpainful, nontender, palpable nodule or mass. In patients in whom the clinical index of suspicion of torsion is high and in those who have gross enlargement of the testis, color Doppler flow imaging should be used early in the examination to make as prompt a diagnosis of torsion as possible. A color or power Doppler examination of the symptomatic testis can usually be performed very quickly. If there is no demonstrable flow within the symptomatic testis, one should quickly make sure that flow is demonstrable in the contralateral asymptomatic testis. This will be discussed in greater detail later.

After the quick color or power Doppler survey, the entire symptomatic testis and epididymis should be scanned in real time gray scale to get an overall picture of the scrotal contents and alignment of the testis and epididymis. The contralateral asymptomatic side should also be quickly surveyed to get an idea about symmetry in size and echogenicity between the two sides and also to assess the position and alignment of the contralateral testis and epididymis. The spermatic cord should be inspected from several centimeters superior to the epididymal head to the tail of the epididymis. The presence of a complex hydrocele and debris or adhesions within it should be noted. Intratesticular nodules or masses should be excluded, and the testes measured. The presence of a solid mass or nodule within the testis suggests the presence of a neoplasm. A complex cystic lesion within the testis may represent an abscess resulting from orchitis or necrosis resulting from infarction or tumor.

One advantage of scrotal–testicular color duplex sonography is that there is almost always a mirror-image contralateral normal structure with which the painful side can be compared. This advantage should be utilized to its fullest extent. When the color Doppler findings do not indicate torsion and the need for immediate surgery, we make this comparison by obtaining split-screen images of corresponding right and left intrascrotal contents in both transverse and longitudinal planes. Split-screen long-axis images of the epididymal heads (**Fig. 5–1**) and long- and short-axis split-screen images of both testes are recorded (**Fig. 5–2**). The epididymal tails are usually best shown on coronal views that are angled from anterosuperior to posteroinferior. Obtaining such a view often requires the patient to temporarily assume a frogleg position. The shape of the epididymis varies from straight (**Fig. 5–3A**) to C-shaped (**Fig. 5–3B**). Imaging the epididymal tails is very important because infection is often most apparent and

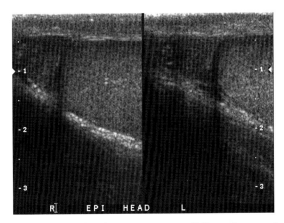

Figure 5–1 Long-axis split-screen images of bilaterally normal epididymal heads. The heads are triangular and symmetrical in size and shape. The transducer position needed to obtain these views varies not only from one patient to another, but from right side to left.

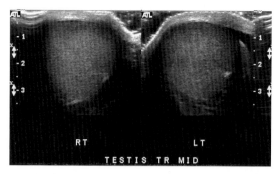

Figure 5–2 Split-screen transverse images through the normal right and left testes—size and echogenicity are symmetrical from right to left.

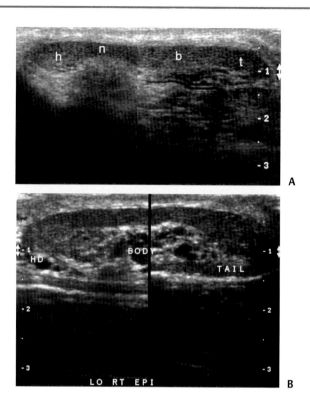

Figure 5–3 (A) Coronal or C view of normal straight epididymis. Combined view of entire length of normal epididymis shows the head (h), neck (n), body (b), and tail (t). **(B)** Coronal or C view of normal curved epididymis.

manifests itself most definitively there. Transverse split-screen images of the spermatic cords just superior to the epididymal heads are also obtained (**Fig. 5–4**). Occasionally, scanning the spermatic cords within the inguinal canals can be helpful. We also obtain an oblique short-axis view through the median raphe of the scrotum to compare the size and echogenicity of the testes on a single image. It is important that the angle of incidence of the beam into the testes be bilaterally symmetrical on this view to minimize the chance that critical angle shadowing will make a testis artifactually look hypoechoic. Usually the left end of the probe must be angled inferiorly because the left testis usually lies lower than the right, but this relationship may be altered in torsion. It is important to make sure that all of the split-screen images are obtained symmetrically through the widest part of the structures being imaged and that the angles of incidence be as close to 90 degrees as possible to minimize artifactual shadowing and errant assessment of relative echogenicities and thicknesses (**Fig. 5–5**). The right and left testes, epididymi, and spermatic cords should be symmetrical in size and echogenicity.

Demonstrating symmetrical sections through right and left sides may require grossly different probe orientations on the right and left sides because the position of the testes within the scrotal sac in normal individuals is often asymmetrical. In torsion, this asymmetry of position is even more pronounced. The relative position of the right and left sides is ascertained at the time of the initial survey.

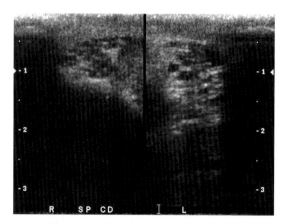

Figure 5–4 Short-axis split-screen images of spermatic cords. These short-axis views were obtained through the spermatic cords just superior to the epididymal heads. The cords are symmetrical in size and echogenicity. Because of tortuosity of the cord, obtaining such views in nonredundant segments of cord can be difficult.

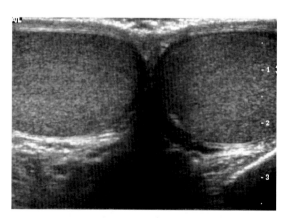

Figure 5–5 Oblique median raphe view through the medial half of each testis. This median raphe view shows the testes to be equal in size and echogenicity. Because the left testis is usually lower than the right, this view cannot be obtained in a true transverse plane and usually requires an oblique view with the left side lower.

Because the testes are freely mobile within the scrotal sac, the alignment of the testis may change during the examination. The goal of this systematic imaging approach is to detect a pattern of swelling or abnormal echogenicity that favors a diagnosis of either infection or torsion. For example, swelling of the epididymal tail and spermatic cord out of proportion to swelling within the epididymal head and testis strongly suggests epididymitis. Furthermore, systematic scanning minimizes the chances of missing the key findings of infection. For example, mild or early epididymitis, or partially treated epididymitis, can affect only the spermatic cord and epididymal tail, sparing the epididymal head and testis. Failure to evaluate the spermatic cords and epididymal tails will cause these findings to be missed.

We are not in favor of using a rolled-up towel to support the testis. Although this may offer symptomatic relief to a patient with epididymitis, it blocks inferior and coronal approaches to the testis and also pushes the scrotal contents superiorly, interfering with the evaluation of the epididymal heads, appendices, and spermatic cords above the testes. Additionally, the rolled-up towel redistributes physiological amounts of fluid within the scrotal sac posteriorly, where it cannot be used to outline small structures such as the appendix testis. Scanning without a rolled-up towel allows the scrotal contents to fall inferiorly and posteriorly and redistributes physiological hydroceles to the upper pole, nicely outlining appendices, epididymal heads, and spermatic cords. It also stretches out the epididymis, facilitating demonstration of the entire epididymis on a single coronal view.

The Doppler examination begins with color or power Doppler interrogation of the testes. We usually quickly evaluate the asymptomatic testis first to make sure that flow is detectable on the side on which torsion is not suspected. If no flow exists in the asymptomatic side, decreased or absent flow in the symptomatic side will have no meaning. If flow cannot be detected within the asymptomatic contralateral testis, velocity scale, wall filter, B-write priority, and Doppler power can be adjusted as needed to demonstrate flow. Increased flow in the symptomatic testis is always important, regardless of the contralateral findings. It indicates inflammatory hyperemia, which is almost always due to infection; in rare cases, it can be a manifestation of reactive hyperemia after spontaneous detorsion.

If flow is present in the asymptomatic testis, but absent or decreased in the symptomatic testis, then torsion is likely. Duplex sonographic interrogation with spectral tracings and complete color Doppler and duplex sonographic studies of the remainder of the intrascrotal contents are usually not performed because it is important for the patient to undergo surgery as soon as possible. Additional examinations in such patients may waste valuable time in which the patient could be prepared for surgery. It should be kept in mind, however, that severe infection, trauma, and inguinal hernia surgery can lead to ischemia of a testis, which appears similar to torsion on color Doppler flow imaging or power Doppler imaging. The pattern of oligemia can be helpful. Spermatic cord torsion tends to cause global absence or decrease in flow within the testis, whereas in ischemia caused by conditions other than torsion, the ischemic changes often appear focal or patchy rather than diffuse.

If flow is present in both testes but increased in the symptomatic testis, or if there appears to be normal and symmetrical flow in both testes, torsion is unlikely. Complete gray-scale imaging with split-screen images and color duplex sonographic examination of intrascrotal contents can then be performed. In some cases, spectral Doppler analysis will show asymmetries in velocities and resistivity indexes, even when color Doppler appears symmetrical. The goal of complete gray-scale and Doppler in assessing testes, epididymi, and spermatic cords is to detect a pattern of hyperemia that suggests a specific diagnosis. For example, abnormally high velocities and low resistivity indexes in the epididymis, but normal velocities in the testes, strongly favor a diagnosis of epididymitis over other causes.

It is very important to assess the intratesticular vessels (centripetal) as well as the more easily seen capsular arteries. In cases of missed torsion, the tunica vaginalis, the lining of the scrotal sac, can be markedly hyperemic. Because the inflamed tunica vaginalis may become adherent to the immediately adjacent tunica albuginea, reactive hyperemia within the tunica vaginalis can be mistaken for flow within a capsular testicular artery, resulting in a missed diagnosis of torsion. By assessing intratesticular arteries rather than capsular arteries, this potential mistake can usually be avoided. As mentioned earlier, it is possible to create an optimal angle of incidence of near 0 degrees without electronically steering the ultrasound beam to maximize Doppler sensitivity.

In most cases the combined pattern of swelling, altered echogenicity, and increased or decreased flow on Doppler ultrasound examination suggest the exact cause of scrotal pain.

Normal Imaging and Doppler Findings

Normal testes, epididymi, and spermatic cords are bilaterally symmetrical in size and texture. The epididymi and testes are normally relatively homogeneous and have mid-level echogenicity. The spermatic cords have heterogeneous texture due to the venous plexus and abundant loose connective tissues they contain. The tortuosity of the spermatic cord makes it difficult to obtain precisely symmetrical images and to precisely measure the spermatic cord, but an eyeball estimate of size and echogenicity is usually possible. Marked asymmetries in size, shape, homogeneity, and echogenicity between right and left sides are abnormal.

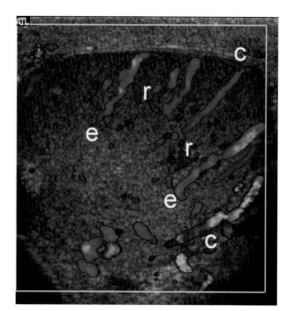

Figure 5–6 Color Doppler image through equator of testis. Capsular arteries (c) course on the outer surface of the testis, centripetal arteries (e) penetrate into the substance of the testis from peripheral to central, and recurrent rami (r) double back toward the surface of the testis. Demonstrating flow in centripetal arteries is important in excluding torsion because vessels within adherent tunica vaginalis can simulate capsular arteries in patients with "missed" torsion.

With current equipment, flow is demonstrable within the capsular arteries, the intratesticular vessels (centripetal and, sometimes, recurrent rami), in almost all adults within the reproductive age groups (**Fig. 5–6**). Demonstrable color Doppler flow should be roughly symmetrical in the right and left testes, with only minimal asymmetry in the number of vessels in right and left testes

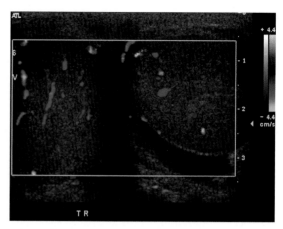

Figure 5–7 Oblique median raphe color Doppler view can be helpful in comparing blood flow in the right and left testes on a single view. In normal individuals, flow should be roughly symmetrical on right and left sides.

shown on oblique transverse median raphe views (**Fig. 5–7**). However, normal intratesticular flow can be more difficult to demonstrate in children, particularly very young children and newborns, and in very elderly men. Additionally, the intratesticular vessels pass through the testis in a few discrete vascular planes. If the ultrasound probe is parallel to the vascular plane on one side, but out of the vascular plane in the contralateral testis, the flow may appear falsely asymmetrical. Every effort should be made to compare comparable tissue planes within the two testes. The vascular planes of the testis are oriented in the long axis of the testis. Therefore, errors in assessment of vascularity are more likely to occur in the longitudinal planes than in transverse plans. The capsular arteries are

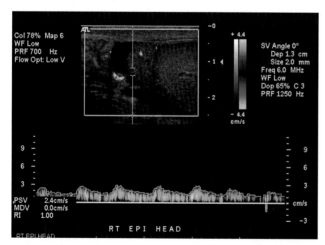

Figure 5–8 Spectral waveforms obtained from a normal epididymal head. Epididymal head waveforms can be obtained in most normal adult patients with current equipment, are low resistance type, and demonstrate rounded systolic peaks. Normal epididymal head peak systolic velocities are ≤5 cm/s and normal end-diastolic velocities are ≤3 cm/s.

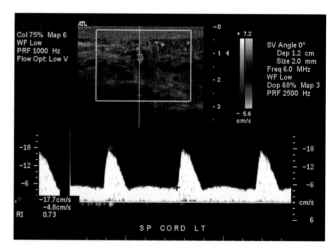

Figure 5–9 Spectral waveform from a normal testicular artery within the spermatic cord superior to the epididymal head. Testicular artery waveforms can be obtained in all normal patients, have a higher resistance pattern than do normal testicular and epididymal waveforms, and have sharp systolic peaks. Peak systolic velocities vary greatly but should be within 50% of contralateral testicular artery peak systolic velocities.

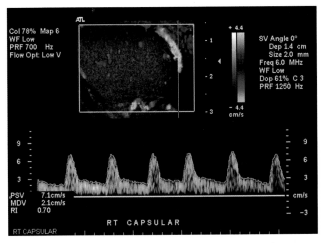

Figure 5–10 Spectral waveform obtained from a capsular artery. These should be obtainable in virtually all normal patients. The waveform resistance index is intermediate between that of the testicular artery within the spermatic cord and those obtained from the epididymis or centripetal arteries within the substance of the testis. Normal peak systolic velocities within capsular arteries are ≤15 cm/s and normal end-diastolic velocities are ≤7 cm/s. Capsular artery velocities are higher than those of the centripetal arteries in most, but not all, patients. Velocities from capsular arteries on one side should not be compared with centripetal arteries on the other side.

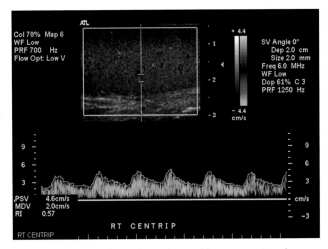

Figure 5–11 Spectral waveform obtained from a centripetal artery. These should be obtainable in almost all adult patients but can be difficult to obtain in infants and young children. Like those from within the epididymal head, waveforms from centripetal arteries are low-resistance type and the systolic peaks are rounded. Normal peak systolic velocities within centripetal arteries vary too greatly to use a fixed number as a cutoff. Comparison should be made with similar contralateral centripetal arteries. There should be less than 50% difference between sides. Centripetal artery velocities are lower than those of the capsular arteries in most, but not all, patients. Velocities from centripetal arteries on one side should not be compared with capsular arteries on the contralateral side.

usually best seen in segments that course at nearly a 0 degree angle of incidence to the beam. This most commonly occurs on the inferomedial surface of the testes. Multiple intratesticular vessels are visible in most adult testes, but may be more or less evident, depending upon the angle of incidence and scan plane.

With current equipment, some flow is demonstrable within the epididymal head in a majority of adult patients. Flow is not demonstrable within the epididymal head in a small percentage of adults and in most children. Flow within the epididymal tail is demonstrable in a larger percentage of adult patients than within the epididymal head but, once again, not always demonstrable in children. On color or power Doppler assessment it can be difficult to determine whether flow that is being detected is within the epididymal head or the adjacent spermatic cord. However, the spectral waveforms obtained from the epididymal head and spermatic cord differ greatly from each other. Waveforms obtained from vessels within the epididymal head have a low impedance pattern, low velocities (peak systolic velocity of ≤ 5 cm/s and end diastolic velocities of ≤ 3 cm/s), and a rounded systolic peak, and they lack an early diastolic notch (**Fig. 5–8**). On the other hand, waveforms obtained from within the spermatic cord (testicular artery or supratesticular artery) have much higher impedance, higher systolic velocities, sharp systolic peaks, and early diastolic notches (**Fig. 5–9**).

Normal spectral waveforms obtained from within the testicular substance should be symmetrical on the right and left sides in most patients, as long as they are obtained

from vessels that appear to be similar in size, angle of incidence, and depth on both sides. One should not compare a capsular artery waveform on one side to a centripetal artery waveform on the other side. The velocities in centripetal and capsular arteries differ from each other in most cases. Velocities are usually, but not always, higher within the capsular than within the intratesticular arteries. Peak systolic velocities in capsular arteries usually range from 5 to 14 cm/s (**Fig. 5–10**). Peak end-diastolic velocities vary from 2 to 6 cm/s (**Fig. 5–11**). Peak systolic velocities obtained from centripetal arteries are far more variable and need to be compared with similar arteries on the contralateral side.

The appearance of pulsed Doppler spectral waveforms obtained from the epididymal tails varies greatly, depending upon the location within the epididymal tail from which the waveforms are obtained. Waveforms obtained farthest from the reflection with the distal spermatic cord have velocities and appearances similar to those obtained from the epididymal head (**Fig. 5–8**). On the other hand, waveforms obtained closer to the reflection with the distal spermatic cord have an appearance more similar to that of the spermatic cord (**Fig. 5–9**).

In normal individuals, peak systolic velocities are much lower in the epididymal head than within the spermatic cord, testes, or epididymal tail, but in cases of severe epididymitis, the velocities in the epididymal head can exceed those within the testes.

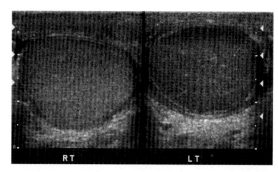

Figure 5–12 Split-screen images in long axis through the midtestes in a patient with acute left spermatic cord torsion show decreased echogenicity in the torsed left testis. In bland infarction, the testicular substance is usually hypoechoic, but in areas that have undergone hemorrhagic infarction, the affected areas usually become hyperechoic.

The velocities within similar vessels on the right and left sides should be symmetrical, but there is enough variability and difficulty in obtaining and measuring spectral waveforms that a 50% or greater difference in velocities between the right and left sides is usually necessary to document a significant difference.

Findings in Testicular Torsion

Imaging Findings

The spermatic cord below the point of spermatic cord torsion, the epididymis, and testis are all abnormally enlarged. The enlargement increases over time, so patients who are very early in the course of torsion may have only minimal enlargement, whereas patients with more severe or longstanding torsion have more severe enlarge-

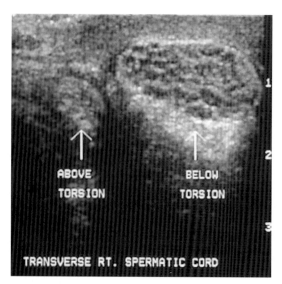

Figure 5–14 Long-axis view of a torsed spermatic cord shows the normal-sized cord above the torsion and the enlarged cord below the torsion. The cord below the torsion contains many distended hypoechoic veins due to either or both venous stasis and thrombosis.

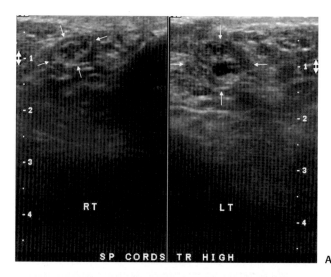

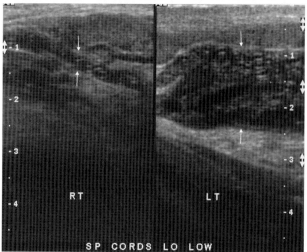

Figure 5–13 (A) Split-screen images of the spermatic cords above the epididymal heads, but below the torsion, in a patient with acute left spermatic cord torsion. Note the left spermatic cord (*arrows*) is larger than the right and that there is a distended pampiniform plexus vein. The distension can be due to stasis early or due to thrombosis late. **(B)** Split-screen long-axis images of the distal spermatic cords and cremasteric plexes (*arrows*) on the right and left side show the cord to be markedly swollen on the left side.

ment. The echogenicity of the testis is usually decreased (**Fig. 5–12**), although very early in the process the echogenicity may be normal, and very late in the process, after infarction has occurred, hemorrhage into the testis may cause heterogeneously increased echogenicity. The echogenicity of the epididymis and spermatic cord also varies, depending on whether hemorrhage has occurred. Enlarged acutely thrombosed pampiniform plexus veins within the spermatic cord can also be demonstrable in some cases and are what make the spermatic cord appear abnormally hypoechoic (**Fig. 5–13**). If the spermatic cord is carefully examined, an abrupt increase in the size and alteration of the spermatic cord may be noted below the point of torsion (**Fig. 5–14**). In other cases, actual twisting

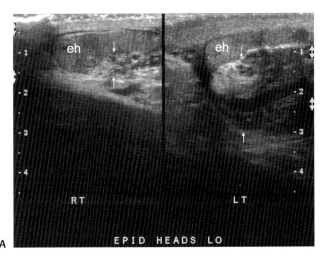

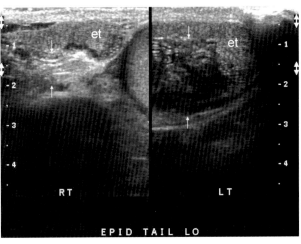

A

B

Figure 5–15 (A) Long-axis, split-screen images of the epididymal heads in a patient with acute left spermatic cord torsion. Note that the spermatic cord and loose areolar tissues (between arrows) that lie posterior to the epididymal head are greatly swollen, but that the

left epididymal head (eh) is only minimally enlarged. **(B)** Long-axis split-screen images of the epididymal tail–spermatic cord junction shows marked enlargement of the left spermatic cord (between arrows), but little swelling in the adjacent epididymal tail (et).

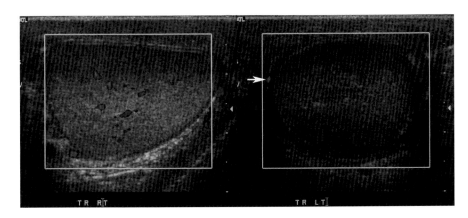

Figure 5–16 Short-axis color Doppler images of the right and left testes in a patient with acute left spermatic cord torsion. There is no demonstrable flow within the torsed left testis, but normal flow within the right testis. Note that a vessel in the medial tunica vaginalis (*white arrow*) could be mistaken for a capsular artery.

of the cord can be seen. The literature mentions enlargement and increased echogenicity within the epididymal head in torsion. However, in our experience, in most cases of torsion the epididymisa head is only minimally enlarged, but the spermatic cord, which passes just superiorly and posteriorly to the epididymal head is grossly enlarged and mistaken for enlargement of the epididymal head. (**Fig. 5–15**).

Doppler Findings

In most cases, flow within the substance of the torsed testis is absent, but there is flow within the contralateral asymptomatic testis demonstrable on split-screen imaging (**Fig. 5–16**) or on the transverse oblique median raphe view (**Fig. 5–17**). However, in cases with lesser degrees of torsion (180 degrees or less), some flow may still be present within the torsed testis (**Fig. 5–18**). In such cases the peak systolic velocities will be abnormally low compared with the contralateral asymptomatic testis. These abnormally low velocities can be associated with resistivity indices that are normal, increased, or decreased. Because of such cases, simply showing some

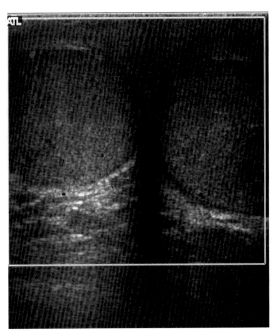

Figure 5–17 Oblique median raphe color Doppler view of both testes in a patient with acute left torsion shows normal flow in the normal right testis, but no demonstrable flow within the torsed left testis.

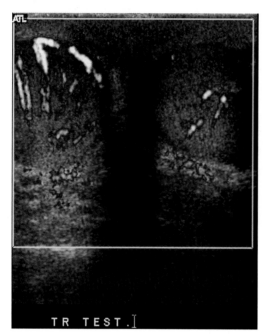

Figure 5–18 Oblique median raphe power Doppler view of both testes in a patient with acute left torsion shows normal flow in the normal right testis and reduced rather than absent flow on the torsed left side. The torsion was less than 360 degrees, allowing some flow past the torsion.

flow within a torsed testis does not completely exclude a diagnosis of torsion. It is still necessary to compare the flow to that in the contralateral side. Flow that appears to be only on the surface of the testis also does not exclude a diagnosis of torsion. Flow must be shown within the intratesticular branches of the testicular artery, the centripetal arteries, and recurrent rami. Demonstrating intratesticular flow is necessary because, in patients with torsion, the tunica vaginalis can adhere to the surface of the testis, and reactive hyperemia within the adherent tunica vaginalis can be mistaken for testicular

capsular artery flow, potentially causing the diagnosis of torsion to be missed (**Fig. 5–16**).

Obviously, no significance can be attributed to a lack of demonstrable flow in the painful testis if flow is not demonstrable in the contralateral asymptomatic testis.

Spermatic cord torsion also results in reduced or absent flow within the swollen spermatic cord and epididymis (**Fig. 5–19**). On the other hand, any evidence of hyperemia within the epididymis and spermatic cord strongly favors a diagnosis of infection over one of torsion.

Occasionally, spontaneous detorsion may occur before the color duplex sonographic examination can be performed. If infarction has already occurred, the findings will be the same as if torsion still exists. However, in patients in whom spontaneous detorsion occurs before infarction, the ultrasound scan and Doppler findings may return to normal or may show residual swelling with reactive hyperemia, findings identical to those seen in patients with epididymo-orchitis. In such patients, the history may be the only way to distinguish infection from spontaneous detorsion. A history of pain rapidly decreasing prior to sonography favors spontaneous detorsion. A history of previous episodes of spontaneously resolving pain might also be elicited from such patients. Most untreated patients with epididymo-orchitis, on the other hand, will not have any abatement of pain before sonography.

Findings in Epididymitis, Orchitis, and Epididymo-orchitis

Imaging Findings

Most cases of infection are sexually transmitted or ascend from the prostate or urinary tract. The infection ascends, in order, through the vas deferens and the spermatic cord, to the epididymal tail, the epididymal body, the epididymal head, and finally the testis. The patient may undergo a

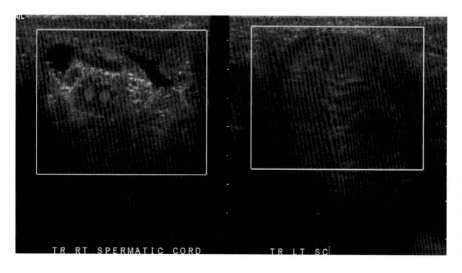

Figure 5–19 Short-axis color Doppler views of the spermatic cords in a patient with acute left torsion shows normal flow within the nontorsed right spermatic cord, but no demonstrable flow within the swollen left spermatic cord below the level of torsion.

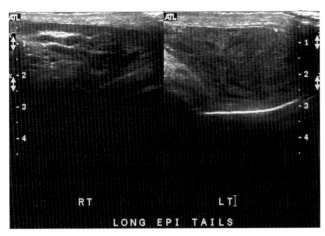

Figure 5–20 Long-axis split-screen images of the epididymal tails in a patient with early acute epididymitis on the left shows focal swelling of the left epididymal tail that is most easily assessed when compared with the contralateral side. Isolated swelling of the epididymal tail is the most common finding in early epididymitis.

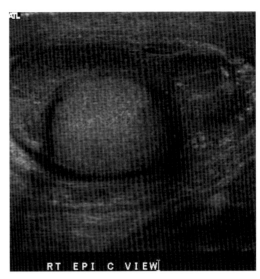

Figure 5–21 Coronal or C view of the epididymis in a patient with later or more severe epididymitis. The entire epididymis is severely swollen.

sonographic examination at any point in this progression. The pattern of swelling and altered echogenicity will reflect the pattern of infectious involvement at the time that the scan is performed.

With isolated vasitis or funiculitis, which occurs very early in the course of ascending infection, only the spermatic cord will be infected and swollen. Later in the process the epididymal tail becomes involved. The pattern of edema and hyperemia isolated to the epididymal tail is actually quite common in patients with epididymitis who present for sonography, making it essential that the epididymal tails be evaluated in all patients with acute scrotal pain who do not show immediate evidence of torsion. The swelling is much more obvious when compared with the contralateral side on split-screen images (**Fig. 5–20**). Finally, the head and tail become involved and the entire epididymis is swollen and hyperemic. This is best shown on coronal or "C" views (**Fig. 5–21**). In some cases, the swelling of the epididymal tail may be so massive that the tail indents and distorts the testis and simulates an epididymal neoplasm (**Fig. 5–22A**). In such cases, liquefactive necrosis and early abscess formation can occur within the epididymal tail (**Fig. 5–22B**). In cases of very severe epididymitis, the venous outflow from the testis can become obstructed, leading to a venous infarction of the testis similar to that caused by torsion.

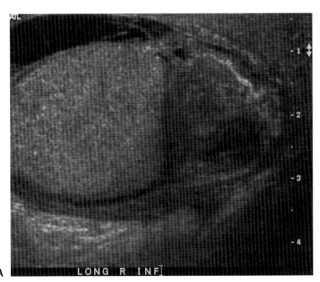

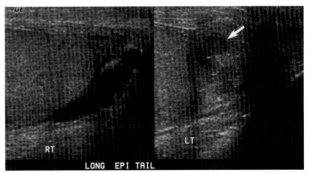

Figure 5–22 (A) Long-axis view of the right epididymal tail in a patient with severe right epididymitis affecting primarily the tail. The tail is so swollen that it appears masslike and flattens and indents the lower pole of the testis. **(B)** Long-axis split-screen images of the epididymal tails shows severe swelling of the left epididymal tail, which is undergoing cystic or hemorrhagic necrosis and early abscess formation (*white arrow*).

Occasional cases of epididymitis will more severely affect the head than the tail. We believe this most commonly occurs in partially, but incompletely, treated cases of epididymitis. It occurs in patients who are treated for epididymitis based upon characteristic clinical findings alone, but who do not respond to antibiotics as quickly as expected. It is our experience that patients with epididymitis are frequently treated with an antibiotic course that is too short—often only 7 days. In many cases this is insufficient to eradicate the infection. It appears that the tail is better vascularized than is the head, and, therefore, it heals more quickly than does the head on antibiotic treatment. Patients who respond completely to short courses of antibiotic treatment are never referred for sonography. We tend to see the highly selected subset of patients who respond suboptimally to treatment, and thus, the subgroup that is more likely to have disproportionate residual swelling of the epididymal head after the swelling in the tail has already cleared.

In cases of epididymitis without associated orchitis, the degree of swelling and hyperemia within the affected part of the epididymis will exceed the swelling and textural abnormality and hyperemia within the ipsilateral testis. This pattern of isolated edema of the epididymis on gray-scale imaging is so typical of epididymitis that it virtually excludes a diagnosis of torsion, even before Doppler ultrasound examination is performed.

Untreated cases of epididymitis may eventually lead to orchitis, resulting in epididymo-orchitis. In such cases, in addition to the spermatic cord and epididymis, the testis will be affected. The ipsilateral testis will be larger and usually more hypoechoic, although the echogenicity can vary (**Fig. 5–23**). This pattern of involvement is so similar to that caused by torsion that Doppler is necessary to distinguish epididymo-orchitis from torsion with certainty.

Hemorrhagic or ischemic necrosis secondary to severe epididymo-orchitis can lead to testicular abscess, which presents as a complex cystic lesion within the testicular

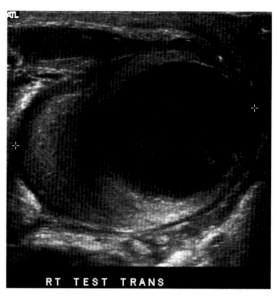

Figure 5–24 Long-axis view of a testicular abscess in a patient with severe epididymo-orchitis who responded poorly to antibiotic treatment.

substance (**Fig. 5–24**). Testicular abscesses can, in turn, rupture through the tunica albuginea into the scrotal sac, leading to a scrotal abscess. Poor or delayed improvement to a priori antibiotic treatment may be the first indication of a developing testicular abscess, so patients who present with a history of many days of pain that is not improving represent a subgroup of scrotal pain patients more likely to have developed a testicular abscess. Treatment of testicular abscess is surgical.

In cases of viral orchitis, the infection spreads to the testis hematogenously and does not ascend through the spermatic cord and epididymis. As would be expected, this causes disproportional swelling and altered echogenicity in the testis, with relative sparing of the spermatic cord and epididymis.

Any infective process can lead to hydrocele, complex hydrocele, or pyocele. Diffuse low-level echoes and fibrinous adhesions within the hydrocele suggest an exudative or inflammatory etiology (**Fig. 5–25**).

Some cases of acute scrotal pain and swelling are the result of scrotal cellulitis. In such cases the scrotal skin and subcutaneous tissues are infected, but the contents of the scrotum inside the tunica vaginalis are spared. This process is usually bilateral. The swelling and tenderness may prevent adequate clinical examination of such cases, making sonography valuable for assessment of intrascrotal contents. Fournier's gangrene is a more serious and potentially life-threatening form of necrotizing scrotal cellulitis. It can involve the tissues of the perineum and the base of the penis as well as the scrotal tissues. It is a necrotizing infection that can be caused by a variety of aerobic and anaerobic bacteria that produce enzymes which allow the infection to break down tissues and spread, cause

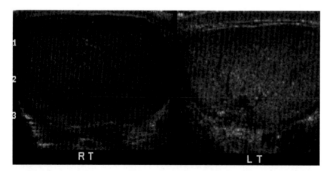

Figure 5–23 Short-axis split-screen images of testes in a patient with acute orchitis shows the infected right testis to be larger and more hypoechoic than the normal contralateral testis. Echotexture of infected testes is usually hypoechoic but can be isoechoic very early, or can demonstrate mixed echogenicity in cases where hemorrhagic necrosis has occurred.

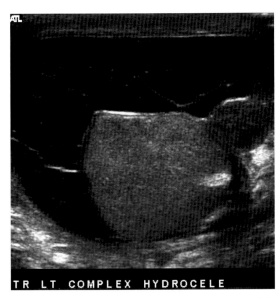

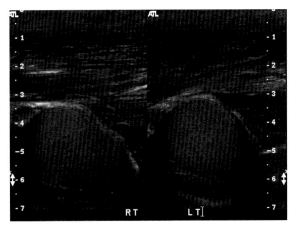

Figure 5–26 Short-axis split-screen images of the midtestes in a quadriplegic patient with acute scrotal cellulitis. Note the marked thickening of the scrotal skin and subcutaneous tissues bilaterally without associated testicular abnormalities. The thickened skin was also markedly hyperemic.

Figure 5–25 Short-axis view of a patient with severe epididymitis and a large complex hydrocele. Fibrinous adhesions bridge the hydrocele, indicating an exudative rather than transudative etiology.

endarteritis and infarction of tissues, and produce gas within the infected tissues. If Fournier's gangrene results in bacteremia, it can be fatal. It is more common in men than in women. Predisposing factors are alcoholism, diabetes, morbid obesity, and immunologic deficiencies. The unusual cases that occur in women are generally related to obstetric trauma or obstetric and gynecologic surgical procedures. We have also found scrotal cellulitis and Fournier's gangrene to be more common in spinal cord injury patients, where a combination of indwelling Foley or suprapubic catheters and decubitus ulcers near the perineum predispose the patient to scrotal cellulitis.

In scrotal cellulitis, sonography shows severe edema and hyperemia within the skin and subcutaneous tissues of the scrotal sac. The testis, epididymis, and spermatic cord are spared (**Fig. 5–26**), but there may be reactive hydrocele. The gray-scale sonographic findings in Fournier's gangrene are similar to those of scrotal cellulitis, but bright echoes with "dirty shadowing" suggestive of air occur within the thickened scrotal tissues (**Fig. 5–27**). The swollen tissues in Fournier's gangrene are typically ischemic, so, unlike inflamed tissues in simple scrotal cellulitis, they will not have demonstrable inflammatory hyperemia.

In summary, the pattern of edema on gray-scale imaging parallels the pattern of inflammation. In epididymo-orchitis the testes, epididymal heads and tails, and spermatic cords are all swollen. However, in epididymitis without associated orchitis, the spermatic cord and all or part of the epididymis is swollen. In vasitis or funiculitis, only the spermatic cord is swollen.

Doppler Findings

Acute inflammation leads to arteriolar, venular, and capillary dilatation. This dilatation, in turn, increases blood flow within vessels supplying the inflamed organ. The inflammatory hyperemia of vasitis, funiculitis, epididymitis, and orchitis is readily demonstrable by color or power Doppler sonography. Compared with the contralateral uninfected

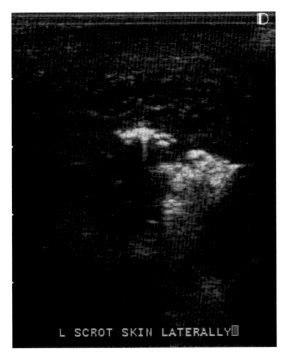

Figure 5–27 Transverse view through the scrotal skin lateral to the left testis in an elderly diabetic male patient with Fournier's gangrene. There is severe edema of the scrotal skin and subcutaneous tissues, and there are bright echoes caused by air within the soft tissues. The bright echo on the right has "dirty shadowing," whereas the bright echo on the left side of the image has ringdown or comet tail artifact.

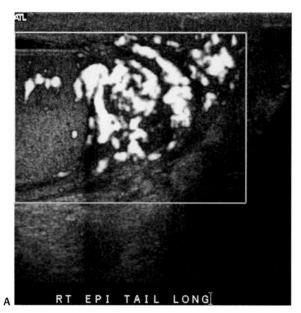

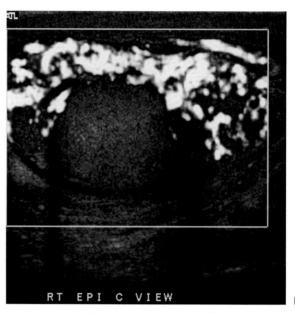

Figure 5–28 (A) Long-axis power Doppler view of the epididymal tail. In early epididymitis there is hyperemia as well as swelling in the epididymal tail. **(B)** Coronal power Doppler view of epididymitis. In severe or later epididymitis, the entire epididymis becomes hyperemic as well as swollen. This power Doppler image is from the same patient as shown in **Fig. 3–21** .

side, the inflamed organ shows more numerous and larger vessels on color or power Doppler imaging and more saturation of color, indicating higher mean velocities.

As is the case for gray-scale evidence of edema, the pattern of hyperemia parallels the pattern of inflammation. When epididymitis primarily affects the epididymal tail, the greatest and most obvious degree of hyperemia will occur within the swollen epididymal tail (**Fig. 5–28A**). When the entire epididymis is infected, the entire epididymis will be hyperemic (**Fig. 5–28B**). In epididymo-orchitis, the ipsilateral testis will be hyperemic in addition to the epididymis (**Fig. 5–29**). In occasional cases, the development of inflammatory hyperemia can precede any demonstrable enlargement (**Fig. 5–30**).

In most cases of infection, the increased flow within the inflamed organ will be so obvious with color or power Doppler alone that duplex sonographic spectral analysis will not be necessary. However, in a few cases, color or power Doppler alone may fail to demonstrate hyperemia.

In such cases, pulsed Doppler spectral analysis can help. A peak systolic velocity within the capsular testicular arteries in an adult reproductive-aged male over 15 cm/s suggests hyperemia, as does peak systolic velocity on the ipsilateral symptomatic side that is 5 cm higher than the velocity on the contralateral side. In infants, young children, and elderly adults, velocities are so low that absolute velocities and velocity differences may be difficult to use. In these patients, ratio peak systolic velocities from mirror image vessels within the symptomatic ipsilateral and asymptomatic contralateral testes of 1.7 or greater suggest the presence of hyperemia on the symptomatic side (**Fig. 5–31**).

Peak systolic velocities in the epididymal head over 5 cm/s and end-diastolic velocities over 3 cm/s usually indicate epididymitis. The peak systolic velocity of the epididymal tail and spermatic cord is more variable, and comparison with contralateral asymptomatic side is more important than the absolute value of the velocity. A ratio of the peak systolic velocity of 1.5 or greater between the

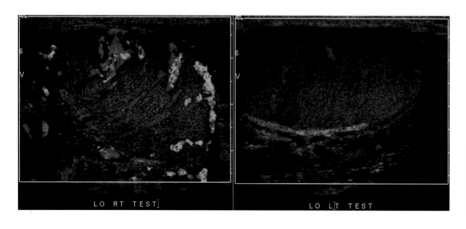

Figure 5–29 Long-axis color Doppler images of the right and left testes in a patient with acute orchitis on the right. The infected right testis is hyperemic compared with the normal left side.

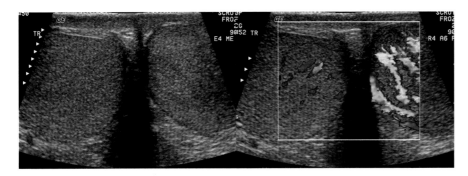

Figure 5–30 Medial raphe gray-scale and color Doppler images of both testes in a patient with acute left orchitis. In a few cases Doppler may become abnormal before the testis enlarges and changes echogenicity. The gray-scale (left image) median raphe image shows symmetrical testicular size and echogenicity on the right and left. The median raphe color image (right image), however, shows obvious hyperemia within the left testis.

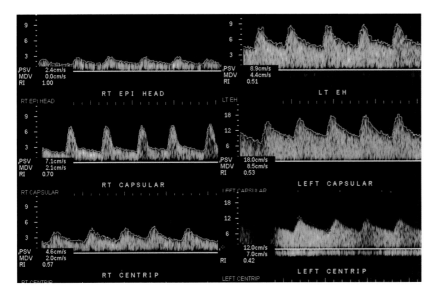

Figure 5–31 Spectral waveforms from the epididymal head, capsular arteries, and centripetal arteries on the right and left sides in a patient with acute left epididymo-orchitis show higher velocities and generally lower resistance on the infected left side. The infected left epididymal head has peak systolic velocity > 5 cm/s and an end-diastolic velocity > 3 cm/s. The capsular artery from the infected left side has a peak systolic velocity > 15 cm/s and an end-diastolic velocity > 7 cm/s. The absolute velocities of the centripetal arteries are more variable and usually require comparison with the opposite side. All the peak systolic velocities on the infected left side are more than 1.7 times greater than the velocities of the corresponding artery on the normal side.

symptomatic and the asymptomatic epididymitis suggests hyperemia on the symptomatic side (**Fig. 5–31**).

Most adults with acute scrotal pain have infection rather than torsion and will show obviously increased color flow. Inflammatory hyperemia is a positive finding, as opposed to torsion-induced oligemia, which is a negative finding. Positive findings are inherently more believable and reliable than negative findings. The presence of hyperemia is, therefore, strongly predictive that the testis is not torsed.

Findings in Torsion of the Appendix Testis

Imaging Findings

In children, torsion of the appendix testis or appendix epididymis is more common than epididymitis and can present with clinical findings indistinguishable from spermatic cord torsion or epididymo-orchitis. The torsed appendix testis will be visible as a small hyperechoic or mixed hyperechoic and hypoechoic nodule medial to the epididymal head. The enlargement and alteration in echotexture of the torsed appendix testis is due to infarction with or without hemorrhage. The epididymal head and spermatic cord immediately adjacent to the torsed appendix testis are usually sympathetically swollen and inflamed (**Fig. 5–32**). The

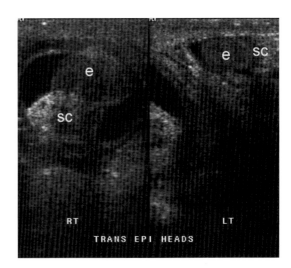

Figure 5–32 Short-axis split-screen images through the epididymal heads in a young boy with acute torsion of the appendix testis on the right. Note that the right epididymal head (e) and spermatic cord (sc) are swollen compared with the left. The reactive inflammation within the epididymal head and spermatic cord are indistinguishable from the primary inflammation caused by acute epididymitis involving the epididymal head unless the appendix testis is specifically evaluated.

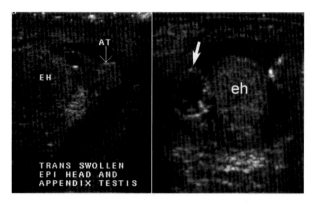

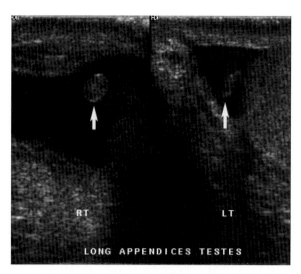

Figure 5–33 The left image shows an enlarged echogenic appendix testis (AT) (*arrow*) that has torsed and undergone bland infarction. Most torsed appendices have this appearance. The right image shows an enlarged complex cystic appendix testis (*arrow*) that has torsed and undergone secondary hemorrhagic infarction. The hemorrhage into the torsed appendix creates the cystic appearance. Only a minority of torsed appendices have this appearance.

Figure 5–34 Long-axis split-screen images of the right and left appendix testes in a patient with an acutely torsed appendix testis. Note that the normal left appendix has a thin, elongated vermiform shape, like that of a grain of rice. The swollen torsed appendix is plumper and rounder, more like the shape of a snow pea.

testis is usually sonographically normal. A small, associated reactive hydrocele often exists. If no specific attempts are made to image the appendix testis, then the diagnosis of torsed appendix will likely be missed and the reactive swelling within the adjacent epididymal head and spermatic cord will be misinterpreted as epididymitis that involves primarily the epididymal head. The sonographic appearance of the torsed appendix depends upon whether infarction is bland or hemorrhagic. Bland infarction results in hyperechoic echotexture, whereas superimposed hemorrhage gives the enlarged appendix a complex cystic appearance (**Fig. 5–33**). Longitudinal split-screen imaging of the appendices testes is definitive, but not always possible (**Fig. 5–34**). As a practical matter, the misdiagnosis of a torsed appendix testis as epididymitis is relatively unimportant—as long as the patient is not taken to surgery for suspected testicular torsion—because both epididymitis and torsion of the appendix testis are managed medically, not surgically. The pain eventually (in a few days) spontaneously abates and the hemorrhagic infarcted appendix testis may slough into the scrotal sac, calcify, and form a "scrotal pearl."

Doppler Findings

No demonstrable flow exists within the enlarged, infarcted, and hemorrhagic torsed appendix testis. Unfortunately, we are so rarely able to demonstrate flow within a normal appendix testis that no importance can be attached to a lack of flow within the enlarged ipsilateral appendix. However, sympathetic or reactive hyperemia will usually be found in the enlarged epididymal head and spermatic cord, immediately adjacent to the torsed appendix testis (**Fig. 5–35**). As is the case for imaging findings, the pattern of inflammatory hyperemia may mimic that of epididymitis that predominantly involves the head. Thus

one must have a clinical index of suspicion for torsion of an appendix to make the diagnosis and to distinguish it from epididymitis involving primarily the epididymal head.

Findings in Testicular Tumors

Imaging Findings

Occasionally, necrosis of or hemorrhage into a testicular tumor causes acute scrotal pain. In fact, ~10% of testicular

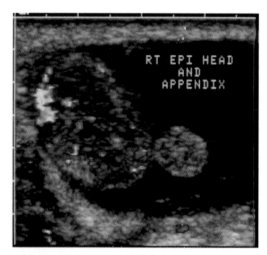

Figure 5–35 Short-axis color Doppler view of torsed appendix testis and adjacent torsed appendix shows no flow in torsed appendix and reactive hyperemia in the adjacent epididymal head. The problem is that we can almost never demonstrate flow in a normal appendix testis. Thus absence of flow in a suspect appendix testis has little value. The diagnosis rests upon clinical suspicion and the gray-scale images.

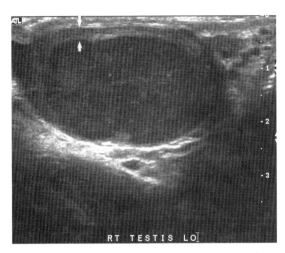

Figure 5–36 Long-axis gray-scale view of a large testicular tumor that presented with acute pain. A small percentage of testicular tumors present with acute pain. In a few cases the tumor may almost completely replace normal tissue, leaving only a thin peripheral rim of normal tissue (between arrows). If the thin rim of normal tissue is not appreciated, there is a risk of misdiagnosing the cause of pain as orchitis.

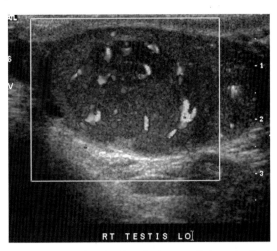

Figure 5–37 Long-axis color Doppler image of a large testicular tumor that replaces nearly all of the substance of the testis. Such large testicular tumors usually have increased vascularity that is more disorganized than hyperemia that occurs within an inflamed testis.

Findings in Testicular Trauma

Imaging Findings

Trauma can increase the risk of torsion, lead to epididymo-orchitis, and result in fracture of the testis, with or without a large hematocele. Because the differential diagnosis for trauma is essentially the same as for acute scrotal pain in the absence of trauma, the standard workup for scrotal pain should be used. The only difference is that a specific attempt should be made to identify testicular fracture. Large hematoceles can make it difficult to determine whether testicular fracture exists. Foci of abnormal echotexture within the substance of the testis can be manifestations of either contusion or occult fracture. Textural abnormalities that extend to the tunica albuginea are more suspicious for occult laceration than are centrally located foci of abnormal echotexture. Macroscopic lacerations can contain liquid blood or echogenic clot (**Fig. 5–38**). One should err on the

tumors present with pain and swelling that simulate those of infection or torsion. Smaller masses or nodules within the testis are usually easily recognized, but very large tumors that almost completely replace the testicular substance can be mistaken for an edematous testis due to orchitis or torsion. However, careful inspection will usually show a thin rim of compressed testicular tissue on one side of the mass (**Fig. 5–36**). Care must also be taken not to mistake a hugely swollen epididymal tail caused by epididymitis for a primary testicular tumor. In some cases, the tail may be so swollen that it compresses and indents the lower pole of the testis sufficiently that it appears to arise from the testis. With a coronal approach, ultrasound imaging can show that the tail is connected to the epididymal body. Additionally, the borders of the indented testis are rounded rather than pointed and claw shaped, as they are when the mass arises from within the testis.

Doppler Findings

Whether abnormally increased flow exists within neoplastic testicular masses depends almost entirely on their size rather than their cell type. Small testicular nodules (< 1.5 cm in maximum diameter) generally do not have any demonstrable flow, and masses larger than 1.5 cm are more likely to have demonstrable tumor flow, regardless of whether the nodules are benign or malignant (**Fig. 5–37**). In general, color Doppler imaging is not as useful in assessing intratesticular masses as it is for evaluating pain.

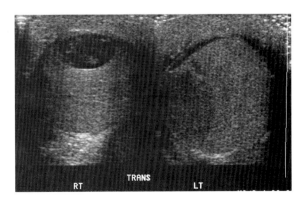

Figure 5–38 Short-axis split-screen images of bilaterally lacerated testes due to blunt trauma. The laceration in the right testis contains liquid blood and appears complex cystic. The laceration in the left testis contains echogenic clot.

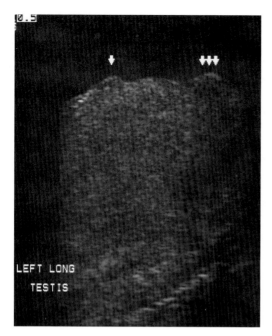

Figure 5–39 Long-axis view of a lacerated testis. The lacerations are not seen. Only mild irregularity of the tunica albuginea gives evidence of underlying lacerations (arrows).

side of aggressiveness when assessing the testis for fracture because early surgical repair improves salvage rate and recovery time. Any irregularity or flap of the tunica albuginea should be viewed as suspicious for a rent in the tunica albuginea with herniation of testicular tissue through the rent or adherent clot (**Fig. 5–39**).

Doppler Findings

The Doppler findings, like the imaging findings of trauma, include the entire gamut of causes of scrotal pain. The

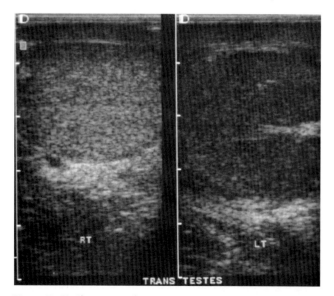

Figure 5–41 Short-axis split-screen images in a patient with an infarcted left testis that is the result of acute spermatic cord compression caused by a postherniorrhaphy hematoma.

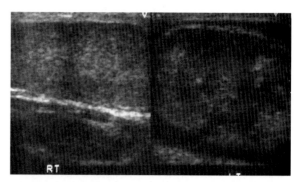

Figure 5–40 Long-axis view of right and left testes in a patient who has undergone ischemic infarction because of venous occlusion caused by severe epididymitis. Notice that the alteration in echogenicity due to venous occlusion is not homogeneous.

Doppler workup should be the same as for any other patient with acute scrotal pain. Doppler can demonstrate inflammatory hyperemia in the days or weeks after trauma in patients who develop posttraumatic orchitis or epididymitis.

Findings in Spermatic Cord Thrombosis from Causes Other than Torsion

Imaging Findings

The imaging findings of spermatic cord compression or thrombosis, whether due to severe epididymitis (**Fig. 5–40**), inguinal hernia surgery (**Fig. 5–41**), trauma, or spontaneous thrombosis (in patients who are hypercoagulable), are similar to those of testicular torsion at a similar temporal stage. The findings are manifestations of venous and lymphatic occlusion. The ultimate result, if not treated promptly, is hemorrhagic venous infarction, the same pathological condition caused by torsion. The testicular and epididymal findings are indistinguishable from those of torsion. The only imaging difference between spermatic cord thrombosis resulting from inguinal herniorrhaphy and torsion is the level at which the spermatic cord

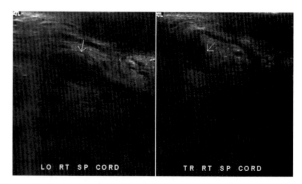

Figure 5–42 Long-axis (left) and short-axis (right) images of the spermatic cord in a patient with acute right-sided pain immediately postvasectomy. There is a small acute hematoma within the spermatic cord just deep to the cremasteric muscle.

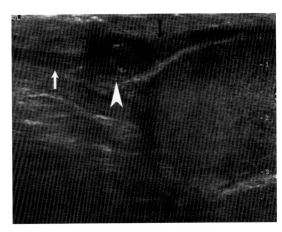

Figure 5–43 Long-axis view of the vas deferens postvasectomy in a patient who developed acute pain postvasectomy. The vas deferens is dilated below the vasectomy site (*white arrow*) There is an acute spermatic cord granuloma (*white arrowhead*). The vas deferens below the sperm granuloma is quite disorganized (*black arrow*).

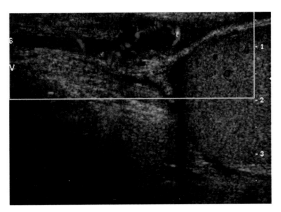

Figure 5–44 Long-axis color Doppler view of the acute sperm granuloma shown in the previous image shows inflammatory hyperemia in the walls of the granuloma. Some degree of inflammation is commonly associated with sperm granulomas, but whether it is due to a chemical inflammation or low-grade infection is difficult to determine.

swelling and hemorrhage arise. In most adult cases of torsion, the level of torsion is in the spermatic cord slightly above the testis, whereas in cases of spermatic cord occlusion due to inguinal hernia repair, the level of obstruction is at the internal inguinal ring or within the inguinal canal. The spermatic cord within the inguinal canal lateral to the penis will, therefore, be normal in size in most cases of spermatic cord torsion but abnormal in cases of testicular venous thrombosis resulting from inguinal hernia surgery. This is because compression of the spermatic cord in such cases occurs either within the inguinal ring or within the inguinal canal. Severe epididymitis may impede venous outflow from the testis, leading to venous infarction. This infarction is usually patchy and inhomogeneous but may be global and uniform. Global, uniform changes are more difficult to distinguish from changes caused by torsion than are patchy inhomogeneous changes. Evaluation of the spermatic cord for flow, twist, or the level of abrupt change in size, and the presence or absence of loose connective tissue edema provide additional clues that help make the distinction.

Doppler Findings

Doppler findings of testicular vein occlusion are identical to those of torsion.

Findings in Postvasectomy Pain

Pain occurring immediately after vasectomy is usually related to spermatic cord hematoma (**Fig. 5–42**) or an immediately developing sperm granuloma. These occur directly in and around the vasectomy site superior to the epididymal head (**Fig. 5–43**). There is usually some hyperemia associated with acute or subacute sperm granulomas (**Fig. 5–44**).

Delayed postvasectomy pain is usually related to chronic ectasia of the vas deferens, chronic epididymitis, and chronic sperm granuloma, which is most likely to occur in the distal spermatic cord near the epididymal tail. Chronic sperm granulomas can be single or multiple, and the echotexture can vary greatly from complex cystic appearance, with and without an echogenic outer rim, to solid and hyperechoic (**Fig. 5–45**). As is the case with acute

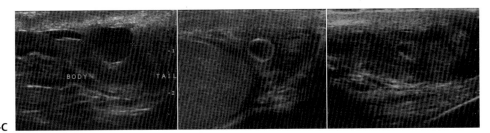

A–C

Figure 5–45 (A) The left image shows a sperm granuloma at the junction of the epididymal tail with the spermatic cord that has the appearance of a complicated cyst. **(B)** The middle image shows a sperm granuloma in a similar location with similar internal texture, but with a bright echogenic rim. **(C)** The image on the right shows multiple sperm granulomas with variable appearances, including

that of a solid hyperechoic nodule. These three patients all presented with low-grade pain years after vasectomy. For unknown reasons, acute sperm granulomas tend to occur superiorly, near the vasectomy site, but chronic sperm granulomas tend to occur within the distal spermatic cord or epididymal tail.

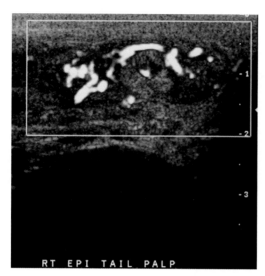

Figure 5–46 Long-axis power Doppler view of the three sperm granulomas shown in the right image of **Fig. 5–42** shows moderate hyperemia, indicating secondary inflammation or infection, just as there is in acute sperm granulomas.

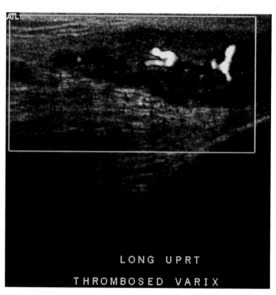

Figure 5–47 Long-axis power Doppler view of the spermatic cord in a patient who has acute thrombosis of a vein within a varicose pampiniform plexus.

sperm granulomas, there is an associated low-grade epididymitis in most cases (**Fig. 5–46**).

Findings in Thrombosis of Varicocele

Varicocele is generally not a cause of acute pain. It can cause infertility, testicular atrophy, and chronic aching, heaviness, or tugging, but usually not acute pain. However, occasionally, because of slow flow, a varicose vein within either the pampiniform plexus or the cremasteric plexus thromboses, causing acute pain. Typically only a single vein thromboses, not the entire plexus.

Gray-scale imaging findings can be helpful if echogenic flow is visible in nonthrombosed veins. Harmonics and "B-flow" can make flow more apparent. Such techniques have an advantage over Doppler in that they are not limited by "slow flow," the typical pattern of flow within varicoceles.

Doppler can be definitive in diagnosing thrombosis within a varicocele. Color Doppler is less sensitive for slow flow and more angle dependent than is power Doppler and thus is more likely than power Doppler to be unable to demonstrate slow flow within a nonthrombosed varicocele, resulting in the false impression of thrombosis where none exists. Thus power Doppler will generally be more effective than color Doppler in evaluating for thrombosis of a varicocele. Additionally, in most patients, especially on the left side, the velocity of flow within a varicocele will increase markedly when the patient is standing rather than lying down. Thus we recommend examining veins within a varicocele for thrombosis while the patient is standing (**Fig. 5–47**). Treatment usually consists only of rest, heat, and antiplatelet therapy, and, perhaps, embolization or ligation of the testicular vein.

Findings in Inguinal Hernia Extending into the Scrotum

Some patients who have large, indirect inguinal herniasm that extend into the scrotum present with pain and swelling in the ipsilateral hemi scrotum. The hernia can contain bowel loops, but most contain only mesenteric and/or omental fat (**Fig. 5–48**). Hernias this large can almost never be reduced completely.

The hernia can cause pain simply by its size and weight, by traction on the omentum or mesentery, or by incarceration or strangulation. Signs of strangulation include abnormally echogenic fat, isoechoic thickening of the hernia sac wall, and abnormal thickening and hypoperistalsis of bowel loops that might be present in the hernia.

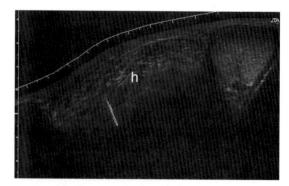

Figure 5–48 Extended field of view of left scrotum and distal left inguinal canal shows large fat-containing indirect inguinal hernia (h), extending into the scrotum to the upper pole of the left testis.

Summary

Color duplex sonography is the procedure of choice for evaluation of acute scrotal pain. The initial goal is to quickly determine whether torsion is the cause of pain. If torsion is present, then the patient immediately undergoes surgery. Once a diagnosis of torsion has been excluded, complete imaging and Doppler evaluation of the testes, epididymi, and spermatic cords will usually enable a specific diagnosis to be made and the most appropriate treatment to be instituted.

Suggested Readings

Benson CB, Doubilet PM, Richie JP. Sonography of the male genital tract. AJR Am J Roentgenol 1989;153:705–713

Bird K, Rosenfield AT. Testicular infarction secondary to acute inflammatory disease: demonstration by B-scan ultrasound. Radiology 1984;152:785–788

Brown JM, Hammers LW, Barton JW, et al. Quantitative Doppler assessment of acute scrotal inflammation. Radiology 1995;197:427–431

Burks DD, Marky BJ, Burkhard TK, et al. Suspected testicular torsion and ischemia: evaluation with color Doppler sonography. Radiology 1990;175:815–821

DeWire DM, Begun FP, Lawson RK, Fitzgerald S, Foley WD. Color Doppler ultrasonography in the evaluation of the acute scrotum. J Urol 1992;147:89–91

Dunn EK, Macchia RJ, Chauhan PS, Laugani GB, Solomon NA. Scintiscan for acute intrascrotal contents. Clin Nucl Med 1986;11:381–388

Fitzgerald SW, Erickson S, DeWire DM, et al. Color Doppler sonography in the evaluation of the adult acute scrotum. J Ultrasound Med 1992;11:543–548

Holder LE, Martire JR, Holmes ER, Wagner HN. Testicular radionuclide angiography and static imaging: anatomy, scintigraphic interpretation and clinical indications. Radiology 1977;125:739–752

Horstman WG, Middleton WD, Melson GL. Scrotal inflammators disease: color Doppler US findings. Radiology 1991;179:55–59

Horstman WG, Middleton WD, Melson GL, Siegel BA. Color Doppler US of the scrotum. Radiographics 1991;11:941–957

Kass EJ, Stone KT, Cacciarelli AA, Mitchel B. Do all children with an acute scrotum require exploration? J Urol 1993;150:667–669

Kissane JM, ed. Anderson's Pathology. 8th ed. Vol 1. St. Louis: CV Mosby; 1985:796–811

Leopold GR, Woo VL, Scheible FW, Nachtsheim D, Gosink BB. High-resolution ultrasonography of scrotal pathology. Radiology 1979;131:719–722

Lerner RM, Mevorach RA, Hulbert WC, Rabinowitz R. Color Doppler US in the evaluation of acute scrotal disease. Radiology 1990;176:355–358

Luker GD, Siegel MJ. Color Doppler sonography of the scrotum in children. AJR Am J Roentgenol 1994;163:649–655

Martin B, Conte J. Ultrasonography of the acute scrotum. J Clin Ultrasound 1987;15:37–44

Mevorach RA, Lerner RM, Greenspan BS, et al. Color Doppler ultrasound compared to a radionuclide scanning of spermatic cord torsion in a canine model. J Urol 1991;145:428–433

Middleton WD, Siegel BA, Melson GL, Yates CK, Andriole GL. Acute scrotal disorders: prospective comparison of color Doppler US and testicular scintigraphy. Radiology 1990;177:177–181

Phillips GN, Schneider M, Goodman JD, Macchia RJ. Ultrasonic evaluation of the scrotum. Urol Radiol 1979–1980;1:157–163

Ralls PW, Jensen MC, Lee KP, et al. Color Doppler sonography in acute epididymitis and orthicitis. J Clin Ultrasound 1990;18:383–386

Rifkin MD, Kurtz AB, Goldberg BB. Epididymitis examined by ultrasound: correlation with pathology. Radiology 1984;151:187–190

See WA, Mack LA, Krieger JN. Scrotal ultrasonography: a predictor of complicated epididymitis requiring orchiectomy. J Urol 1988;139:55–56

Symmers WStC, ed. Systemic Pathology. 2nd ed. Vol 4. London: Churchill Livingstone; 1979

Tumeh SS, Benson CB, Richie JP. Acute diseases of the scrotum. Semin Ultrasound CT MR 1991;12:115–130

Wilbert DM, Schaerfe CW, Stern WD, Strohmaier WL, Bichler KH. Evaluation of the acute scrotum by color-coded Doppler ultrasonography. J Urol 1993;149:1475–1477

6 Erectile Dysfunction

Harvey L. Nisenbaum and Steven C. Horii

- *Clinical Scenario 1* (**Fig. 6–1**) A 23-year-old male who has had erectile dysfunction (ED) for ~2 years. Patient states that his problem is difficulty in getting and maintaining an erection. The remainder of the medical history is noncontributory.

- *Clinical Scenario 2* (**Fig. 6–2**) A 75-year-old male who has had erectile dysfunction since radiation therapy for prostate cancer 3 years ago. Patient is hypertensive and is on oral medication. There is a question of heart disease, but no history of diabetes, smoking, Peyronie's disease, or pelvic trauma.

- *Clinical Scenario 3* (**Fig. 6–3**) A 45-year-old male who has had difficulty in getting and maintaining an erection for the last 6 or 7 years. It has increased in severity recently. The patient has a history of prior alcohol and drug abuse and prior episode of prostatitis, which was treated with antibiotics. When he was younger, he did a considerable amount of bicycle riding and did develop transient numbness in the genital area.

- *Clinical Scenario 4* (**Fig. 6–4**) A 56-year-old male who has had erectile dysfunction progressing for several years. The patient denies hypertension, smoking, coronary artery disease, diabetes, Peyronie's disease, pelvic trauma, or prostate cancer.

- *Clinical Scenario 5* (**Fig. 6–5**) A 71-year-old male who has had erectile dysfunction for 20 years. Patient has had two previous transurethral resections of the prostate. Patient has unstable angina. There is no history of hypertension, smoking, diabetes, Peyronie's disease, pelvic trauma, or prostate cancer.

- *Clinical Scenario 6* (**Fig. 6–6**) A 51-year-old male who has had erectile dysfunction for ~5 years associated with Peyronie's disease. The patient denies hypertension, smoking, coronary artery disease, diabetes, pelvic trauma, or prostate cancer.

Differential Diagnosis

Prevalence

In July 1999, the First International Consultation on Erectile Dysfunction (ED) convened in Paris. It was cosponsored by the World Health Organization, International Consultation on Urological Diseases, and Société Internationale d'Urologie. ED was redefined as the consistent or recurrent inability to attain and/or maintain penile erection sufficient for sexual performance. A 3-month duration of ED is required to meet the criteria of consistency; the exceptions are cases of trauma or surgically induced ED. The term *ED* should not be used to describe penile curvatures, prolonged erection, painful erection, premature ejaculation, anorgasmia, or lack of desire.[1]

In 1995, it was estimated that there were over 152 million men worldwide who experienced ED; it is projected there will be ~322 million with ED in 2025, an increase of nearly 170 million men. The largest projected increases will be in the developing world (i.e., Africa, Asia, and South America).[2]

In 1994, the Massachusetts Male Aging Study (MMAS) reported that the prevalence of minimal, moderate, and complete impotence was 52%. The prevalence of complete impotence tripled from 5 to 15% between subject ages 40 and 70 years.[3] An update of the MMAS in 2000 indicated the incidence rate for erectile dysfunction was 25.9 cases per 1000 man-years [95% confidence interval (CI) 22.5 to 29.9]. The annual incidence rate increased with each decade of age and was 12.4 cases per 1000 man-years (95% CI 9.0 to 16.9), 29.8 (24.0 to 37.0), and 46.4 (36.9 to 58.4) for men 40 to 49, 50 to 59, and 60 to 69 years old, respectively. The age-adjusted risk of ED was higher for men with lower education, diabetes, heart disease, and hypertension. Population projections for men 40 to 69 years old are 17,781 new cases of ED in Massachusetts and 617,715 in the United States (white males only) annually.[4]

Anatomy of the Penis

The penis is composed of three cylindrical structures: two dorsally located corpora cavernosa, and one ventrally located corpus spongiosum. The corpus spongiosum contains the anterior urethra. Distally, the corpus spongiosum expands to become the glans penis. The proximal ends of the corpora cavernosa, the crura, originate at the undersurface of the puboischial rami as two separate structures, but merge under the pubic arch and remain attached up to the glans. The septum between the two corpora cavernosa is incomplete in men. Blood supply to the corpus spongiosum and glans is through bilateral dorsal arteries (**Fig. 6–1C,D**), which arise on each side from the common

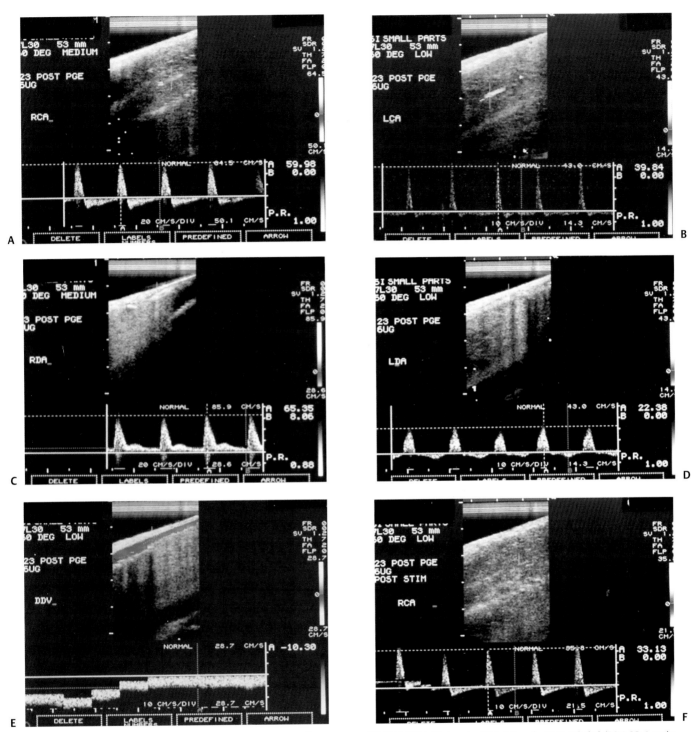

Figure 6–1 Clinical scenario 1. **(A–E)** Following intracavernosal injection of 6 μg of prostaglandin-E1 (Caverject), erectile response was 5/5. **(A)** RCA (PSV, 60 cm/s; EDV, 0 cm/s; RI, 1.0; reversal of diastolic flow). **(B)** LCA (PSV, 39.8 cm/s; EDV, 0 cm/s; RI, 1.0; reversal of diastolic flow). **(C)** RDA (PSV, 65.4 cm/s; EDV, 8.1 cm/s; RI, 0.88). **(D)** (PSV, 22.4 cm/s; EDV, 0 cm/s; RI, 1.0). **(E)** DDV (Peak velocity, 10.3 cm/s). **(F–J)** Following self-stimulation, erectile response was 5/5. **(F)** RCA (PSV, 33.1 cm/s; EDV, 0 cm/s; RI, 1.0; reversal of diastolic flow). (*Continued*)

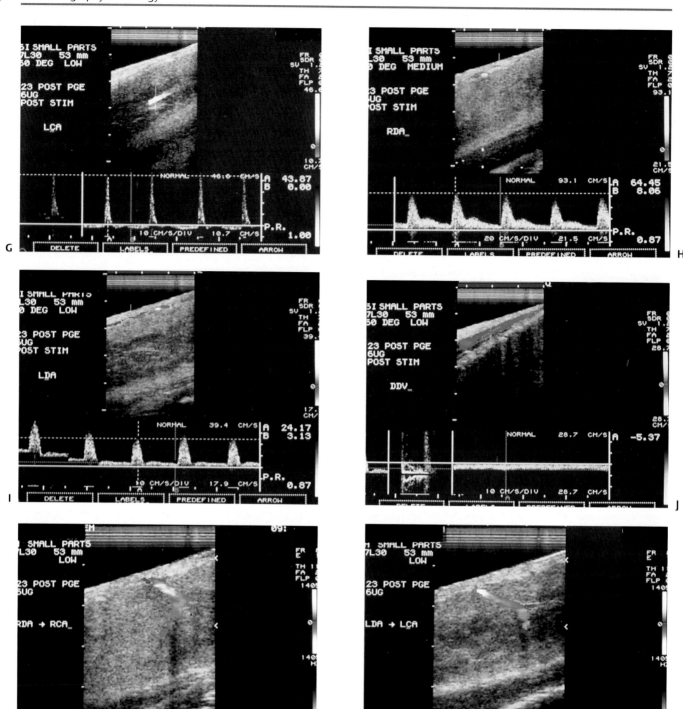

Figure 6–1 (*Continued*) **(G)** LCA (PSV, 43.9 cm/s; EDV, 0 cm/s; RI, 1.0; reversal of diastolic flow). **(H)** RDA (PSV, 64.5 cm/s; EDV, 8.1 cm/s; RI, 0.87). **(I)** LDA (PSV, 24.2 cm/s; EDV, 3.1 cm/s; RI, 0.87). **(J)** DDV (Peak velocity, 5.4 cm/s). **(K)** RDA to RCA collateral. **(L)** LDA to LCA collateral. Results: normal study. Diagnosis: Psychogenic erectile dysfunction. RCA, right cavernous artery; LCA, left cavernous artery; RDA, right dorsal artery; LDA, left dorsal artery; DDV, deep dorsal vein; PSV, peak systolic velocity; EDV, end-diastolic velocity; RI, resistive index.

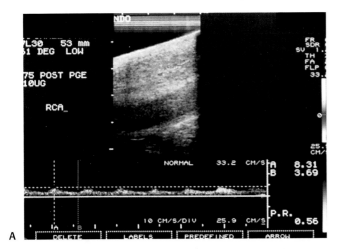

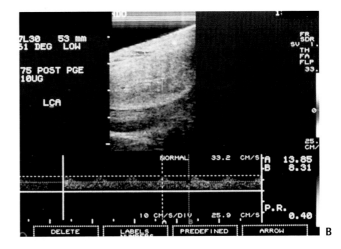

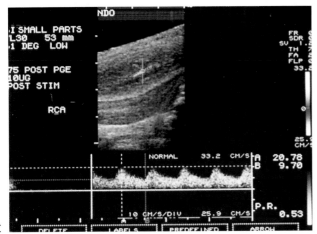

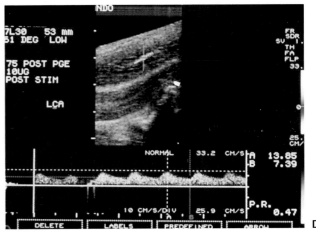

Figure 6–2 Clinical Scenario 2. **(A,B)** Following intracavernosal injection of 10 μg of prostaglandin-E1, (Caverject), erectile response was 1/5. **(A)** RCA (PSV, 8.3 cm/s; EDV, 3.7 cm/s; RI, 0.56). **(B)** LCA (PSV, 13.9 cm/s; EDV, 8.3 cm/s; RI, 0.40). **(C,D)** Following self-stimulation, erectile response was 1/5. **(C)** RCA (PSV, 20.8 cm/s; EDV, 9.7 cm/s; RI, 0.53).

(D) LCA (PSV, 13.9 cm/s; EDV, 7.4 cm/s; RI, 0.47). Results: Bilateral cavernosal arterial insufficiency; cannot exclude cavernosal venous occlusive dysfunction. Diagnosis: Arteriogenic erectile dysfunction. RCA, right cavernous artery; LCA, left cavernous artery; PSV, peak systolic velocity; EDV, end-diastolic velocity; RI, resistive index.

penile artery, itself a branch of the internal pudendal artery. The primary blood supply to each corpus cavernosum is through a cavernous artery (**Fig. 6–1A,B**), a branch of the common penile artery. The cavernous artery is responsible for tumescence of the corpus cavernosum and the dorsal artery for engorgement of the glans penis during erection. Each corpus cavernosum is a conglomeration of sinusoids, larger in the center and smaller in the periphery. The spongy tissues of the corpora cavernosa are encapsulated by a two-layered fibrous sheath called the tunica albuginea. The tunica affords great flexibility, rigidity, and tissue strength to the penis. Along its course, the cavernous artery gives off many helicine arteries, which supply the trabecular erectile tissue and the sinusoids. These helicine arteries are contracted and tortuous in the flaccid state and become dilated and straight during erection.[5]

The venous drainage from the corpora originates in tiny venules leading from the peripheral sinusoids immediately beneath the tunica albuginea. These venules travel in the trabeculae between the tunica and the peripheral sinusoids to form the subtunical venous plexus before exiting as the emissary veins. The emissary veins usually take an oblique course between the two layers of the tunica albuginea. Emissary veins draining the proximal corpora cavernosa join to form cavernous and crural veins. These veins join the periurethral veins from the urethral bulb to form the internal pudendal veins. The emissary veins from the more distal corporus cavernosum and spongiosum drain dorsally to the deep dorsal vein, laterally to the circumflex vein, and ventrally to the periurethral vein. Beginning at the coronal sulcus, the prominent deep dorsal vein (DDV) (**Fig. 6–1E**) constitutes the main venous drainage of the glans penis, corpus spongiosum, and distal two thirds of the corpora cavernosa. Usually one, but sometimes more than one, DDV runs upward behind the symphysis pubis to join the periprostatic venous plexus. Variations in the number, distribution, and termination of the venous systems are common.[5]

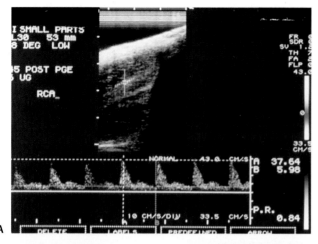
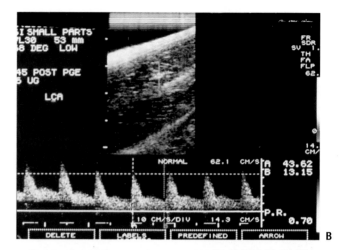
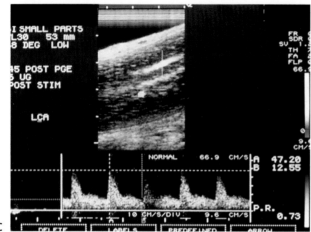
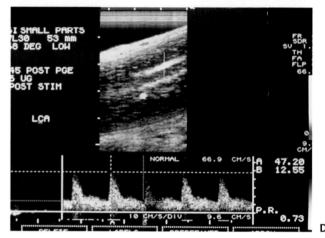

Figure 6–3 Clinical Scenario 3. **(A,B)** Following intracavernosal injection of 6 μg of prostaglandin-E1 (Caverject), erectile response was 2/5. **(A)** RCA (PSV, 37.6 cm/s; EDV, 6 cm/s; RI, 0.84). **(B)** LCA (PSV, 43.6 cm/s; EDV, 13.2 cm/s; RI, 0.70). **(C,D)** Following self-stimulation, erectile response was 3/5. **(C)** RCA (PSV, 38.2 cm/s; EDV, 7.8 cm/s; RI, 0.80). **(D)** LCA (PSV, 47.2 cm/s; EDV, 12.6 cm/s; RI, 0.73). Results: Cavernosal venous occlusive dysfunction. Diagnosis: venogenic erectile dysfunction. RCA, right cavernous artery; LCA, left cavernous artery; PSV, peak systolic velocity; EDV, end-diastolic velocity; RI, resistive index.

The innervation of the penis is both autonomic (sympathetic and parasympathetic) and somatic (sensory and motor). The parasympathetic (S2–S4) activity is responsible for tumescence and the sympathetic (T11–L2) activity causes detumescence.[5]

Physiology of Erection

The penile erectile tissue, specifically the cavernous smooth musculature and the smooth muscles of the arteriolar and arterial walls, plays a key role in the erectile process. In the flaccid state, these smooth muscles are chronically contracted by the sympathetic discharge, allowing only for a small amount of arterial flow for nutritional purposes.[5] Sexual stimulation triggers the release of neurotransmitters from the cavernous nerve terminals. This results in relaxation of the smooth muscles and the following events: (1) dilatation of the arterioles and arteries with increased blood flow in both the diastolic and systolic phases; (2) trapping of the incoming blood by the expanding sinusoids; (3) compression of the subtunical venous plexuses between the tunica albuginea and the peripheral sinusoids, reducing the venous outflow; (4) stretching of the tunica to its capacity, which encloses the emissary veins between the inner circular and the outer longitudinal layers of the tunica and further decreases the venous outflow to a minimum; (5) an increase in intracavernous pressure (maintained at around 100 mm Hg), which raises the penis from the dependent position to the erect state (the full erection phase); and (6) a further pressure increase (to several hundred mm Hg) with contraction of the ischiocavernosus muscles (rigid erection phase).[5]

There are three types of erection: psychogenic, reflexogenic, and nocturnal.[5] Psychogenic erection is the result of

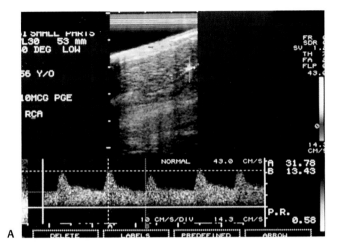

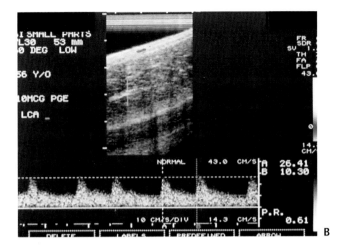

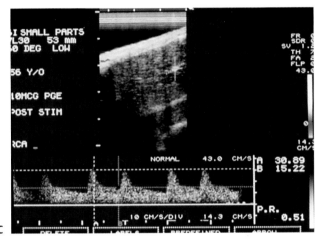

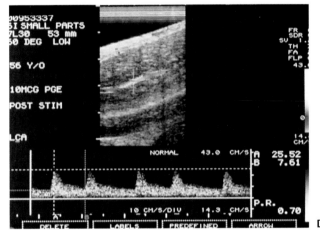

Figure 6–4 Clinical Scenario 4. **(A,B)** Following intracavernosal injection of 10 μg of prostaglandin-E1 (Caverject), erectile response was 2/5. **(A)** RCA (PSV, 31.8 cm/s; EDV, 13.4 cm/s; RI, 0.58). **(B)** LCA (PSV, 26.4 cm/s; EDV, 10.3 cm/s; RI, 0.61; irregular heart rhythm). **(C,D)** Following self-stimulation, erectile response was 2/5. **(C)** RCA (PSV, 30.9 cm/s; EDV, 15.2 cm/s; RI, 0,51). **(D)** LCA (PSV, 25.5 cm/s; EDV, 7.6 cm/s; RI, 0.70). Results: Mild bilateral cavernosal arterial insufficiency with cavernosal venous occlusive dysfunction. Diagnosis: venogenic erectile dysfunction with mild arteriogenic component and cardiac arrhythmia. RCA, right cavernous artery; LCA, left cavernous artery; PSV, peak systolic velocity; EDV, end-diastolic velocity; RI, resistive index.

audiovisual stimulation or fantasy. Impulses from the brain modulate the spinal erection centers (T11–L2 and S2–S4) to activate the erectile process. There is an increased formation of nitric oxide (NO) by the nonadrenergic/noncholinergic neurons and endothelial cells, which stimulates the production of cyclic guanosine monophosphate (cGMP), resulting in the depletion of intracellular calcium and relaxation of smooth muscle resulting in erection. To return to the flaccid state, cGMP is broken down by phosphodiesterase type 5 (PDE5). Sildenafil (Viagra, Pfizer, New York, New York) is the first oral medication to inhibit PDE5 and prolong the effects of cGMP. It was also the first oral medication to receive Food and Drug Administration (FDA) approval. Currently, there are three oral medications on the market that inhibit PDE5 [sildenafil (Viagra); tadalafil (Cialis, Lilly ICOS, Indianapolis, Indiana); vardenafil (Levitra, Schering, Kenilworth, New Jersey)], which are used to treat ED.

Reflexogenic erection is produced by tactile stimuli to the genital organs. The impulses reach the spinal erection centers; some of them follow the ascending tract, resulting in sensory perception, whereas others activate the autonomic nuclei to send messages via the cavernous nerves to the penis to induce erection. This type of erection is preserved in patients with upper spinal cord injuries.[5]

Nocturnal erections occur mostly during rapid-eye-movement (REM) sleep. The mechanism that triggers REM sleep is located in the pontine reticular formation. During REM sleep, the cholinergic neurons in the lateral pontine tegmentum are activated, whereas the adrenergic neurons in the locus caeruleus and the serotonergic neurons in the midbrain raphe are silent. This differential activation may be responsible for the nocturnal erections during REM sleep.[5]

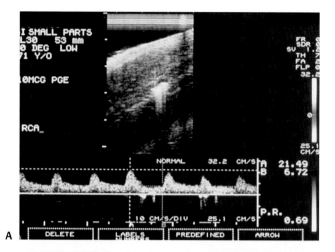

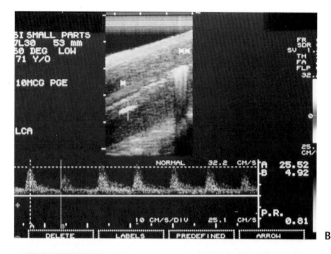

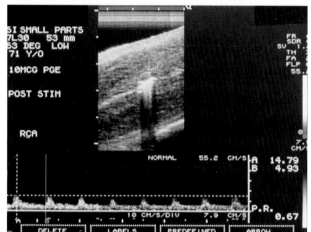

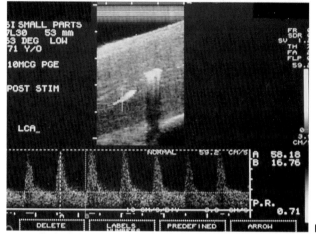

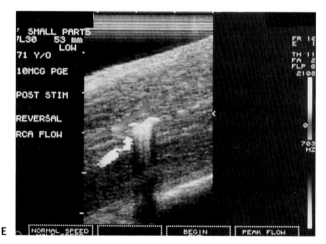

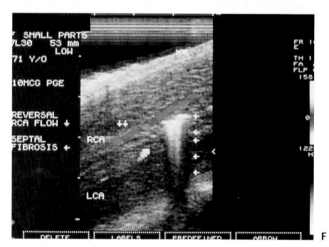

Figure 6–5 Clinical Scenario 5. **(A,B)** Following intracavernosal injection of 10 µg of prostaglandin-E1 (Caverject), erectile response was 1/5. **(A)** RCA (PSV, 21.5 cm/s; EDV, 6.7 cm/s; RI, 0.69). **(B)** LCA (PSV, 25.5 cm/s; EDV, 4.9 cm/s; RI, 0.81). **(C,D)** Following self-stimulation, erectile response was 3/5. **(C)** RCA (PSV, 14.8 cm/s; EDV, 4.9 cm/s; RI, 0.67). **(D)** LCA (PSV, 58.2 cm/s; EDV, 16.8 cm/s; RI, 0.71). **(E)** LCA to RCA collateral.

(F) Reversal of flow in proximal RCA (double arrow) and septal fibrosis (single arrow) without Peyronie's deviation. Results: Right cavernosal arterial insufficiency with cavernosal venous occlusive dysfunction. Diagnosis: Mixed arteriogenic and venogenic erectile dysfunction. RCA, right cavernous artery; LCA, left cavernous artery; PSV, peak systolic velocity; EDV, end-diastolic velocity; RI, resistive index.

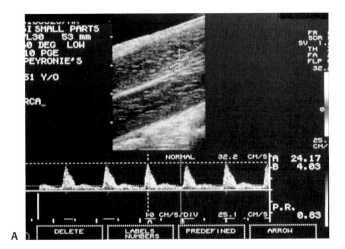

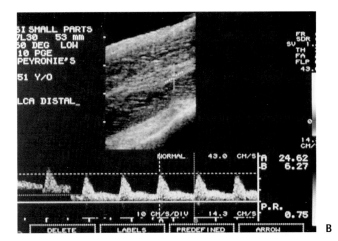

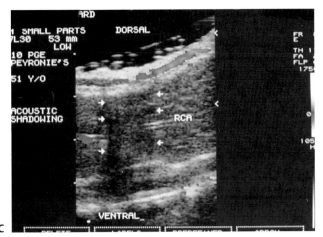

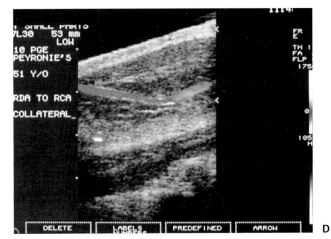

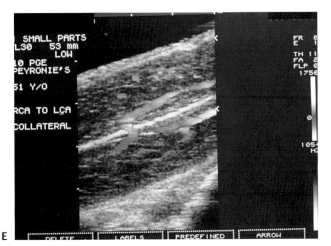

Figure 6–6 Clinical Scenario 6. **(A,B)** Following intracavernosal injection of 10 μg of prostaglandin-E1 (Caverject), erectile response was 3/5. No self-stimulation study was performed. **(A)** RCA (PSV, 24.2 cm/s; EDV, 4 cm/s; RI, 0.83). **(B)** LCA (PSV, 24.6 cm/s; EDV, 6.3 cm/s; RI, 0.75). **(C)** Distal dorsal plaque with acoustic shadowing (*arrows*) causing a dorsal penile curvature of ~45 degrees. **(D)** RDA to

RCA collaterals. **(E)** RCA to LCA collaterals. Results: Penile curvature with dorsal plaque; mild bilateral cavernosal arterial insufficiency. Diagnosis: Peyronie's disease. RCA, right cavernous artery; LCA, left cavernous artery; PSV, peak systolic velocity; EDV, end-diastolic velocity; RI, resistive index.

Classification of Erectile Dysfunction

Erectile dysfunction can be classified as psychogenic, neurogenic, endocrinologic, vasculogenic (arteriogenic, venogenic, mixed), or drug-induced.[5]

Psychogenic

Sexual behavior and penile erection are controlled by the hypothalamus, limbic system, and cerebral cortex. Therefore, stimulatory or inhibitory messages can be related to the spinal erection centers to facilitate or inhibit erection. Two possible mechanisms have been proposed to explain the inhibition of erection in psychogenic dysfunction: direct inhibition of the spinal erection center by the brain as an exaggeration of the normal suprasacral inhibition and excessive sympathetic outflow or elevated peripheral catecholamine levels, which may increase penile smooth muscle tone and thus prevent the relaxation necessary for erection.

Neurogenic

Because erection is a neurovascular event, any disease or dysfunction affecting the brain, spinal cord, cavernous and pudendal nerves, or receptors in the terminal arterioles and cavernous smooth muscles can induce dysfunction. Pathological processes involving the brain such as Parkinson's disease, stroke, tumors, Alzheimer's disease, and trauma can be associated with partial or complete erectile dysfunction. Spinal cord injuries, spina bifida, disk herniation, syringomyelia, tumor, and multiple sclerosis can affect the afferent or efferent neural pathways involving the spine and be associated with erectile dysfunction.

Because of the close relationship between the cavernous nerves and the pelvic organs, surgery on these organs is a frequent cause of impotence. The incidence of iatrogenic ED resulting from radical prostatectomy has ranged from 43 to 100%; abdominal perineal resection, 15 to 100%; and external sphincterotomy at the 3 and 9 o'clock positions, 2 to 49%. The introduction of nerve-sparing radical prostatectomy has dramatically reduced the incidence of impotence from nearly 100% to between 30 and 50%.

Alcoholism, vitamin deficiency, or diabetes may affect the cavernous nerve terminals, resulting in a deficiency of neurotransmitters. In diabetics, impairment of neurogenic and endothelium-dependent relaxation results in inadequate nitric oxide (NO) release.

Endocrinologic

The endocrine disorders that are associated with ED are androgen ablation therapy for prostate cancer, dysfunction of the hypothalamic–pituitary axis resulting in hypogonadism, prolactin-secreting pituitary tumors, hyperthyroidism, and hypothyroidism. Hyperprolactinemia, whether resulting from a pituitary adenoma or drugs, leads to both reproductive and sexual dysfunction. Symptoms may include loss of libido, ED, galactorrhea, gynecomastia, and infertility. Hyperprolactinemia is associated with low circulating levels of testosterone, which appear to be secondary to inhibition of gonadotropin-releasing hormone secretion by the elevated prolactin levels.

Hyperthyroidism is commonly associated with diminished libido, which may be due to the increased circulating estrogen levels and less often with erectile dysfunction. In hypothyroidism, low testosterone secretion and elevated prolactin levels contribute to ED.

Diabetes mellitus, although the most common endocrinologic disorder, causes ED through its vascular, neurological, endothelial, and psychogenic complications rather than through hormone deficiency per se.

Vasculogenic

Arteriogenic

Atherosclerotic or traumatic arterial occlusive disease of the hypogastric-cavernous-helicine arterial tree can decrease the perfusion pressure and arterial flow to the sinusoidal spaces, thus increasing the time needed to attain maximal erection and decreasing the rigidity of the erect penis. In the majority of patients with arteriogenic ED, the impaired penile perfusion is a component of the generalized atherosclerotic process. One study found that the incidence and age at onset of coronary disease and ED are parallel. Common risk factors associated with arterial insufficiency include hypertension, hyperlipidemia, cigarette smoking, diabetes mellitus, blunt perineal or pelvic trauma, and pelvic irradiation. Focal stenosis of the common penile or cavernous artery is most often seen in young patients who have sustained pelvic fracture or direct perineal trauma. Long-distance cycling is also a risk factor for vasculogenic and neurogenic ED.

Venogenic

Veno-occlusive dysfunction has been proposed as one of the most common causes of vasculogenic impotence. Veno-occlusive dysfunction may result from several possible pathophysiological processes: (1) the presence or development of large venous channels draining the corpora cavernosa, frequently seen in patients with primary ED; (2) degenerative changes (Peyronie's disease, old age, and diabetes) or traumatic injury to the tunica albuginea (penile fracture), resulting in inadequate compression of the subtunical and emissary veins; (3) structural alterations in the fibroelastic components of the trabeculae, cavernous smooth muscle, and endothelium; (4) insufficient trabecular smooth muscle relaxation, causing inadequate sinusoidal expansion and insufficient compression of the subtunical venules, occurring in an anxious individual with excessive adrenergic tone or in a patient with inadequate neurotransmitter release from the parasympathetic nerves; and (5) acquired venous shunts (the result of operative correction of priapism), causing persistent glans-cavernosum or cavernosum-spongiosum shunting.

Peyronie's disease is characterized by a lesion in the tunica albuginea of the corpora cavernosa (**Fig. 6–6C**). During erection, this lesion causes functional shortening and curvature of the involved aspect of the tunica. The lesion has commonly been called a plaque. Peyronie's disease is seen in ~1% of white men. Although the disease has been reported in younger patients, there is a clear predominance between the ages of 45 and 60 years. The plaque is a focal scar that may result in susceptible individuals from an inflammatory response to microtrauma from bending and buckling of the erect penis during sexual intercourse. In the flaccid penis, the plaque is usually palpable as a nodule or thickening, often on the dorsal aspect of the penis.

Peyronie's disease is also associated with the development of ED in some patients. It appears that in most cases, however, ED precedes the development of Peyronie's disease.

Drug-Induced

In general, drugs that interfere with central neuroendocrine or local neurovascular control of penile smooth muscle have a potential for causing ED. Central neurotransmitter pathways and dopaminergic pathways involved in sexual function may be disturbed by antipsychotics, antidepressants, and some centrally acting antihypertensive drugs.

Centrally acting sympatholytics, including methyldopa, clonidine, and reserpine, are known to cause sexual dysfunction. Alpha-adrenergic blocking agents such as phenoxybenzamine and phentolamine may cause ejaculatory failure or retrograde ejaculation. Beta-adrenergic blockers have been implicated in sexual dysfunction. Thiazide diuretics have been credited with widely differing effects on potency, and spironolactone produces erectile failure in 4 to 30% of patients and has been associated with decreased libido, gynecomastia, and mastodynia. Major tranquilizers or antipsychotics can decrease libido, causing erectile failure and ejaculatory dysfunction. The mechanisms involved may include sedation, anticholinergic action, a central antidopaminergic effect, α-adrenergic antagonist action, and release of prolactin. Among antidepressants, tricyclic and heterocyclic antidepressants and selective serotonin reuptake and monamine oxidase inhibitors reportedly cause ED and ejaculatory disorders. The sexual side effects seen in patients taking minor tranquilizers may well be a result of the central sedative effects of these agents.

Cigarette smoking may induce vasoconstriction and penile venous leakage because of its contractile effect on the cavernous smooth muscle. In a study of nocturnal penile tumescence in cigarette smokers, there was an inverse correlation between nocturnal erection, both rigidity and duration, and the number of cigarettes smoked per day. Men who smoked more than 40 cigarettes a day had the weakest and shortest nocturnal erections.

Alcohol in small amounts improves erection and sexual drive because of its vasodilatory effect and suppression of anxiety; however, large amounts can cause central sedation, decreased libido, and transient ED. Chronic alcoholism may result in liver dysfunction, decreased testosterone, and increased estrogen levels and alcoholic polyneuropathy, which also effects penile nerves.

Cimetidime, a histamine H2 receptor antagonist, has been reported to suppress the libido and produce erectile failure. It is thought to act as an antiandrogen and to increase prolactin levels.

Other drugs known to cause ED are estrogens and drugs with antiandrogenic actions such as ketoconazole and cyproterone acetate. Finally, many anticancer drugs may be associated with a progressive loss of libido, peripheral neuropathy, azospermia, and erectile failure.

Erectile Dysfunction Associated with Systemic Disease and Other Causes

ED has been estimated to occur in 35 to 75% of men with diabetes mellitus, with onset occurring at an earlier age than those without diabetes. The incidence of ED in diabetes has been found to be age dependent: 15% at age 30 years and 55% at age 34 to 60 years. Diabetes may cause ED through its effects on central nervous system and peripheral nerve function, androgen production, psychological factors, vascular integrity, and endothelial and smooth muscle function.

Hyperlipidemia and atherosclerosis are major contributors to ED. Hyperlipidemia is a well-known risk factor for arteriosclerosis. It enhances the deposition of lipid in the vascular lesions, causing atherosclerosis and eventual occlusion. The atherosclerotic lesions can extend to the internal pudendal or cavernous arteries to reduce inflow. Additionally, the hyperlipidemia may also cause dysfunction of the cavernous smooth muscle and the endothelium.

Hypertension is another well-recognized risk factor for arteriosclerosis; a prevalence of ~45% has been noted in one series of impotent men. The associated arterial stenotic lesions are thought to be the cause of ED. In addition to increased peripheral vascular resistance, alteration in the vessel architecture, resulting in an increased wall:lumen ratio and reduced dilatory capacity, may also contribute to impotence in hypertensive patients.

Chronic renal failure has frequently been associated with diminished erectile function, impaired libido, and infertility. In one study, by the time patients with uremia began maintenance dialysis, 50% were impotent. The mechanism is probably multifactorial: depressed testosterone levels, diabetes mellitus, vascular insufficiency, multiple medications, autonomic and somatic neuropathy, and psychological stress. After successful renal transplantation, 50 to 80% of patients have returned to their pre-illness potency.

Patients with severe pulmonary disease often fear aggravating dyspnea during sexual intercourse. Patients with angina, heart failure, or myocardial infarction can have ED from anxiety, depression, or arterial insufficiency. Other systemic diseases such as cirrhosis of the liver, scleroderma, chronic debilitation, and cachexia are also known to cause ED.

Diagnostic Evaluation

Nonimaging Tests

With the recent introduction of effective oral agents like sildenafil (Viagra), tadalafil (Cialis), and vardenafil (Levitra) for the treatment of ED, questions have been raised about the need for more sophisticated diagnostic tests. Broderick and Lue propose a two-level diagnostic approach, depending on the patient's and the partner's goal and the patient's age, general health, and medical condition.[1] The first level consists of a detailed medical and psychosexual history, physical examination, and hormonal and laboratory testing followed by a discussion of treatment options and further diagnostic tests. The patient is then given the choice of either a therapeutic trial (with oral medication, a vacuum constriction device, or intracavernous injection) or a second level of evaluation. The latter level is designed to elucidate the cause of the dysfunction and entails one or more of the following tests: psychological consultation, nocturnal penile tumescence and rigidity testing, advanced neurological testing, and functional arterial and venous studies.

The objectives of diagnostic evaluation, whether limited or extensive, are to (1) identify medical and psychosexual causes of ED, (2) assess the degree and reversibility of the dysfunction, and (3) formulate a treatment strategy that is consistent with the specific diagnosis of ED and meets the goals of the patient and his partner.

To begin the evaluation, a careful medical history with knowledge of concurrent illnesses and medications is essential. Because ED may have multiple causes, a detailed history and physical examination may help determine whether the dysfunction is a result of anatomical, psychogenic, endocrinologic, neurological, or vascular abnormalities and/or is medication induced.

The psychosexual history is a very important part of the diagnostic evaluation and should include the duration of ED and level of libido. The presence of morning or night-time erection, the quality of the erection, and the presence of any psychological conflict may help determine whether the dysfunction is mostly psychogenic or organic.

Because ED is known to be associated with many common medical conditions and medications, careful questioning may yield insights. A history of peripheral vascular or coronary artery disease, diabetes, renal failure, tobacco and alcohol use, and psychological, neurological, or chronic debilitating disease can direct further evaluation.

Similarly, the patient's past surgical history is important. Pelvic surgery (prostatectomy, distal colectomy, abdominoperineal resection), radiation therapy, and pelvic trauma may be associated with impotence.

Careful physical examination with particular attention to sexual and genital development may occasionally reveal an obvious cause such as micropenis or Peyronie's plaque. The finding of small, soft, atrophic testes or gynecomastia should prompt an endocrine evaluation for hypogonadism or hyperprolactinemia. Patients with certain genetic syndromes, such as Klinefelter's syndrome, may present with obvious physical signs of hypogonadism or distinctive body habitus. A careful neurological examination should also be performed. Patients with diabetes or degenerative neurological disorders may show evidence of peripheral neuropathy. Testing for genital or perineal sensation and the bulbocavernosus reflex is also useful in assessing possible neurogenic impotence. One study showed that a careful history and physical examination had a 95% sensitivity, but only a 50% specificity in diagnosing organic ED.

The laboratory investigation is directed at identifying treatable conditions or previously undetected metabolic illnesses that may be contributory (e.g., metabolic disturbances such as renal insufficiency, diabetes, and endocrine abnormalities such as hypogonadism and hyperprolactinemia). A complete laboratory evaluation includes serum chemistries, renal function, complete blood count, urinalysis, and hormonal evaluation (generally, serum testosterone, prolactin, and thyroid function). Prostate specific antigen (PSA) level is recommended in all men 50 years of age or older or younger than 40 years of age if there is a family history of prostate cancer or if the patient is African American.

After the patient has had a careful history and physical and laboratory testing, the results are discussed with the patient (and partner), and available treatment options are discussed. If further testing is performed, they may include psychological consultation, nocturnal penile tumescence and rigidity testing, advanced neurological testing, and functional arterial and venous studies.

Psychometry and Psychological Interview

There are three groups of psychometric instruments available for the evaluation of ED: (1) the personality questionnaires, (2) depression inventories, and (3) questionnaires for sexual dysfunction and relationship factors.[1] A skillful diagnostic interview remains the mainstay of psychological evaluation. The interview should be focused on the following: (1) the current sexual problem and its history, (2) deeper causes of sexual dysfunction, (3) the relationship with the partner, and (4) psychiatric symptoms.

Nocturnal Penile Tumescence and Rigidity Testing

Nocturnal penile erection or sleep-related erection is a recurring cycle of penile erections associated with rapid eye movement sleep in virtually all potent men. Patients documented to have normal nocturnal penile tumescence and rigidity testing (NPTR) are presumed to have normal capacity for spontaneous erotically induced erections. The primary goal of NPTR testing is to distinguish psychogenic from organic impotence. This study consists of nocturnal monitoring devices that measure the number of erectile episodes, maximum penile rigidity, tumescence (circumference), and duration of the nocturnal erections. Traditionally, NPTR is recorded in conjunction with electroencephalography, electro-oculography, and electromyography (EMG), with nasal air flow, and with oxygen saturation to document REM sleep and the presence or absence of hypoxia (sleep apnea). Laboratories also monitor sleep movement patterns because periodic limb movement disorders are associated with abnormal NPTR.

Some feel the greatest value of NPTR is for the patient with no neurovascular risk factors who present with a history suggestive of a psychogenic cause.[1]

Sexual Stimulation (Audiovisual and Vibratory)

Another alternative to NPTR testing for differential diagnosis is the use of vibrotactile or visual sexual stimulation, or both. This test is designed to elicit penile responses during visual and vibrotactile stimulation in conjunction with cognitive tasks (distraction and monitoring of erections). It has been found that about one third of patients with purely psychogenic ED have an average increase in penile girth of more than 30 mm as a response to combined vibration and film. None of the patients with organic involvement exceeded this 30 mm criteria; however, one study analyzed the scientific community's attitude toward sexual stimulation video testing and warned that many factors may affect the outcome such as the physician's fear of being accused of voyeurism, the physician's feelings about his or her own erotic fantasies and about pornography, and the castrating effects of a hospital environment. This type of testing is helpful in the evaluation and management of the patient with complex ED.[1]

Neurological Testing

Neurological testing should assess peripheral, spinal, and supraspinal centers and both somatic and autonomic pathways associated with erection.

Biothesiometry for Somatic Nervous System Evaluation

This test is designed to measure the sensory perception threshold to various amplitudes of vibratory stimulation produced by a handheld electromagnetic device (biothesiometer) placed on the pulp of the index fingers, both sides of the penile shaft, and the glans penis. At least one study found no relationship between results of penile glans biothesiometry and neurourophysiological tests of the dorsal penile nerve, probably owing to the fact that vibration is not an adequate stimulus to the glandular skin, which contains free nerve endings only and hardly any vibration receptors. The biothesiometric investigation of penile glans innervation is probably unsuited for the evaluation of penile innervation and cannot replace neurourophysiological tests.[1]

Sacral Evoked Response-Bulbocavernosus Reflex Latency for Somatic Nervous System Evaluation

This test is performed by placing two stimulating ring electrodes around the penis, one near the corona, and the other 3 cm proximal. Concentric needle electrodes are placed in the right and left bulbocavernosus muscles to record the response. Square-wave impulses are delivered via direct current stimulator. The latency period for each stimulus-response is measured from the beginning of the stimulus to the beginning of the response. An abnormal bulbocavernosus reflex (BCR) latency time, defined as a value greater than 3 standard deviations above the mean (30 to 40 msec), carries a high probability of neuropathology. In a study of diabetic patients, a significant clinical and neurophysiological correlation between the absence of the BCR on clinical examination and its prolonged latency on electrophysiological measurements was shown.[1]

Dorsal Nerve Conduction Velocity

In patients with adequate penile length, it is possible to use two BCR latency measurements, one from the glans and one from the base of the penis, to determine the conduction velocity of the dorsal nerve (i.e., by dividing the distance between the two stimulating electrodes by the difference in latency between the base and the glans). One study determined an average conduction velocity of 23.5 m/s with a range of 21.4 to 29.1 m/s in normal subjects.[1]

Genitocerebral-Evoked Potential Studies

This test involves electrical stimulation of the dorsal nerve of the penis, as described with a BCR latency test. Instead of recording electromyogram (EMG) responses, the study records the evoked potential waveforms overlying the sacral spinal cord and cerebral cortex. The cerebral response to peripheral nerve stimulation is one of the potentials of extremely low amplitude, and complex electronic equipment is used to store and average data of thousands of waveforms recurring as often as every 10th of a msec. The first latency recorded is the time of stimulation to the first replicated spinal response—the peripheral conduction time. The second is from the time of the stimulation to the first replicated cerebral response—the total conduction time. The difference between the two is the central conduction time. Unlike BCR latency, this is a purely sensory evaluation. This study is not useful as a routine test, but it can provide an objective assessment of the presence, location, and nature of afferent penile sensory dysfunction in patients with subtle abnormalities on neurological examination.[1]

Heart Rate Variability for Autonomic Nervous System Evaluation

Although autonomic neuropathy is an important cause of ED, direct testing is not available. However, many diseases that involve the autonomic nervous system affect innervation to multiple organ systems, and many tests have been developed to assess the integrity of the sympathetic and parasympathetic nervous system.

The test of heart rate control (mainly parasympathetic) consists of measuring heart rate variations during quiet breathing, during deep breathing, and as one stands up. The normal parameters are (1) the heart rate variation coefficient of the mean RR variation during quiet breathing should be less than 1.88 in 41- to 60-year-olds and 2.52 for those less than 40 years old; (2) the maximal average difference between the minimal heart rate of inspiration and maximal rate of expiration during three successive breathing cycles should be higher than 15 beats per minute in the younger group and nine beats per minute in the older group; and (3) the ratio of the longest RR interval of the bradycardiac phase and the shortest RR interval of the tachycardiac phase should be greater than 1.11.[1]

The test of blood pressure control (mainly sympathetic) measures the blood pressure response to standing up. The decrease in systolic blood pressure should be less than 13 mm Hg. Because heart rate and blood pressure responses can be affected by many external factors, these tests must be conducted under standardized conditions.

Sympathetic Skin Response for Autonomic Nervous System Evaluation

Sympathetic skin response (SSR) measures the skin potential evoked by electric shock stimuli. For example, the electrical stimuli can be applied to the median or tibial nerve and the evoked potential recorded at the contralateral hand, foot, or penis. One study evaluated 50 men with ED with the SSR and other neurophysiological tests and found that the SSR was absent in 11 of 30 cases, but was normal in all patients with nonneurogenic ED. The SSR, especially

if recorded from the penis, seems to be a useful method of testing penile autonomic innervation.[1]

Corpus Cavernosum Electromyography for the Autonomic Nervous System Evaluation

Direct recording of cavernous electrical activity with a needle electrode during flaccidity and with visual sexual stimulation was first reported by Wagner and coworkers. The normal resting flaccid electrical activity from the corpora cavernosa was a rhythmic slow wave with an intermittent burst of activity. These bursts virtually ceased during visual sexual stimulation or after intracavernous injection of a smooth muscle relaxant. The electrical activity returned during the detumescence phase. Patients with suspected autonomic neuropathy demonstrated a discoordination pattern with continuing electrical activity during visual sexual stimulation or after intracavernous injection of a smooth muscle relaxant. The cavernous EMG is characterized by highly reproducible waveforms (potentials) in the individual subject. More studies are needed to find the clinical utility of cavernous EMG.[1]

Vascular Evaluation

Penile Brachial Pressure Index

The penile brachial index (PBI) represents penile systolic blood pressure divided by the brachial systolic blood pressure. The technique involves applying a small pediatric blood pressure cuff to the base of the flaccid penis and measuring the systolic blood pressure with a continuous-wave Doppler probe. Penile brachial index of 0.7 or less has been used to indicate arteriogenic impotence. This test has many inherent limitations. Measurement in the flaccid state does not reveal the full functional capacity of the cavernous arteries in the erect state, and errors may also occur from improper fitting of the blood pressure cuff. Also, the continuous-wave Doppler probe does not discriminately select the arterial flow of the paired cavernous arteries, which are primarily involved in producing erections. In the flaccid state, the probe detects all pulsatile flow within its path and usually detects the higher blood flow of the dorsal artery, which is located superficially and supplies the glans penis, rather than the deeper flow of the cavernous arteries. This error sometimes leads to the finding of a normal PBI in a patient with true arteriogenic impotence (false-negative). Therefore, a normal PBI cannot be relied upon to exclude arteriogenic impotence.[1]

Penile Plethysmography (Penile Pulse Volume Recording)

This test is performed by connecting a 2.5 or 3 cm cuff to an air plethysmograph. The cuff is inflated to a pressure above brachial systolic pressure, which is then decreased by 10 mm Hg increments, and tracings are obtained at each level. The pressure demonstrating the best waveform is recorded. The normal waveform is similar to a normal arterial waveform obtained from a finger: a rapid upstroke, a sharp peak, a lower downstroke, and occasionally, a dicrotic notch. In patients with arteriogenic ED, the waveform shows a slow upstroke, a low, rounded peak, slow downstroke, and no dicrotic notch. The proponents of this method argue that because penile pulse volume recording measures contributions of all the vessels at the root of the penis, it is more accurate than recording the pressure in individual arteries (as in PBI). However, this study is performed with the penis in the flaccid state and cannot distinguish whether the dorsal or the cavernous artery is impaired.[1]

Combined Intracavernous Injection and Stimulation Test

Differentiation among psychogenic, neurogenic, and vascular causes is often difficult, even with a complete history, physical exam, and endocrine evaluation. Intracorporeal injection of a vasodilating agent is a useful diagnostic tool, both inexpensive and minimally invasive, in patients with suspected vasculogenic impotence. The pharmacological screening test allows the clinician to bypass neurogenic and hormonal influences and evaluate the vascular status of the penis directly and objectively.

To produce a normal erection, arterial vasodilatation, sinusoidal relaxation, and decreased venous outflow must all occur in response to a vasodilating agent. In the past, several agents were used, including papaverine, a smooth muscle relaxant, and phentolamine, an α-adrenergic blocking agent. Currently, the most commonly used agent is alprostadil [prostaglandin-E1 (PGE$_1$)], a potent vasodilating agent that is metabolized locally in the penis. The technique involves injecting 10 to 20 µg through a 27 to 29 gauge needle into the corpus cavernosum. The needle site is compressed manually to prevent hematoma formation. Erectile response is periodically evaluated for both rigidity and duration. If full erection has not occurred within 15 minutes, the patient performs manual self-stimulation.

The pharmacological test yields important information regarding penile vascular status. A normal erectile response (unbending rigidity of at least 15 min duration) following pharmacological testing rules out veno-occlusive dysfunction and severe arterial insufficiency and, generally, increases suspicion for psychogenic or neurogenic ED.

An abnormal pharmacological test suggests penile vascular disease and warrants further evaluation. The patient's fear of injection often produces a heightened sympathetic response, which inhibits the response of the cavernous smooth muscle to the intracavernous agent. This problem may produce a false-positive result. To avoid this error, we have found it helpful to give patients as much privacy as possible during the study. They are also instructed to perform self-stimulation if a rigid erection does not result within 15 minutes. This technique is known

as the combined injection and stimulation (CIS) test. In our experience, many patients (~75%) who initially have a subnormal response to an intracavernous injection have significant improvement in erection after self-stimulation. Some physicians, using audiovisual sexual stimulation after pharmacologically induced erection, also reported that 56.5% of the patients experience improved erection with their technique.[1]

Cavernosometry

The standard nonimaging diagnostic study for veno-occlusive dysfunction is pharmacological cavernosometry. Cavernosometry involves simultaneous saline infusion and intracorporeal pressure monitoring. A more physiological refinement is the addition of intracavernous injection of a vasodilating agent such as papaverine or PGE$_1$. The saline infusion rate necessary to maintain an erection is thus directly related to the degree of venous leakage. One study compared plain and pharmacological cavernosometry and reported that plain cavernosometry gave false-positive results in 6% and false-negative results in 16% of patients, and that pharmacological cavernosometry was much more reproducible. Veno-occlusive dysfunction is indicated by either the inability to increase intracorporeal pressure to the level of the mean systolic blood pressure with saline infusion or a rapid drop of intracorporeal pressure at the cessation of infusion.

In 1990, a modification of the pump infusion cavernosometry technique by replacing the infusion pump mechanism with a gravity saline infusion set (gravity cavernosometry) was introduced. The infusion source is placed ~160 cm above the penis (equivalent to 120 mm Hg pressure). With an intact veno-occlusive mechanism, the steady-state intracavernous pressure will closely approximate the pressure of the infusion source (above 110 cm water); with a defective mechanism, it will remain significantly lower. Gravity infusion cavernosometry correlates well with pump infusion cavernosometry and may provide a more economic alternative.

Cavernosography (radiography of the corporeal bodies) is performed after cavernosometry.[1]

Imaging Tests Other than Ultrasound

Arteriography

Penile arteriography was introduced in 1978. At present, selective pudendal arteriography performed with the aid of intracavernous injection is considered by many the gold standard for evaluating penile arterial anatomy. The study is performed by intracavernous injection of a vasodilating agent (e.g., papaverine, papaverine and phentolamine, or PGE$_1$), followed by selective cannulation of the internal pudendal artery and injection of a diluted contrast solution of low osmolarity. Anatomy and radiograph appearance of the cavernous arteries are then evaluated according to an established criteria.

Confounding interpretation is the anatomical fact that deviations from paired common penile arteries have been documented in 50% of normally potent volunteers. Arteriography is more useful in providing anatomical rather than functional information.[1]

Cavernosography

The standard imaging study to better define veno-occlusive dysfunction is pharmacological cavernosography. Cavernosography involves infusion of radiocontrast solution into the corpora cavernosa during an artificial erection to visualize the site of venous leakage. It should always be performed after activation of the veno-occlusive mechanism by intracavernous injection of a vasodilator. Various leakage sites to the glans, corpus spongiosum, superficial and deep dorsal veins, cavernous and crural veins can be detected. In a majority of patients more than one site can be visualized by cavernosography. Although many impotent men studied with this technique are found to have venous leakage, initial enthusiasm for venous ligation procedures have waned because of poor long-term results. The development of collateral leakage sites is presumably one reason for the high failure rate. Also, it is becoming increasingly clear that venous leakage is also the consequence of intrinsic sinusoidal disease.[1]

Radioisotopic Penography

The original studies used xenon 133 washout technique during visual sexual stimulation. Several investigators have modified the technique and use pharmacological erection as well as different radioisotopes with a measurement of blood flow. A method was developed for measuring flow to the dependent portion of the penis with technetium-labeled red blood cells. None of the subjects with arterial disease achieved flows greater than 20 mL per min per 100 mg of tissue, whereas flow in patients without arterial disease exceeded this value. Hwang et al reported a technique combining penography with intracavernous injection. The skin test and corporeal xenon 133 penile washout test were conducted on each patient before and 5 and 60 minutes after the intracavernous injection of alprostadil (PGE_1). The authors found the xenon 133 penile washout test helpful in assessing the hemodynamics of the cavernous and dorsal arteries.[1]

Magnetic Resonance Imaging/Magnetic Resonance Angiography

Magnetic resonance imaging/magnetic resonance angiography (MRI/MRA) should follow office pharmacotesting and penile Doppler assessment and should be restricted to patients with a history of pelvic trauma who are candidates for vascular reconstruction. Contrast-enhanced digital-subtraction magnetic resonance angiography (CE-DS-MRA) can delineate small vessels such as the internal pudendal and penile arteries and thus has the potential to become a noninvasive angiography method in the workup of ED.[1]

Ultrasound Imaging

Penile Blood Flow Study Using Color Duplex Doppler Ultrasound

In 1980, during the course of a vascular reconstructive procedure, Ronald Virag noted that infusion of papaverine into the hypogastric artery produced erection.[6] In 1983, a dramatic demonstration of the efficacy of penile self-injection was offered by Charles Brindley, who injected himself.[7] Brindley subsequently popularized the use of α blockers (phenoxybenzamine and phentolamine) and intracorporeal injection in the management of organic and psychogenic ED. In 1985, Lue et al introduced the technique of high-resolution sonography and quantitative Doppler spectrum analysis.[8] Duplex Doppler allowed real-time imaging of the central cavernous arteries with measurement of dynamic changes in cavernous arterial diameter and flow following intracorporeal injection of papaverine.

Zorgnioti and Lefleur promoted penile self-injection with the drug combination papaverine and phentolamine.[9] In 1986, Ishii et al published the first clinical series on PGE_1 for self-injection.[10] Clinicians subsequently turned to the benefits of combination therapy: exploiting the specific pharmacorelaxing properties of different intracavernous agents, reducing the pain sometimes associated with PGE_1 (20 to 33%), reducing the risk of corporal fibrosis and hepatic dysfunction (8%) associated with papaverine, and minimizing the cost and volume of penile injections. Bennett et al (1991) first described the clinical efficacy of trimix: papaverine, phentolamine, and PGE_1.[11] In July 1995, Upjohn Company (Kalamazoo, Michigan) received Food and Drug Administration approval to market injectable PGE_1 (Caverject) specifically for the diagnosis and treatment of "male impotence." PGE_1, because of its efficacy and safety (low priapism rates), is the drug of choice for the first penile injection. The demonstration that vasoactive injections could produce penile erection without benefit of psychic or tactile stimuli revolutionized the diagnosis and treatment of ED by providing a direct test of end organ integrity and offering an etiology-specific therapy.

The formula for resistive index is RI = peak systolic velocity (PSV) minus end-diastolic velocity (EDV) divided by PSV. The value of RI depends on the resistance to arterial inflow, and in the context of corporal physiology, is a function of changing intracorporeal pressure during the various phases of erection following either natural or pharmacological stimulation. As penile pressure equals or exceeds diastolic systemic pressure, diastolic flow in the corpora will approach zero and the value for RI approaches 1.0; in full rigidity the diastolic flow may reverse (flow is transiently retrograde). During tumescence or with a partial erection, diastolic flow persists and the value for RI remains < 1.0. The RI correlates very well with visual rating of erectile responses. Both EDV and RI are useful parameters in predicting adequacy of veno-occlusion.

The hemodynamic parameters of a normal erection on color duplex Doppler ultrasound (CDDU) vary with age. In a retrospective review of over 600 cases, 150 were documented in patients of various ages where intracavernous challenge with PGE$_1$ produced excellent, well-sustained rigidity of at least 20 minutes. Penile blood flow study parameters were recorded 5 to 10 min following PGE$_1$ injection and repeated following privacy and self-stimulation. Mean PGE$_1$ dosages producing excellent erections by age group were 5 µg, (20 to 49 years); 6 µg, (50 to 59 years); 10 µg, (60 to 79 years). Rigid erection following privacy and self-stimulation was associated with RI/PSV of 0.95/54 (cm/s) in men 20 to 29 years old; 0.93/45 (cm/s) in men 30 to 49 years old; 0.94/33 (cm/s) in men 50 to 69 years old; and 0.96/32 (cm/s) in men 70 to 79 years old. The data suggest that cavernous arterial flow may decrease with age, but normal corporal dynamics permit penile rigidity across a wide range of PSVs. RI parameters did not statistically vary with age, suggesting the dynamics of veno-occlusion are the critical factor in the aging erection.[12,13]

Technique

The examination should be performed in a secure setting to reduce patient anxiety and to reduce sympathetic cavernous smooth muscle tone. Following the intracavernosal injection of PGE$_1$ (6 µg if < 50 years old; 10 µg if ≥ 50 years old), the erection is graded at 10 min as follows: 1, no erection; 2, slight tumescence; 3, full volume without rigidity; 4, incomplete rigidity but sufficient for sexual intercourse; and 5, full erection with unbending rigidity. The penis is scanned using color Doppler imaging with a 7 to 10 MHz linear transducer, and Doppler waveforms are obtained from both cavernous arteries in their longitudinal plane with the sampling angle being 60 degrees or less. The peak systolic velocity is a good indicator of arterial function. Peak velocities below 25 cm/s indicate severe arterial insufficiency (**Fig. 6–2**). Velocities of 25 to 34 cm/s indicate some degree of arterial compromise. Peak velocities of 35 cm/s and above indicate normal arterial function.[14]

The dorsal arteries are not subjected to the intracorporeal pressure changes of each progressive erection phase and therefore, antegrade diastolic flow persists even in well-sustained rigidity (**Fig. 6–1C,H**). Dorsal to cavernous (**Fig. 6–1K,L, Fig. 6–6D**) and cavernous to cavernous (**Fig. 6–5E, Fig. 6–6E**) arterial collaterals are common normally and are important in the presence of cavernous arterial insufficiency. Deep dorsal vein (**Fig. 6–1J**) flow persists during rigid erection as a function of dorsal arterial flow and should not be interpreted as evidence of corporal venous leakage.[14]

In patients with normal venous competence, the cavernous arterial waveform has significant diastolic flow as the erection is developing. Once an erection is achieved, diastolic flow ceases or may become reversed (**Fig. 6–1A,B,F,G**). In cases of significant venous leakage, there is persistent diastolic flow in the cavernosal artery despite expansion of the sinusoids.

Failure of the veno-occlusive mechanism is reflected in the Doppler waveforms of the cavernous arteries. EDV greater than 5 cm/s is abnormal (**Fig. 6–3, Fig. 6–4**). The suspicion of venous leakage is raised when the patient has an excellent arterial response (≥ 30 to 35 cm/s, PSV), but with a well-maintained EDV (3 to 5 cm/s), accompanied by partial erection after self-stimulation. Among patients with PSV > 25 cm/s, venous leakage on cavernosometry was predicted with a sensitivity of 90% and specificity of 56% when end-diastolic flow was > 5 cm/s. In Japan, Naroda et al found RI > 0.9 was associated with normal dynamic infusion cavernosometry in 90% and RI < 0.75 was associated with venous leakage in 95% of patients.[15]

If the patient does not achieve a full erection (grade 5), the measurements are repeated following 5 minutes of privacy and self-stimulation. Evaluation of veno-occlusive dysfunction requires intact arterial inflow.

The corporeal bodies should be scanned in the transverse plane from the base to the tip. The echotecture should be homogeneous with fibrotic areas being relatively hyperechoic. Peyronie's plaques will appear as linear echogenic thickenings of the tunica and if associated with acoustic shadowing may be calcified. If there is evidence of Peyronie's disease, the degree of curvature is estimated, and the plaque is evaluated (**Fig. 6–6**).

Percent Arterial Dilatation

An increase in penile arterial blood flow velocity after the intracavernous injection is accompanied by an increase in cavernous arterial diameter. Lue and associates[8] have determined that a mean increase in diameter of the cavernous artery following injection should exceed 75%.[8] Patients with arterial insufficiency will show minimal or no vasodilatation.

The accuracy of this particular criterion has been disputed by other investigators. Some have found poor correlation between the percentage of arterial vasodilatation and arteriographic evidence of arterial insufficiency.[1]

New Techniques

Lencioni et al[16] used contrast-enhanced power Doppler in addition to conventional CDDU. In normal volunteers, dynamic contrast-enhanced power Doppler imaging enabled accurate demonstration of the arteriolar structures of the penis (helicine arteries). Following the intracavernosal injection of PGE$_1$, the diagnosis of arteriogenic ED in a group of patients was confirmed by low-peak systolic velocity in the cavernous arteries by standard CDDU. These patients were also studied with power Doppler following the intravenous injection of an ultrasound contrast agent (Levovist, Schering AG, Berlin, Germany). Among these patients, two different subgroups were identified by contrast-enhanced power Doppler imaging: group A showed normal or almost normal helicine arteries, and group B showed marked reduction of these vessels. In group B, a significantly higher number of patients had a history of diabetes, smoking, and hypertension. Lencioni et al concluded that the identification of patients with relatively intact arteriolar structures might help select patients for revascularization procedures.[16]

Benefits of Ultrasound

In contrast to pudendal arteriography, duplex sonography is not invasive and can be performed in the office setting. Second, the high-resolution duplex ultrasound probe allows the sonographer to image the individual cavernous arteries selectively and perform Doppler blood flow analysis simultaneously within these vessels. Color Doppler imaging provides an additional advantage of easier assessment of direction of blood flow (**Fig. 6–5F**) and collaterals among the cavernous and dorsal arteries, which are crucial in penile vascular and reconstructive surgeries.

High-resolution sonography is used to image the corpora cavernosa, corpus spongiosum, and tunica albuginia. The cavernous body should have a homogeneous, uniform echogenicity. The finding of echogenic areas or calcification within the corporal bodies or the tunica albuginea may represent intrinsic sinusoidal disease, fibrosis, or Peyronie's disease.

Pulsed Doppler analysis of the cavernous arteries provides a quantifiable functional assessment of the penile arterial flow during pharmacological erection. In this respect, duplex sonography is superior to arteriography, which relies on radiographic criteria and provides mainly anatomical rather than functional information. Arteriography is most useful as a detailed road map of the penile arterial system in patients who are candidates for penile revascularization. Duplex sonography, on the other hand, when properly employed, provides the clinician with useful objective criteria with respect to blood flow velocity and arterial vasodilatation, both of which have been demonstrated to correlate with arterial health.

Pitfalls of Ultrasound

Although sonography has been shown to be perhaps the most versatile technique for evaluating vasculogenic ED, significant limitations have been pointed out. The fact that, like all radiographic testing, it is performed in a nonsexual setting with little privacy can increase the patient's anxiety level and cause a sympathetic response that will inhibit the response to injection. This may then reduce both the peak systolic blood flow velocity and arterial vasodilatation and lead the clinician to discern an incorrect diagnosis of arteriogenic impotence. It is recommended that manual stimulation in a private setting after intracavernous injection be part of the test or a repeat injection be given.

The results of the sonographic study may also be influenced by the temporal response to the intracavernous injection. Arterial flow decreases significantly during the full erection phase, and sonography performed during this time will yield a deceptively low peak velocity. On the other hand, other investigators have found a small but significant number of patients who will show a delayed and eventually normal arterial response to intracavernous injection. Some have suggested that a sonographic examination be extended for up to 30 minutes after injection to detect these late responders. However, it is unclear if the delayed arterial response represents a normal variant or, more likely, a mild form of arteriogenic impotence.[1]

Although a few studies have used normal volunteers in a standardized technique to establish a normal arterial response, most criteria regarding peak systolic velocity and vasodilatation have been established with patients with nonarteriogenic impotence. Lee et al studied a group of potent volunteers to arrive at similar criteria for their subjects.[16]

Lastly, sonography is operator dependent. A thorough understanding of erectile physiology and anatomy is necessary to perform and interpret the examination properly. The experience of the clinician is critical to arriving at the correct diagnosis and avoiding pitfalls.

Summary

Patients with ED should consult with a physician who is knowledgeable about the subject. They should have a complete evaluation, including a detailed medical and psychosexual history, physical examination, and hormonal and laboratory testing. This should be followed by a discussion of treatment options and further diagnostic tests. The patient is then given the choice of either a therapeutic trial (with oral medication, a vacuum constriction device, or intracavernous injection) or a second level of evaluation. The latter level is designed to elucidate the cause of the dysfunction and entails one or more of the following tests: psychological consultation, nocturnal penile tumescence and rigidity testing, advanced neurological testing, and functional arterial and venous studies.

References

1. Broderick GA, Lue TF. Evaluation and nonsurgical management of erectile dysfunction and priapism. In: Walsh PC, Retik AB, Vaughan ED Jr, Wein AJ, eds. Campbell's Urology. 8th ed. Vol 2. Philadelphia: Saunders; 2002:1619–1671

2. Ayta IA, McKinlay JB, Krane RJ. The likely worldwide increase in erectile dysfunction between 1995 and 2025 and some possible policy consequences. BJU Int 1999;84:50–56

3. Feldman HA, Goldstein I, Hatzichristou DG, Krane RJ, McKinlay JB. Impotence and its medical and psychosocial correlates: results of the Massachusetts male aging study. J Urol 1994;151: 54–61

4. Johannes CB, Araujo AB, Feldman HA, Derby CA, Kleinman KP, McKinlay JB. Incidence of erectile dysfunction in men 40 to 69 years old: longitudinal results from the Massachusetts male aging study. J Urol 2000;163:460–463

5. Lue TF. Physiology of penile erection and pathophysiology of erectile dysfunction and priapism. In: Walsh PC, Retik AB, Vaughan ED Jr, Wein AJ, eds. Campbell's Urology. 8th ed. Vol 2. Philadelphia: Saunders; 2002:1591–1618

6. Virag R. Intracavernous injection of papaverine for erectile failure. Lancet 1982;2:918

7. Brindley GS. Cavernosal alpha-blockade: a new technique for investigating and treating erectile impotence. Br J Psychiatry 1983; 143:332–337

8. Lue TF, Hricak H, Marich KW, Tanagho EA. Vasculogenic impotence evaluated by high resolution ultrasonography and pulsed Doppler spectrum analysis. Radiology 1985;155:777–781

9. Zorgniotti AW, Lefleur RS. Auto-injection of the corpus cavernosum with a vasoactive drug combination for vasculogenic impotence. J Urol 1985;133:39–41

10. Ishii N, Watanabe H, Irisawa C, et al. Intracavernous injection of prostaglandin E1 for the treatment of erectile impotence. J Urol 1989;141:323–325

11. Bennett AH, Carpenter AJ, Barada JH. An improved vasoactive drug combination for a pharmacological erection program. J Urol 1991;146:1564–1565

12. Broderick GA, Arger PA. Penile blood flow study: age specific reference ranges [abstract]. J Urol 1994;151:A371

13. Broderick GA, Arger PA. Normal values for penile blood flow studies: distinguishing prepenile from intrapenile disease [abstract]. J Urol 1997;157:A694

14. Benson CB, Aruny JE, Vickers MA. Correlation of duplex sonography with arteriography in patients with erectile dysfunction. AJR Am J Roentgenol 1993;160:71–73

15. Lencioni RA, Paolicchi A, Sarteschi M, et al. Dynamic contrast-enhanced power Doppler imaging in the assessment of arteriogenic impotence. Radiology 1997;205(P)(Suppl):335

16. Lee B, Sikka SC, Randrup ER, et al. Standardization of penile blood flow parameters in normal men using intracavernous prostaglandin E1 and visual sexual stimulation. J Urol 1993;149: 49–52

7 Urinary Tract Infections in Children

Harriet J. Paltiel

Epidemiology

Urinary tract infection (UTI) is a common problem in childhood as well as an important cause of morbidity. Chronic or recurrent UTI can ultimately result in hypertension and renal failure, particularly when associated with obstructive uropathy or vesicoureteral reflux (VUR). Most UTIs are bacterial in origin. Diagnosis is made by documenting significant bacteriuria, defined as greater than 100,000 colony-forming units (cfu)/mL of a single organism, in one or more clean-voided specimens of urine. When the urine is obtained by suprapubic puncture or bladder catheterization, less than 100,000 cfu/mL can be considered significant.[1-3] The incidence of neonatal bacteriuria has been reported as ranging from 1 to 1.4%,[4-6] with a male-to-female ratio of between 2.8 and 5.4:1.[7,8] The sex ratio for bacteriuria in preschool and school-age children is reversed from that seen in infancy, ranging from 0.7 to 1.9% of girls, and 0.2 to 0.4% of boys.[9-13]

UTI in children can be asymptomatic or symptomatic. The true incidence of UTI is unknown because of the nonspecificity or absence of symptoms in young children. The term *asymptomatic bacteriuria* denotes the presence of two consecutive clean-voided urine specimens, both yielding positive cultures of the same uropathogen, in a patient without urinary symptoms.[14] Poor feeding, failure to thrive, irritability, vomiting, or diarrhea may be the only signs indicative of an underlying problem. Symptomatic infections may be confined to the urethra (urethritis) or bladder (cystitis), or may involve the ureter (ureteritis), the collecting system (pyelitis), or the renal parenchyma (pyelonephritis). Fever occurs in most infants with symptomatic UTIs, but is often absent in neonates.[15] Once children develop speech and are toilet trained, symptoms of UTI are more readily detected. Disturbances of micturition often signal lower-tract UTI.[16] Symptoms and signs of lower UTI include dysuria, frequency, and cloudy, foul-smelling urine. Pyelonephritis often results in an acute, febrile illness, associated with malaise, chills, vomiting, and flank pain. An infant with urosepsis may be critically ill, whereas in young children with less severe symptoms, it may be difficult to distinguish cystitis from pyelonephritis solely on the basis of clinical presentation.

The incidence of symptomatic UTI in boys and girls under 2 years of age was shown to be the same (1.6%) in a Swedish prospective, multicenter study.[17] In a study of children living in Göteborg, Sweden, published in 1974, Winberg et al estimated that the aggregate risk for symptomatic UTI up to the age of 11 years was at least 3% for girls and 1.1% for boys.[15] In a more recent report from the same city, the prevalence of culture-documented, symptomatic UTIs in children up to the age of 7 years was higher than the previous estimate, with 8.4% of girls and 1.7% of boys affected.[18]

The majority of UTIs are caused by the family of gram-negative, aerobic bacilli known as *Enterobacteriaceae* that includes *Escherichia, Klebsiella, Enterobacter, Citrobacter, Proteus, Providencia, Morganella, Serratia*, and *Salmonella* species. Of these, *Escherichia (E.) coli* is by far the most frequently isolated organism, being responsible for ~80% of UTIs. *Pseudomonas* is a gram-negative, aerobic bacillus, unrelated to the *Enterobacteriaceae*, which may be isolated from the urine of patients with impaired immunologic defense mechanisms. The most common gram-positive organisms found in UTIs are *Staphylococcus* and *Enterococcus*. Gram-negative organisms usually infect the urinary tract by ascent from the perineum, whereas gram-positive organisms often reach the kidney hematogenously. Ascending infection occurs in ~97% of cases.[19]

Pathogenesis

Bacterial Virulence

UTI occurs when bacterial virulence factors overwhelm host resistance.[20-22] Some of the most important bacterial virulence factors include adherence to uroepithelial cells, large amounts of K-antigen in the bacterial capsule, production of hemolysin and colicin, the ability to incorporate iron, and resistance to serum bactericidal activity.

Bacterial adherence is an essential step in the initiation of UTI. Uropathogenic bacteria attach both to specific receptor sites on the uroepithelium and in a nonspecific fashion by electrostatic hydrophobic means. As a consequence of this attachment, virulent bacteria may ascend into the upper urinary tract in the absence of VUR or structural abnormalities. Adhesion is mediated by surface glycoprotein projections known as pili or fimbriae, which serve as ligands for glycoprotein and glycolipid receptors on uroepithelial cells. Fimbriated *E. coli* are categorized as either mannose-sensitive or mannose-resistant, according to their ability to agglutinate erythrocytes in the presence of mannose. *E. coli* expressing type I (or common) fimbriae are mannose-sensitive and are thought to be ubiquitous among UTI-causing *E. coli* strains. Mannose-resistant pili on *E. coli* can be further categorized as P- or X-fimbriated, based on their ability to agglutinate human erythrocytes expressing P (or other) blood group antigens. P-fimbriated *E. coli* are associated with the development of upper tract infection, probably because the major glycolipid component of renal cell membranes is the receptor for P fimbriae.[23] Other bacterial virulence factors include K or capsular antigens that inhibit phagocytosis; hemolysin, which lyses phagocytes and erythrocytes resulting in the release of iron; colicin, a substance produced by some strains of *E. coli* that kills competing strains; and the aerobactin system, which chelates urinary iron and offers a growth advantage to bacteria that possess it.[23,24]

Host Factors

Many host resistance factors protect the urinary tract from infection, including the presence of antibodies, male sex, a low density of bacterial receptor sites on host epithelial cells, lack of perineal colonization by virulent fecal bacteria, and unimpeded flow of urine.

Immunity to UTI is boosted in the neonatal period by the maternal transmission of immunoglobulin (Ig)A antibodies and other protective factors such as lactoferrin and oligosaccharides through breastfeeding that impede microbial mucosal attachment.[25] The short urethra in girls appears to be the most obvious explanation for the increased relative incidence of UTIs in girls beyond the first year of life compared with boys. There is significantly increased risk of UTIs in uncircumcised male infants in the first year of life, which is believed to be due to colonization of the prepuce by uropathogenic bacteria.[26–28]

A genetic predisposition to childhood UTI is suggested by studies that demonstrate increased adherence of uropathogens to the uroepithelial cells of children who have had a UTI,[29] as well as by a recent study that demonstrated a mutation in the neutrophil interleukin (IL)-8 receptor (CXCR1) in children with recurrent pyelonephritis.[30]

Anatomical/Functional Abnormalities

Frequent and complete bladder emptying eliminates bacteria and prevents UTI. The predisposition to recurrent UTIs and VUR in children with dysfunctional voiding is related to overdistention from infrequent voiding, residual volume due to inadequate emptying, and increased intravesical pressure caused by uninhibited bladder contrac-

tions. Development of normal voiding patterns in these children reduces the incidence of recurrent UTIs.[31,32] A correlation has also been shown between constipation and recurrent UTIs in children.[33,34] Improvement in bowel habits often results in a decrease in the incidence of recurrent UTIs.

Resistance to bacterial infection may be compromised by impedance to the unidirectional flow of urine out of the urinary tract, as may occur with VUR, obstruction, or both. Obstruction can occur at any site within the urinary tract. Children with obstruction of the distal end of the ureter [either primary ureterovesical junction (UVJ) obstruction or ectopic ureterocele] or the urethra (posterior urethral valves) often present with infection. Although the most common site of obstruction of the pediatric urinary tract occurs at the ureteropelvic junction (UPJ), children with this condition do not usually present with UTI.

Vesicoureteral Reflux

VUR is an abnormality that is frequently associated with UTI. With VUR, urine flows in a retrograde fashion into the ureter. VUR is almost always a primary phenomenon due to incompetence of the UVJ and is not secondary to infection or obstruction.[35,36] VUR is especially common in neonates and infants. It occurs in families,[37] is less common in black children,[38,39] and decreases in severity or resolves as the child gets older. Resolution is less likely to occur if the degree of VUR is severe or is associated with other abnormalities such as voiding dysfunction.

VUR provides a pathway for bacteria within the bladder to reach the kidney. Due to the phenomenon of "aberrant micturition," part of the urine expelled from the bladder refluxes up the ureter and flows back into the bladder. The resulting stagnation of urine encourages bacterial overgrowth.[40] Secondary VUR is usually due either to an abnormality of micturition, such as dysfunctional voiding (a neurogenic bladder abnormality), or to the presence of a diverticulum at the UVJ.[32,41] When VUR is present, it is the most significant host factor in the etiology of childhood pyelonephritis. The risk for acute pyelonephritis and subsequent renal scarring is related to the severity of VUR.[42,43]

Pyelonephritis may result in the destruction of nephrons and their replacement by fibrous tissue. Once lost, these renal units are never regenerated or replaced. The destruction of renal parenchyma is directly proportional to the severity and frequency of episodes of infection. The increased burden placed on the remaining nephrons is thought to result in hyperfiltration injury and glomerulosclerosis.[44–46] The term *reflux nephropathy* is used to describe both the acute damage to the kidney as well as the long-term sequelae caused by reflux of infected urine.[47] Chronic pyelonephritis refers to the process of fibrosis and scar formation that follows bacterial infection.[48] The medulla is initially affected, but eventually the full thickness of renal parenchyma is involved. Scars are focal and frequently polar in location.

When VUR and ipsilateral obstruction coexist, infection is much more common and its clinical presentation and renal sequelae tend to be more severe. This is presumably due to the fact that pressure in the collecting system is elevated and drainage of infected urine is impeded.[49]

Clinical Outcome

Infants and young children are at higher risk than older children for the development of acute renal injury with UTI. In addition to acute morbidity, potential long-term consequences of UTI include renal scarring as well as the rarer complications of hypertension and renal failure.[50] The risk for renal damage increases with recurrent UTIs.[51] The significance of asymptomatic or covert bacteriuria is poorly understood. Although some authorities believe that asymptomatic children should be treated, others have postulated that the bacteria may, in fact, be nonpathogenic. These bacteria may actually protect the patient from potentially more virulent organisms by blocking epithelial receptor sites.[51,52]

Diagnostic Evaluation

Nonimaging Tests

Evaluation of children with UTI begins with a history of voiding and bowel habits in those who are toilet trained. Family history should also be obtained because heredity appears to be a factor in an individual's predisposition to bacteriuria and VUR.[37,53] Physical examination includes abdominal palpation to detect bladder distention, bowel distention from fecal impaction, and flank masses. Circumcision status is important in boys because of the increased risk of UTIs in uncircumcised boys. Abnormal findings in girls include the presence of labial adhesions or vulvovaginitis, both of which may predispose to perineal colonization by bacteria.

In children with a significant history of voiding dysfunction associated with encopresis or constipation, an evaluation of perineal sensation and lower extremity reflexes and an examination of the lower back for sacral dimpling or cutaneous abnormalities suggestive of underlying spinal abnormalities should be performed. Rectal examination for fecal impaction is indicated if there is a history of encopresis or severe constipation.

UTI can be diagnosed reliably only by urine culture. Thus, specimens for urine culture should be obtained in all patients in whom suspicion for infection is high. In chil-

dren who are not toilet trained, an initial urine specimen is often obtained by placing a collection bag on the perineum. Although this technique has been correctly criticized for producing a high rate of contaminated specimens, the method is reliable when the culture is negative. Contamination is directly related to the length of time the bag remains on the perineum. Confirmation of all positive urine specimens obtained in this fashion is advisable prior to treatment. Bladder catheterization or suprapubic aspiration should be performed whenever the clinical situation dictates immediate treatment or confirmation of a positive urine bag specimen. In older children who are toilet trained, significant bacteriuria in a single properly collected midstream, clean-catch urine specimen is reliable for diagnostic purposes.[54]

Imaging Tests

Current guidelines of the American Academy of Pediatrics recommend obtaining a voiding cystourethrogram (VCUG) and a renal sonogram for infants and young children after a first febrile UTI.[55] In many centers, including our own, an imaging evaluation is performed in all children who present after their first documented UTI. This approach assumes that renal scarring is both acquired and preventable, that a combination of infection and VUR is the cause of renal damage, and that high-risk cases can be clearly identified at an early stage with imaging. These assumptions have been recently challenged by reports of children with VUR and congenitally small or scarred kidneys that cannot be treated with ureteral reimplantation or prophylactic antibiotics,[56,57] and at least one study that showed that treatment of VUR in childhood did not prevent end-stage renal disease attributable to reflux nephropathy.[58] Another publication concluded that ultrasonography performed at the time of acute illness is of limited value, and that a VCUG for the identification of VUR is useful only if antimicrobial prophylaxis is effective in reducing reinfections and renal scarring.[59] As stated by Dick and Feldman in 1996, methodologically sound, prospective studies are ultimately necessary to assess whether children with their first urinary tract infection who have routine diagnostic imaging are better off than children who have imaging for specific indications.[60]

Recommendations for particular radiological studies in children with culture-documented UTI are, to a certain extent, based on the availability of various imaging modalities and the experience and expertise of the imager. Most children are not studied during the acute phase of a UTI, although children hospitalized for febrile infections may be screened with ultrasound before discharge. Ultrasound is the initial examination of choice for imaging all children with a history of UTI. The role of ultrasound is to rule out urinary tract obstruction. VCUG by bladder catheterization is also performed to detect the presence of VUR. VCUG is usually reserved for children with a history of febrile UTI. Some imagers prefer a conventional, fluoroscopically monitored VCUG, whereas others prefer nuclear cystography. Conventional contrast VCUG allows more precise determination of the severity of VUR and assessment of bladder and urethral anatomy. Nuclear cystography is associated with reduced gonadal radiation and permits continuous monitoring throughout the study, which increases its sensitivity to transient VUR.[61] Nuclear cystography is generally accepted to be the best examination for following children with known reflux, for documenting the result of antireflux surgery, and for screening children whose siblings have reflux.[62,63] No further imaging is necessary in most cases if the cystogram and ultrasound of the kidneys and bladder are normal.

Additional imaging evaluation of the upper urinary tract in children with UTI varies from institution to institution. Planar scintigraphy or single photon emission computed tomography (SPECT) of the renal parenchyma with either technetium-(Tc) 99m-labeled dimercaptosuccinic acid (DMSA) or glucoheptonate (GH) have been used to detect acute pyelonephritis and renal scarring.[64–66] Tc-99m DMSA binds to the proximal renal tubules and provides excellent images of the parenchyma. Tc-99m GH also binds to tubular epithelial cells, but a large amount is filtered, allowing evaluation of the pelvicaliceal system, ureters, and bladder on early images, as well as the renal cortex on delayed images. Although both agents can show cortical involvement, Tc-99m DMSA is preferred over Tc-99m GH because of a lower gonadal dose. Renal cortical scanning may be of particular value when the diagnosis of pyelonephritis is unclear based on clinical and laboratory findings alone. For instance, neonates and young infants may present with nonspecific signs and symptoms. Urine cultures may not have been obtained in an appropriate fashion or before antibiotic treatment. Another example is of children with myelodysplasia who are managed by clean intermittent catheterization, where chronic asymptomatic bacteriuria is common. Thus, the diagnostic significance of a positive urine culture is limited when these patients present with unexplained fever.[62,67] Tc-99m DMSA scintigraphy is considered preferable to computed tomography (CT) for renal cortical imaging in the pediatric population due to its lower radiation dose. However, CT may be of value in selected patients to determine the extent of the inflammatory process and the presence of abscess, ureteral or parenchymal calcifications, and gas. Urinary obstruction can also be confirmed.[68,69]

When hydronephrosis or hydroureter or both are depicted by ultrasound, and VUR is absent, a quantitative assessment of renal function and drainage of the dilated collecting system and ureter may be obtained with diuretic renography using Tc-99m-labeled mercaptoacetyltriglycine (MAG-3).[70] In most instances, nonobstructive dilation can be reliably differentiated from true obstruction.

Magnetic resonance imaging (MRI) is not currently employed in the routine investigation of UTI. Several recent publications have compared its efficacy to that of Tc-99m-DMSA scintigraphy in the diagnosis of pyelonephritis and have advocated its use as a rapid, accurate, and minimally invasive technique for the detection of renal scarring that does not involve ionizing radiation.[71,72]

Ultrasound Imaging

The sonographic examination of the pediatric urinary tract includes images of the kidneys, ureters (if visible), and urinary bladder. The child may be given fluids to drink, and cooperative children are asked not to void for several hours before the study. In a young child who is not toilet trained, the bladder must be checked first and often during the course of the examination because it may fill and empty suddenly. The highest-frequency transducer that will penetrate the area to be studied is used. Routine examination includes longitudinal and transverse images of the kidneys and bladder. Scans are performed with the patient in both supine and prone positions. Supine images are best obtained with sector or convex transducers that can be positioned between the ribs, whereas prone images are performed with a convex or linear transducer.

Coronal images are obtained with the patient supine. The liver and spleen act as acoustic windows, thereby permitting optimal visualization of the upper renal poles and comparison of the echogenicity of the renal parenchyma with that of the adjacent liver and spleen. Sagittal views obtained with the child prone are used to optimize visualization of the lower renal poles. Images of the bladder are obtained with the child supine and are best performed when the bladder is moderately distended, so that abnormalities such as bladder wall thickening can be appreciated, but the patient is not uncomfortable. The proximal ureter is evaluated at the level of the renal pelvis as well as distally at the level of the bladder to detect dilation and ureterocele. Postvoid images of the kidneys and bladder are useful in children with hydronephrosis, hydroureter, and/or neurogenic bladder dysfunction to determine the effect of bladder distension on the degree of hydronephrosis. Renal length measurements should be compared with standards for patient age, height, weight, or body surface area.[73–76] Color and pulsed Doppler ultrasound imaging is used in evaluating renal perfusion.

Cystitis

Acute cystitis in children is rarely associated with significant long-term morbidity. The recurrence rate of lower UTI is relatively high.[77] Many children with recurrent UTI suffer from dysfunctional voiding. When inflamed, the bladder

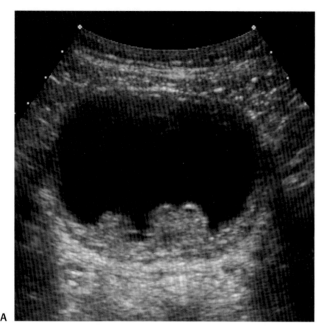

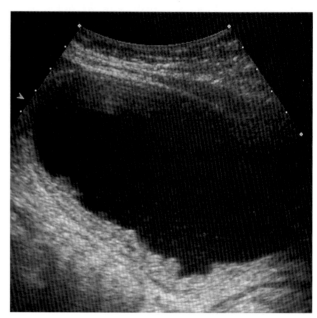

Figure 7–1 **(A)** Transverse and **(B)** sagittal sonograms of the pelvis in a patient with cystitis demonstrate irregular thickening of the bladder wall.

wall becomes thickened and irregular (**Fig. 7–1**). Blood clot or echogenic debris may be seen within the bladder lumen.[78,79]

Acute Pyelonephritis

The acutely infected kidney often appears normal by ultrasound.[80,81] However, in severe infections, gray-scale ultrasound can demonstrate diffuse renal enlargement; loss of corticomedullary differentiation; submucosal edema of the renal pelvis and/or ureter; and calyceal, pelvic, and/or ureteral dilatation (**Fig. 7–2**).[80-85] The term *acute focal pyelonephritis* (formerly called *acute lobar nephronia*) refers to localized renal swelling caused by acute focal infection without liquefaction (**Fig. 7–3**).[86] Ultrasound can also be used to detect renal calculi, which may predispose to infection (**Fig. 7–4**). Conventional gray-scale ultrasound fares poorly in comparison with CT and Tc-99m-DMSA scintigraphy, the current imaging standards.[87-91] A study of 91 children with culture-documented febrile UTI studied by DMSA scintigraphy and conventional ultrasound showed changes consistent with pyelonephritis in 63% of the DMSA scans but in only 24% of the sonograms.[90]

There are few studies comparing the sensitivity and specificity of state-of-the-art ultrasound in the diagnosis of acute pyelonephritis to other imaging modalities. Several recent studies have shown that power Doppler imaging improves the detection of acute pyelonephritis compared with conventional gray-scale imaging, although it is still inferior to CT and Tc-99m-DMSA scintigraphy.[92-94] The recent development of Doppler contrast agents holds promise for improving our ability to diagnose acute pyelonephritis with ultrasound technology.[95,96]

Complications of Acute Pyelonephritis

Complications of acute pyelonephritis include renal and perirenal abscesses and pyonephrosis.

Abscess

When children with UTI do not respond rapidly to antibiotic treatment, repeat sonograms are warranted to detect

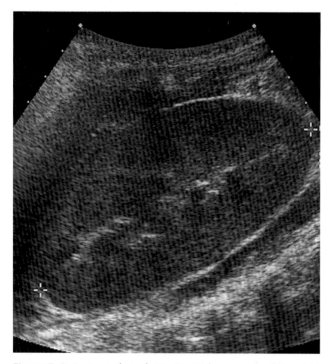

Figure 7–2 Acute pyelonephritis. Sagittal sonogram of the right flank reveals a swollen, echogenic kidney with decreased corticomedullary differentiation.

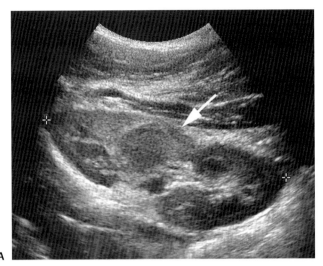

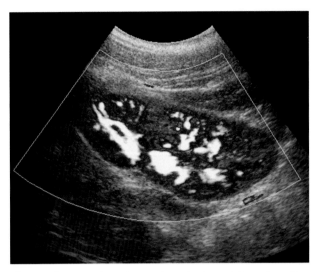

A   B

Figure 7–3 Acute focal pyelonephritis. **(A)** Sagittal sonogram reveals a central zone of increased renal parenchymal echogenicity and swelling (arrow). **(B)** Power Doppler sonogram depicts decreased perfusion to this area.

complications that may require drainage. Renal abscesses are relatively uncommon in the pediatric population. They occur either from progression of acute pyelonephritis or as a result of hematogenous spread from a remote location. *E. coli* and *Staphylococcus aureus* are the usual causative organisms. Renal abscesses tend to be multiple and bilateral when of hematogenous origin. With ultrasound, a mature abscess appears as a well-circumscribed mass with an irregular, relatively echogenic wall and a hypoechoic or anechoic center due to liquefied pus.

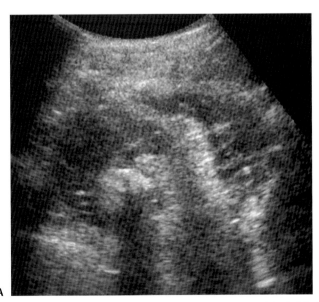

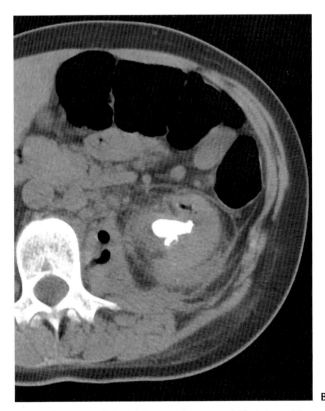

A   B

Figure 7–4 Staghorn calculus. **(A)** Sagittal sonogram of the left kidney demonstrates foci of increased echogenicity in the renal sinus associated with distal acoustic shadowing. **(B)** Unenhanced computed tomographic scan of the abdomen shows a calcified, branching stone in the left renal pelvis.

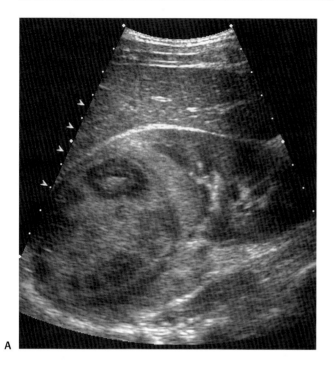

A

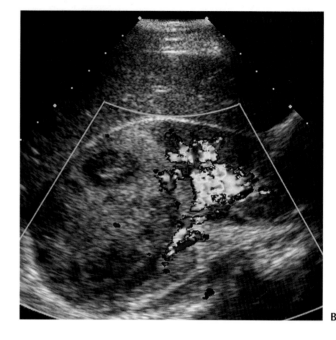

B

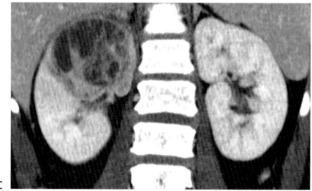

C

Figure 7–5 Renal abscess. **(A)** Sagittal sonogram reveals a heterogeneous, well-circumscribed mass in the right upper renal pole. **(B)** Color Doppler image shows no perfusion of the lesion. **(C)** Coronal reformat of a contrast-enhanced computed tomographic scan confirms the right upper pole renal abscess that contains multiple necrotic, low-attenuation foci.

Doppler ultrasound reveals absence of perfusion (**Fig. 7–5**).

Perinephric Abscess

Perinephric abscess is usually unilateral and results from inflammation of the soft tissues adjacent to the kidney. Infection of the perinephric space most often develops following rupture of a renal cortical abscess, but may follow seeding from bloodborne infections or after renal trauma (**Fig. 7–6**). Ultrasound may be used to guide percutaneous aspiration and drainage in children with renal and perirenal abscesses.

Pyonephrosis

Pyonephrosis is a complication of pyelonephritis that consists of pus within a dilated renal collecting system. The diagnosis is suspected when fever and flank pain are associated with radiological demonstration of urinary tract obstruction. The most common sonographic findings include hydronephrosis with a fluid–debris level (**Fig. 7–7**). However, the collecting system can be completely anechoic, contain only low-level echoes, or demonstrate very strong echoes due to the presence of gas-forming microorganisms. Ultrasound may be used to guide aspiration and drainage of the collecting system. The sensitivity and specificity of ultrasound in the diagnosis of pyonephrosis have varied in different series from 25 to 67% and 96 to 100%, respectively. False-positive results occur with severe obstruction, where the collecting system is filled with proteinaceous material or debris. False-negative results can occur when purulent material is not echogenic.[97–101]

Vesicoureteral Reflux

Conventional gray-scale ultrasound is a poor screening method for the detection of VUR because the study is frequently normal, particularly in patients with lesser degrees of reflux.[102–104] In the study of Alon et al, ultrasound

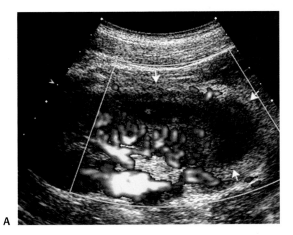

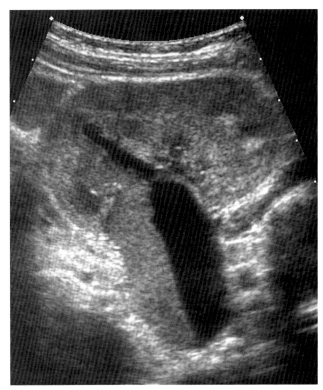

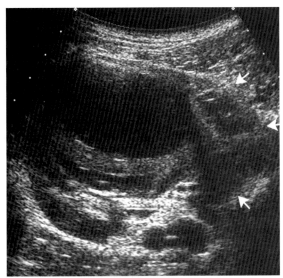

Figure 7–7 Pyonephrosis in a young boy with left ureteropelvic junction obstruction. Sagittal sonogram of the left kidney obtained with the patient prone shows a markedly dilated renal pelvis with a fluid–debris level.

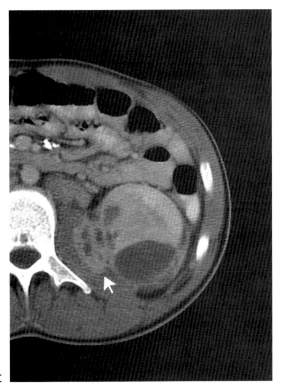

was normal in 38 of 44 urinary systems with low-grade reflux (86%).[104] In the presence of long-standing, severe VUR, marked dilation of the renal collecting system needs to be differentiated from obstructive hydronephrosis and hydroureter. In an effort to improve the sensitivity of ultrasound in the detection of VUR, contrast agents have been instilled into the bladder. Visualization of contrast material within the renal pelvis is indicative of VUR. Although this technique is used with some frequency in Europe as a primary imaging modality for VUR in girls and as a follow-up examination, it is not currently employed in the United States.[105,106]

Figure 7–6 Renal abscess with perinephric extension. **(A)** Sagittal power Doppler sonogram of the left kidney reveals a swollen, avascular lower pole (arrows). **(B)** Prone transverse sonogram demonstrates a band of echogenic material along the medial aspect of the kidney (arrows) and adjacent to the anechoic abscess. **(C)** The perinephric abscess interposed between the psoas muscle and the kidney is well depicted by computed tomography (arrow). Multiple low attenuation foci are present within the kidney.

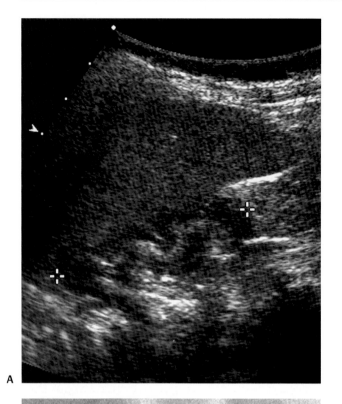

A

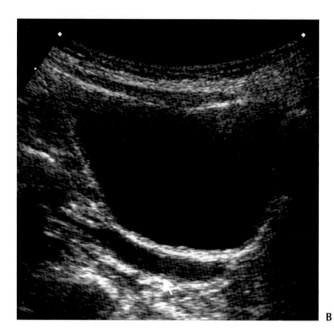

B

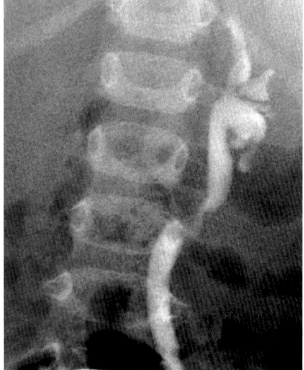

C

Figure 7–8 Chronic pyelonephritis. **(A)** Sagittal sonogram reveals a small left kidney (between calipers) with an irregular contour. The parenchyma is thin and there is poor corticomedullary differentiation. **(B)** Sagittal sonogram of the pelvis depicts dilation of the distal left ureter posterior to the bladder (arrow). **(C)** Voiding cystourethrogram demonstrates left-sided vesicoureteral reflux. Note calyceal crowding and distorted morphology due to marked parenchymal loss.

Chronic Pyelonephritis

Chronic pyelonephritis results from repeated episodes of acute pyelonephritis. Sonographic findings include a small kidney with an irregular contour due to focal parenchymal loss. Compensatory hypertrophy of the contralateral kidney can develop. The renal cortex may be more echogenic than normal and there is frequently loss of normal corticomedullary differentiation. Conventional gray-scale ultrasound can demonstrate renal atrophy and large scars, but it is not as sensitive or specific as 99m-Tc-DMSA scintigraphy in depicting milder degrees of scarring (**Fig. 7–8**).[89,107,108] Likewise, in a recent study by Hitzel et al, the predictive value of color and power Doppler sonography was not thought to be sufficiently high for use in routine clinical practice.[109] A recent experimental study by Farhat et al suggests that contrast-enhanced sonography may be of potential utility in the diagnosis of postpyelonephritic renal scarring.[110]

Fungal Infection

Fungal infection of the urinary tract is most often due to *Candida albicans*. Immunodeficiency states, indwelling catheters, and prolonged antibiotic or immunosuppressive therapy are risk factors. Premature infants with diminished cellular immunity are especially susceptible to fungal infection. Seeding of the kidney is followed by the development of cortical abscesses and extension of inflammation into the interstitium and tubules. Complications include mycelial collections in the tubules, collecting system, and urinary bladder, as well as necrotizing papilli-

tis. Sonographic abnormalities include renal enlargement and a generalized increase in parenchymal echogenicity with loss of normal corticomedullary differentiation. Mycelial clumps (fungus balls) in the collecting system and bladder appear as nonshadowing, echogenic masses that may cause obstruction (**Fig. 7–9**).[111-114]

Summary

Ultrasound imaging in the child with a UTI is useful in depicting underlying anatomical abnormalities that may predispose to infection, identifying renal structural damage as a consequence of infection, and providing a baseline for subsequent evaluation of renal growth.

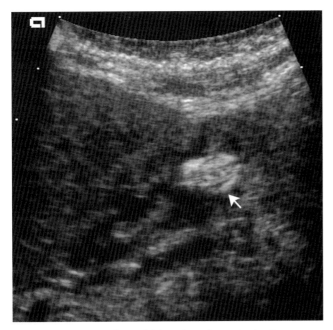

Figure 7–9 Infant with candidal pyelonephritis. Sagittal sonogram demonstrates a large echogenic fungus ball in the lower pole collecting system of a duplex right kidney (arrow).

References

1. Ginsburg CM, McCracken GH. Urinary tract infections in young infants. Pediatrics 1982;69:409–412
2. Hoberman A, Wald ER, Reynolds EA, Penchansky L, Charron M. Is urine culture necessary to rule out urinary tract infection in young febrile children? Pediatr Infect Dis J 1996;15:304–309
3. Nelson JD, Peters PC. Suprapubic aspiration of urine in premature and term infants. Pediatrics 1965;36:132–134
4. Abbott GD. Neonatal bacteriuria: a prospective study in 1460 infants. BMJ 1972;1:267–269
5. Littlewood JM, Kite P, Kite BA. Incidence of neonatal urinary tract infection. Arch Dis Child 1969;44:617–620
6. O'Doherty NJ. Urinary tract infection in the neonatal period and later infancy. In: O'Grady F, Brumfitt W, eds. Urinary Tract Infection. London: Oxford University Press; 1968:113–122
7. Bergström T, Larson H, Lincoln K, Winberg J. Studies of urinary tract infections in infancy and childhood. J Pediatr 1972;80: 858–866
8. Drew JH, Acton CM. Radiological findings in newborn infants with urinary infection. Arch Dis Child 1976;51:628–630
9. Kunin CM, Deutscher R, Paquin A. Urinary tract infection in children: an epidemiologic, clinical and laboratory study. Medicine 1964;43:91–130
10. Lindberg U, Claësson I, Hanson L, Jodal U. Asymptomatic bacteriuria in schoolgirls, I: Clinical and laboratory findings. Acta Paediatr Scand 1975;64:425–431
11. Newcastle Symptomatic Bacteriuria Research Group. Asymptomatic bacteriuria in schoolchildren in Newcastle upon Tyne. Arch Dis Child 1975;50:90–102
12. Savage DC, Wilson MI, McHardy M, Dewar DA, Fee WM. Covert bacteriuria of childhood: a clinical and epidemiological study. Arch Dis Child 1973;48:8–20
13. Saxena SR, Collis A, Laurance BM. Bacteriuria in preschool children [letter]. Lancet 1974;2:517–518
14. Kass EH. Asymptomatic infections of the urinary tract. Trans Assoc Am Physicians 1956;69:56–64
15. Winberg J, Andersen HJ, Bergström T, et al. Epidemiology of symptomatic urinary tract infection in childhood. Acta Paediatr Scand 1974;252(Suppl):1–20
16. Johnson CE, Shurin PA, Marchant CD, et al. Identification of children requiring radiologic evaluation for urinary infection. Pediatr Infect Dis 1985;4:656–663
17. Hansson S, Bollgren I, Esbjorner E, Jakobsson B, Marild S. Urinary tract infections in children below two years of age: a quality

assurance project in Sweden. The Swedish Pediatric Nephrology Association. Acta Paediatr 1999;88:270–274

18. Hellström A, Hanson E, Hansson S, Hjälmas K, Jodal U. Association between urinary symptoms at 7 years old and previous urinary tract infection. Arch Dis Child 1991;66:232–234

19. Practice parameter. The diagnosis, treatment, and evaluation of the initial urinary tract infection in febrile infants and young children. American Academy of Pediatrics. Committee on Quality Improvement. Subcommittee on Urinary Tract Infection. Pediatrics 1999;103(4 Pt 1):843–852

20. Torres VE, Kramer SA, Holley KE, et al. Interaction of multiple risk factors in the pathogenesis of experimental reflux nephropathy in the pig. J Urol 1985;133:131–135

21. Roberts JA. Factors predisposing to urinary tract infections in children. Pediatr Nephrol 1996;10:517–522

22. Ogata RT. Factors determining bacterial pathogenicity. Clin Physiol Biochem 1983;1:145–159

23. Johnson JR. Virulence factors in *Escherichia coli* urinary tract infection. Clin Microbiol Rev 1991;4:80–128

24. Kunin CM. Urinary tract infections in females. Clin Infect Dis 1994;18:1–12

25. Hanson LA, Korotkova M, Haverson L, et al. Breast-feeding, a complex support system for the offspring. Pediatr Int 2002;44: 347–352

26. To T, Agha M, Dick PT, Feldman W. Cohort study on circumcision of newborn boys and subsequent risk of urinary-tract infection. Lancet 1998;352:1813–1816

27. Craig JC, Knight JF, Sureshkumar P, Mantz E, Roy LP. Effect of circumcision on incidence of urinary tract infection in preschool boys. J Pediatr 1996;128:23–27

28. Nayir A. Circumcision for the prevention of significant bacteriuria in boys. Pediatr Nephrol 2001;16:1129–1134

29. Svanborg-Eden C, Jodal U. Attachment of *Escherichia coli* to urinary sediment epithelial cells from urinary tract infection-prone and healthy children. Infect Immun 1979;26:837–840

30. Frendeus B, Godaly G, Hang L, Karpman D, Svanborg C. Interleukin-8 receptor deficiency confers susceptibility to acute pyelonephritis. J Infect Dis 2001;183(Suppl 1):S56–S60

31. Snodgrass W. Relationship of voiding dysfunction to urinary tract infection and vesicoureteral reflux in children. Urology 1991;38: 341–344

32. Koff SA, Murtagh DS. The uninhibited bladder in children: effect of treatment on recurrence of urinary infection and on vesicoureteral reflux resolution. J Urol 1983;130:1138–1141

33. Neumann PZ, deDomenico IJ, Nogrady MB. Constipation and urinary tract infection. Pediatrics 1973;52:241–245

34. O'Regan S, Yazbeck S, Schick E. Constipation, bladder instability, urinary tract infection syndrome. Clin Nephrol 1985;23:152–154

35. Hutch JA. Theory of maturation of the intravesical ureter. J Urol 1961;86:534–538

36. Gross GW, Lebowitz RL. Infection does not cause reflux. AJR Am J Roentgenol 1981;137:929–932

37. Noe HN, Wyatt RJ, Peeden JN, Rivas ML. The transmission of vesicoureteral reflux from parent to child. J Urol 1992;148:1869–1871

38. Askari A, Belman AB. Vesicoureteral reflux in black girls. J Urol 1982;127:747–748

39. Skoog SJ, Belman AB. Primary vesicoureteral reflux in the black child. Pediatrics 1991;87:538–543

40. Hutch JA. Aberrant micturition. J Urol 1966;96:743–745

41. Hernanz-Schulman M, Lebowitz RL. The elusiveness and importance of bladder diverticula in children. Pediatr Radiol 1985;15: 399–402

42. Majd M, Rushton HG, Jantausch B, Wiedermann BL. Relationship among vesicoureteral reflux, P-fimbriated *Escherichia coli,* and acute pyelonephritis in children with febrile urinary tract infection. J Pediatr 1991;119:578–585

43. Bisset GS, Strife JL, Dunbar JS. Urography and voiding cystourethrography: findings in girls with urinary tract infection. AJR Am J Roentgenol 1987;148:479–482

44. Steinhardt GF. Reflux nephropathy. J Urol 1985;134:855–859

45. Matsuoka H, Oshima K, Sakamoto K, Taguchi T, Takebayashi S. Renal pathology in patients with reflux nephropathy: the turning point in irreversible renal disease. Eur Urol 1994;26:153–159

46. Kincaid-Smith P. Glomerular lesions in atrophic pyelonephritis and reflux nephropathy. Kidney Int 1975;8:S81–S83

47. Risdon RA. Reflux nephropathy. Diagn Histopathol 1981;4:61–70

48. Hodson CJ. The radiological contribution toward the diagnosis of chronic pyelonephritis. Radiology 1967;88:857–871

49. Hodson CJ. Neuhauser lecture: reflux nephropathy: a personal historical review. AJR Am J Roentgenol 1981;137:451–462

50. Wennerstrom M, Hansson S, Jodal U, Sixt R, Stokland E. Renal function 16 to 26 years after the first urinary tract infection in childhood. Arch Pediatr Adolesc Med 2000;154:339–345

51. Hansson S, Martinell J, Stokland E, Jodal U. The natural history of bacteriuria in childhood. Infect Dis Clin North Am 1997;11: 499–512

52. Chan RC, Reid G, Irvin RT, Bruce AW, Costeron JW. Competitive exclusion of uropathogens from human uroepithelial cells by Lactobacillus whole cells and cell wall fragments. Infect Immun 1985; 47:84–89

53. Fennell RS, Wilson SG, Garin EH, et al. Bacteriuria in families of girls with recurrent bacteriuria: a survey of 112 family members showed similar infections in 14 percent of the female siblings. Clin Pediatr 1977;16:1132–1135

54. Hellerstein S. Urinary tract infections: old and new concepts. Pediatr Clin North Am 1995;42:1433–1457

55. American Academy of Pediatrics, Committee on Quality Improvement, Subcommittee on Urinary Tract Infection. The diagnosis, treatment, and evaluation of the initial urinary tract infection in febrile infants and young children. Pediatrics 1999;103:843–852 [Errata, Pediatrics 1999;103:1052, 1999;104:118, 2000;105:141

56. Buonomo C, Treves ST, Jones B, Summerville D, Bauer S, Retik A. Silent renal damage in symptom-free siblings of children with vesicoureteral reflux: assessment with technetium Tc 99m dimercaptosuccinic acid scintigraphy. J Pediatr 1993;125:721– 723

57. Risdon RA. The small scarred kidney in childhood. Pediatr Nephrol 1993;7:361–364

58. Craig JC, Irwig LM, Knight JF, Roy LP. Does treatment of vesicoureteric reflux in childhood prevent end-stage renal disease attributable to reflux nephropathy? Pediatrics 2000;105:1236–1241

59. Hoberman A, Charron M, Hickey RW, Baskin M, Kearney DH, Wald ER. Imaging studies after a first febrile urinary tract infection in young children. N Engl J Med 2003;348:195–202

60. Dick PT, Feldman W. Routine diagnostic imaging for childhood urinary tract infections: a systematic overview. J Pediatr 1996; 128:15–22

61. Brendstrup L, Carlsen N, Nielsen SL, et al. Micturition cystourethrography using x-ray or scintigraphy in children with reflux. Acta Paediatr Scand 1983;72:559–562

62. Rushton HG. Urinary tract infections in children: epidemiology, evaluation, and management. Pediatr Clin North Am 1997;44: 1133–1169

63. Lebowitz RL, Mandell J. Urinary tract infection in children: putting radiology in its place. Radiology 1987;165:1–9

64. Ilyas M, Mastin ST, Richard GA. Age-related radiological imaging in children with acute pyelonephritis. Pediatr Nephrol 2000;17: 30–34

65. Piepsz A, Blaufox MD, Gordon I, et al. Consensus on renal cortical scintigraphy in children with urinary tract infection: Scientific Committee of Radionuclides in Nephrourology. Semin Nucl Med 1999;29:160–174

66. Arnold RW, Subramanian G, McAfee JG, Blair RJ, Thomas FD. Comparison of Tc-99m complexes for renal imaging. J Nucl Med 1975;16:357–367

67. Schlager TA, Dilks S, Trudell J, Whittam TS, Hendley JO. Bacteriuria in children with neurogenic bladder treated with intermittent catheterization: natural history. J Pediatr 1995;126:490–496

68. Kawashima A, Sandler CM, Goldman SM, Raval BK, Fishman EK. CT of renal inflammatory disease. Radiographics 1997;17:851–866

69. Klar A, Hurvitz H, Berkun Y, et al. Focal bacterial nephritis (lobar nephronia) in children. J Pediatr 1996;128:850–853

70. Bubeck B, Brandau W, Steinbächer M, et al. Technetium-99m labeled renal function and imaging agents, II: Clinical evaluation of 99m Tc MAG 3 (99m Tc mercaptoacetylglycine). Nucl Med Biol 1988;15:109–118

71. Lonergan GJ, Pennington DJ, Morrison JC, et al. Childhood pyelonephritis: comparison of gadolinium-enhanced MR imaging and renal cortical scintigraphy for diagnosis. Radiology 1998; 207:377–384

72. Kavanagh EC, Ryan S, Awan A, McCourbrey S, O'Connor R, Donoghue V. Can MRI replace DMSA in the detection of renal parenchymal defects in children with urinary tract infections? Pediatr Radiol 2005;35:275–281

73. Rosenbaum DM, Korngold E, Teele RL. Sonographic assessment of renal length in normal children. AJR Am J Roentgenol 1984;142: 467–469

74. Han BK, Babcock DS. Sonographic measurements and appearance of normal kidneys in children. AJR Am J Roentgenol 1985;145: 611–616

75. Carrico CW, Zerin JM. Sonographic measurement of renal length in children: does the position of the patient matter? Pediatr Radiol 1996;26:553–555

76. De Sanctis JT, Connolly SA, Bramson RT. Effect of patient position on sonographically measured renal length in neonates, infants, and children. AJR Am J Roentgenol 1998;170:1381–1383

77. Kunin CM. The natural history of recurrent bacteriuria in schoolgirls. N Engl J Med 1970;282:1443–1448

78. Friedman EP, de Bruyn R, Mather S. Pseudotumoral cystitis in children: a review of the ultrasound features in four cases. Br J Radiol 1993;66:605–608

79. Gooding GA. Varied sonographic manifestations of cystitis. J Ultrasound Med 1986;5:61–63

80. Sty JR, Wells RG, Starshak RJ, Schroeder BA. Imaging in acute renal infection in children. AJR Am J Roentgenol 1987;148:471–477

81. Mackenzie JR, Fowler K, Hollman AS, et al. The value of ultrasound in the child with an acute urinary tract infection. Br J Urol 1994;74:240–244

82. Dinkel E, Orth S, Dittrich M, Schulte-Wissermann H. Renal sonography in the differentiation of upper from lower urinary tract infection. AJR Am J Roentgenol 1986;146:775–780

83. Pickworth FE, Carlin JB, Ditchfield MR, et al. Sonographic measurement of renal enlargement in children with acute pyelonephritis and time needed for resolution: implications for renal growth assessment. AJR Am J Roentgenol 1995;165:405–408

84. Avni EF, Van Gansbeke D, Thoua Y, et al. US demonstration of pyelitis and ureteritis in children. Pediatr Radiol 1988;18:134–139

85. Morehouse HT, Weiner SN, Hoffman JC. Imaging in inflammatory disease of the kidney. AJR Am J Roentgenol 1984;143:135–141

86. Klar A, Hurvitz H, Berkun Y, et al. Focal bacterial nephritis (lobar nephronia) in children. J Pediatr 1996;128:850–853

87. Lavocat MP, Granjon D, Allard D, et al. Imaging of pyelonephritis. Pediatr Radiol 1997;27:159–165

88. Mastin ST, Drane WE, Iravani A. Tc-99m DMSA SPECT imaging in patients with acute symptoms or history of UTI. Comparison with ultrasonography. Clin Nucl Med 1995;20:407–412

89. Smellie JM, Rigden SP, Prescod NP. Urinary tract infection: a comparison of four methods of investigation. Arch Dis Child 1995;72: 247–250

90. Björgvinsson E, Majd M, Eggli KD. Diagnosis of acute pyelonephritis in children: comparison of sonography and 99mTc-DMSA scintigraphy. AJR Am J Roentgenol 1991;157:539–543

91. Verber IG, Strudley MR, Meller ST. 99mTc dimercaptosuccinic acid (DMSA) scan as first investigation of urinary tract infection. Arch Dis Child 1988;63:1320–1325

92. Majd M, Nussaum-Blask AR, Markle BM, et al. Acute pyelonephritis: comparison of diagnosis with 99mTc-DMSA SPECT, spiral CT, MR imaging, and power Doppler ultrasound in an experimental pig model. Radiology 2001;218:101–108

93. Dacher J-N, Pfister C, Monroc M, Eurin D, Le Dosseur P. Power Doppler sonographic pattern of acute pyelonephritis in children: comparison with CT. AJR Am J Roentgenol 1996;166: 1451–1455

94. Halevy R, Smolkin V, Bykov S, Chervinsky L, Sakran W, Koren A. Power Doppler ultrasonography in the diagnosis of acute childhood pyelonephritis. Pediatr Nephrol 2004;19:987–991

95. Kim B, Lim HK, Choi MH, et al. Detection of parenchymal abnormalities in acute pyelonephritis by pulse inversion harmonic imaging with or without microbubble ultrasonographic contrast agent: correlation with computed tomography. J Ultrasound Med 2001;20:5–14

96. Riccabona M, Uggowitzer M, Klein E, Lindbichler F, Ebner F. Fotter echo-enhanced color Doppler sonography in children and adolescents. J Ultrasound Med 2000;19:789–796

97. Jeffrey RB Jr, Laing FC, Wing VW, Hoddick W. Sensitivity of sonography in pyonephrosis: a reevaluation. AJR Am J Roentgenol 1985; 144:71–73

98. Schneider K, Helmig FJ, Eife R, et al. Pyonephrosis in children–is ultrasound sufficient for diagnosis? Pediatr Radiol 1989;19:302–307

99. Wu TT, Lee YH, Tzeng WS, et al. The role of C-reactive protein and erythrocyte sedimentation rate in the diagnosis of infected hydronephrosis and pyonephrosis. J Urol 1994;152:26–28

100. St. Lezin M, Hofmann R, Stoller ML. Pyonephrosis: diagnosis and treatment. Br J Urol 1992;70:360–363

101. Colemen BG, Arger PH, Mulhern CB Jr, Pollack HM, Banner MP. Pyonephrosis: sonography in the diagnosis and management. AJR Am J Roentgenol 1981;137:939–943

102. Riccipetitoni G, Chierici R, Tamisari L, et al. Postnatal ultrasound screening of urinary malformations. J Urol 1992;148:604–605

103. Jequier S, Forbes PA, Nogrady MB. The value of ultrasonography as a screening procedure in a first-documented urinary tract infection in children. J Ultrasound Med 1985;4:393–400

104. Alon U, Berant M, Pery M. Intravenous pyelography in children with urinary tract infection and vesicoureteral reflux. Pediatrics 1989;83:332–336

105. Darge K, Moeller RT, Trusen A, Butter F, Gordjani N, Riedmiller H. Diagnosis of vesicoureteric reflux with low-dose contrast-enhanced harmonic ultrasound imaging. Pediatr Radiol 2005;35: 73–78

106. Berrocal T, Gava F, Arjonilla A, Lonergan GJ. Vesicoureteral reflux: diagnosis and grading with echo-enhanced cystosonography versus voiding cystourethrography. Radiology 2001;221: 359–365

107. Stokland E, Hellstrom M, Hansson S, et al. Reliability of ultrasonography in identification of reflux nephropathy in children. BMJ 1994;309:235–239

108. Moorthy I, Wheat D, Gordon I. Ultrasonography in the evaluation of renal scarring using DMSA scan as the gold standard. Pediatr Nephrol 2004;19:153–156

109. Hitzel A, Liard A, Vera P, Manrique A, Menard JF, Dacher JN. Color and power Doppler sonography versus DMSA scintigraphy in acute pyelonephritis and in prediction of renal scarring. J Nucl Med 2002;43:27–32

110. Farhat W, Traubici J, Sherman C, Williams T, Babyn P, McLorie G. Reliability of contrast enhanced sonography with harmonic imaging for detecting early renal scarring in experimental pyelonephritis in a porcine model: preliminary results. J Urol 2002;168:1114–1117

111. Karlowicz MG. Candidal renal and urinary tract infection in neonates. Semin Perinatol 2003;27:393–400

112. Bryant K, Maxfield C, Rabalais G. Renal candidiasis in neonates with candiduria. Pediatr Infect Dis J 1999;18:959–963

113. Tung KT, MacDonald LM, Smith JC. Neonatal systemic candidiasis diagnosed by ultrasound. Acta Radiol 1990;31:293–295

114. Baetz-Greenwalt B, Debaz B, Kumar ML. Bladder fungus ball: a reversible cause of neonatal obstructive uropathy. Pediatrics 1988;81:826–829

8 Right Lower Quadrant Pain: Ruling Out Appendicitis

Lawrence C. Chow and R. Jeffrey Brooke Jr.

Although the incidence of appendicitis appears to be declining slightly in the Western world, it nonetheless remains the most common cause of acute abdominal pain requiring surgery.[1,2] In the United States each year, ~250,000 patients undergo appendectomies for presumed appendicitis.[1,2] The differential diagnosis 1of acute appendicitis is extremely broad, and appendicitis often mimics the presentation of many other gastrointestinal, genitourinary, or gynecologic abnormalities. Historically, clinical misdiagnosis is common; ~20% of patients presumed to have appendicitis undergo a nontherapeutic laparotomy with removal of a normal appendix. The rate of negative appendectomy is even higher in women of reproductive age, in whom 30 to 40% of surgeries yield normal appendices.[3,4]

Surgeons have traditionally relied almost entirely on the patient's history and physical examination to determine the need for surgery.[1–13] However, during the past decade imaging studies have played an increasingly important role in the diagnostic evaluation of patients with

possible appendicitis.[8,9] Several large clinical series have documented a high degree of sensitivity and specificity for computed tomography (CT) and sonography in the evaluation of patients with right lower quadrant pain and possible acute appendicitis.[8,9] The accurate noninvasive imaging of acute appendicitis now makes obsolete the complete reliance upon the patient's history and physical examination to determine the need for surgery.

Differential Diagnosis

In patients with acute right lower quadrant pain, appendicitis is only one of a large number of gastrointestinal, genitourinary, and gynecologic disorders. Common clinical mimics of acute appendicitis include mesenteric adenitis (**Fig. 8–1**), ureteral calculi, right-sided diverticulitis, acute gynecologic disorders, and viral gastroenteritis. In his classic monograph on the early diagnosis of the acute abdomen, Sir Zachary Cope listed 34 different disorders that

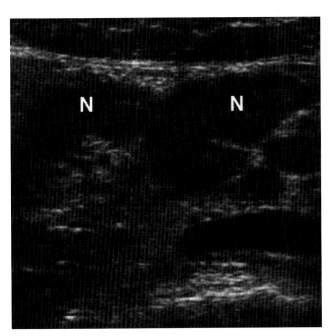

Figure 8–1 Mesenteric adenitis. Note multiple enlarged mesenteric lymph nodes (N) on sagittal sonogram of right lower quadrant in a patient with a normal appendix (not shown).

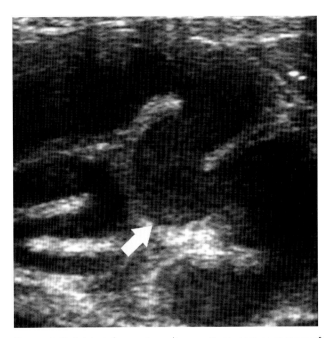

Figure 8–2 Pelvic inflammatory disease. Transverse sonogram of right lower quadrant demonstrates dilated and tortuous fallopian tube (*arrow*) containing intraluminal low-level echoes representing pus.

may clinically mimic acute appendicitis.[13] This list has greatly expanded in the past several decades, with advances in medical knowledge and newer disease entities, such as acquired immunodeficiency syndrome (AIDS), associated with immunosuppressive states. One factor contributing to the overall complexity of acute right lower quadrant pain as a clinical problem is that the differential diagnosis ranges from benign self-limited disorders (e.g., mesenteric adenitis or viral gastroenteritis) to lesions that carry significant morbidity if not treated promptly, including bowel obstruction, perforation, infarction, or abscesses of various etiologies.

In women of reproductive age, it is often difficult to clinically differentiate appendicitis from acute gynecologic disorders. Pelvic inflammatory disease (**Fig. 8–2**), degenerating myomas (**Fig. 8–3**), ovarian torsion, and ruptured or hemorrhagic functional cysts may all mimic the clinical presentation of acute appendicitis at times.[4] In patients over 50 years of age, perforated cecal neoplasm should also be considered in the differential diagnosis.[14]

Clinical Presentation

The "classic history" for acute appendicitis is the onset of diffuse abdominal or midepigastric pain that after a period of time localizes to the right lower quadrant.[1,2] Pain is frequently accompanied by anorexia and at times nausea and vomiting. Of note is the fact that this classic history is present in only 55% of patients with acute appendicitis.[2] The most characteristic physical finding is guarding and rebound tenderness over the McBurney point in the right iliac fossa. The early diagnosis of acute appendicitis is often

difficult in pediatric patients due to problems in obtaining an adequate history. Some elderly or immunocompromised patients may have relatively minimal pain with acute appendicitis.

The location of the appendiceal tip is highly variable and may be a major factor in contributing to the patient's symptoms and localization of pain. Flank pain may be the most striking finding in a patient with a retrocecal appendix that extends along the right lateral flank. In patients with a pelvic appendix, suprapubic tenderness or deep pelvic pain may be the most predominant clinical symptom. In female patients, this may closely mimic symptoms of salpingitis, ovarian torsion, or other acute gynecologic abnormalities. Endovaginal sonography may be quite useful to demonstrate pelvic appendicitis in women (**Fig. 8–4**).

Diagnostic Evaluation

Laboratory values in appendicitis are highly variable and often nonspecific.[15] Although leukocytosis with left shift is common, up to one third of adult patients with acute appendicitis have a normal leukocyte count.[15] Elderly patients, in particular, are known to have relatively normal laboratory values with acute appendicitis. A high fever with leukocytosis is characteristic of, but not always present with, a periappendiceal abscess.

Although it seems reasonable that patients with clear-cut clinical evidence of acute appendicitis be managed surgically without preoperative imaging, patients with atypical presentations and patients who are poor surgical candidates can benefit from preoperative imag-

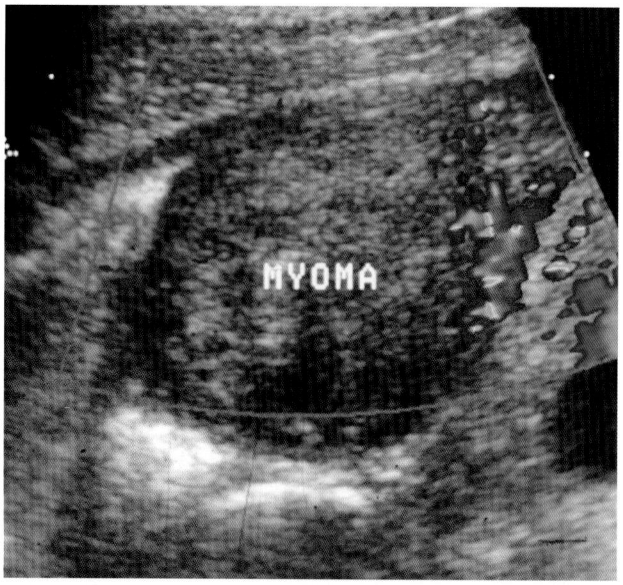

Figure 8–3 Degenerating myoma in pregnancy. Transverse color Doppler sonogram demonstrates avascular myoma in patient with 20 week gestation.

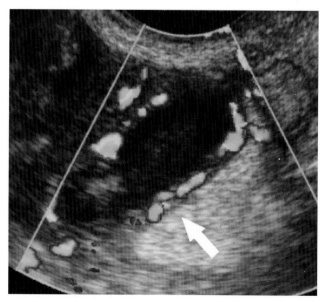

Figure 8–4 Pelvic appendicitis on endovaginal color Doppler sonogram. Note dilated appendix (*arrow*) with mural hyperemia.

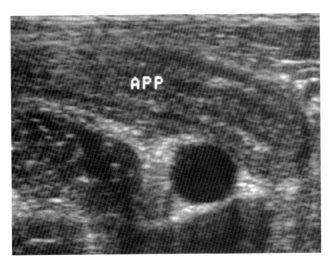

Figure 8–5 Early acute appendicitis. Enlarged noncompressible appendix (APP) is noted anterior to external iliac artery (A) and iliopsoas muscle (M).

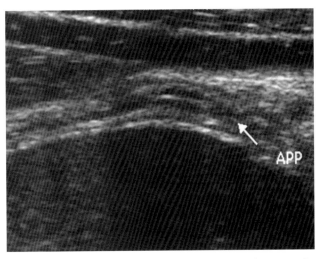

Figure 8–6 Normal appendix visualized by sonography. Appendix (APP) is identified in its long axis with maximal diameter of 5 mm.

ing.[16] Due to the extensive differential diagnoses in women of child-bearing age, including numerous gynecologic entities for right lower quadrant pain, these patients benefit most from preoperative imaging. Bendeck et al showed that the negative appendectomy rate was significantly lower (8 vs 28%) in women who underwent preoperative sonography versus those who had no preoperative imaging.[16] Other studies have also documented a reduction in the negative appendectomy rate with preoperative imaging.[17]

Ultrasound

Imaging

Graded compression sonography is based on the principle that when pressure is applied to a normal bowel loop with a transducer, it will readily compress.[9] Any inflammatory or neoplastic process infiltrating the bowel wall alters its compliance, making it relatively noncompressible. Whenever possible, it is important to use the highest-resolution linear array transducer that affords adequate penetration to visualize the key anatomical landmarks of the psoas muscle and external iliac artery and vein (**Fig. 8–5**). The study should be considered nondiagnostic if these normal structures cannot be visualized. In general, a 6 to 8 MHz linear or curved array transducer is adequate for most pediatric and adult patients. Endovaginal sonography is a valuable tool in female patients of reproductive age to evaluate the adnexal areas and detect pelvic appendicitis.[18]

At the outset of the examination, the patient is asked to point with a single finger to the site of maximal pain or tenderness. This maneuver is often helpful in identifying a potentially aberrantly located appendix. Sonographic imaging is then initiated in the transverse plane using light

pressure to first identify the abdominal wall musculature and the right colon. The right colon is the largest structure in the right flank with the typical sonographic bowel signature (echogenic submucosal layer) that has no peristalsis. The right colon is then followed caudally to its termination as a cecal tip. Pressure is gradually applied to the cecal tip to express all the gas and fecal contents from its lumen and enhance visualization of the noncompressible appendix. It is very important to vary the acoustic window to obtain the optimal view to demonstrate the appendix. Sometimes, as in the setting of a deep pelvic appendix, a full urinary bladder can be used as an acoustic window to visualize an otherwise inaccessible appendix. This technique, however, obviates graded compression. In the situation of a retrocecal appendix, placing the patient in a left lateral decubitus position may aid visualization by displacing the cecum and terminal ileum medially. With the patient in this position, scanning the right flank can sometimes be helpful by reducing the transducer–target distance. Finally, in women of childbearing age, transvaginal sonography can play an important role in the visualization of a pelvic appendix or in the identification of alternative diagnoses. In one study of sonographically detected appendicitis, transabdominal sonography detected 76% of cases, whereas transvaginal sonography added 24%.[18]

Although other published reports have suggested that the normal appendix can be visualized in a high percentage of patients (**Fig. 8–6**), the point is somewhat controversial.[19] At our own institution, we are able to image the normal appendix in only ~15 to 20% of patients. In general, the normal appendix measures 5 mm or less in maximal anteroposterior diameter and is readily compressible.[20] Often there is a small amount of echogenic residual fecal debris and gas within the normal appendix.

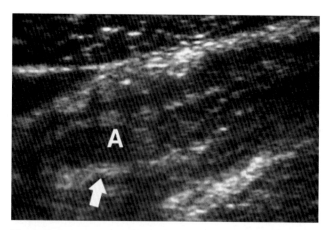

Figure 8–7 Acute nonperforated appendicitis. Note enlarged appendix (A). Echogenic submucosa is still preserved (*arrow*), indicating lack of perforation.

Diagnostic Criteria for Sonographic Diagnosis of Appendicitis

The appendix can be confidently identified when a nonperistaltic, blind-ending, tubular structure is seen arising from the base of the cecum. The diagnosis of acute appendicitis can be established with confidence if a noncompressible appendix with a maximal outer diameter of 7 mm or greater is identified[20] (**Fig. 8–7**). An appendix that measures in the range of 5 to 6 mm should be considered equivocal.[21] These patients may be observed clinically because there is no risk of morbidity from perforation. Some of these patients will not prove to have appendicitis and, therefore, a trial period of observation is clearly warranted. Short-interval follow-up imaging of these patients during the observation period may reveal positive findings in those patients with early developing appendicitis.[16] Pa-

tients with right lower quadrant pain and a visualized appendicolith are often taken to surgery, even with a borderline-sized appendix, due to concern for the potential morbidity of perforation in such patients.

For the most part, the diagnosis of acute appendicitis is based on gray-scale imaging findings. In equivocal cases, hyperemia of the inflamed appendix demonstrated by color Doppler sonography may be helpful in establishing the diagnosis, with reported sensitivities and specificities of 50 to 88% and 96 to 100%, respectively (**Fig. 8–8**).[22–24] Microbubble contrast agents used in conjunction with power and spectral Doppler imaging have recently been reported to improve the sensitivity of this finding.[25] However, false-negatives can result from gangrenous appendices with necrosis of appendiceal vessels. It is important to use low-volume-flow settings to visualize the small intramural appendiceal blood vessels. Other potential uses of color Doppler sonography are in evaluation of focally thickened bowel wall segments or other entities that may simulate appendicitis. These include inflammatory bowel disease (**Fig. 8–9**), thrombosis of the ovarian vein (**Fig. 8–10**), degenerating myomas, and other focal gastrointestinal abnormalities (**Fig. 8–11**).

Several other ancillary findings that support the diagnosis of acute appendicitis can be helpful. An appendicolith may be seen as an associated echogenic shadowing focus (**Fig. 8–12**), and its identification in the setting of other findings of appendicitis strengthens the sonographic diagnosis. Hyperechoic periappendiceal fat representing inflamed mesentery or omentum is a frequent finding in the presence of appendicitis with high specificity, but low sensitivity.[26] Although in our experience this is often an early sign of appendicitis, at least one study suggests that this finding may be an indicator of more advanced disease.[27]

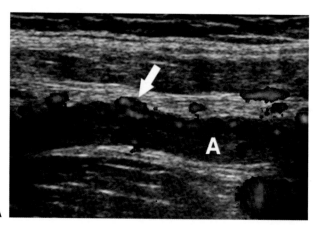

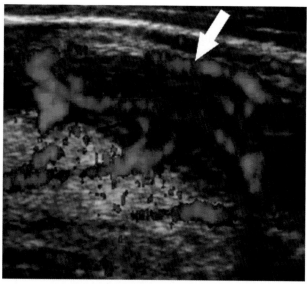

A

B

Figure 8–8 Hyperemia in early appendicitis. **(A)** Power Doppler sonogram demonstrates enlarged increased mural flow (*arrow*) within a minimally enlarged appendix (A), borderline in size. **(B)** The more advanced stage of appendicitis; note marked mural flow in appendix (*arrow*).

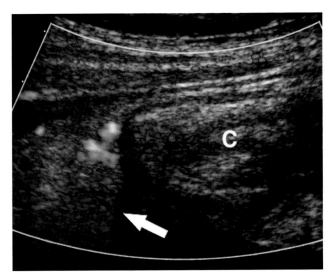

Figure 8–9 Cecal Crohn's disease. Note mural thickening of cecum (C) and prominent adjacent fibrofatty mass (*arrow*) with increased mural flow indicating hyperemia.

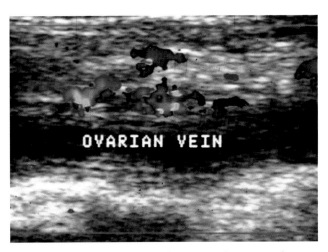

Figure 8–10 Ovarian vein thrombosis mimicking appendicitis in postpartum patient. Sagittal color Doppler sonogram demonstrates absent flow from occluded ovarian vein.

The presence or absence of luminal gas within the appendix as a criterion to exclude or diagnose appendicitis has been a topic of some controversy.[28] Although at least one study suggests an excellent negative predictive value for acute appendicitis (94%) with the identification of luminal gas,[29] even in that study gas *was* observed in 12% of cases of severe appendicitis and 31% of cases of mild or moderate appendicitis. In this same study, the absence of gas had only a 57% positive predictive value for the presence of appendicitis.

Limitations of Sonographic Diagnosis of Appendicitis

The entire length of the appendix must be visualized to its termination as a blind tip to avoid incorrect diagnoses. Unless the tip is identified, one cannot conclude that the structure in question truly represents the appendix because a segment of distal ileum may be misinterpreted as a dilated appendix. Ileum, however, does not arise from the cecal base, is not blind-ending, and often demonstrates peristalsis. Additionally, when the distal tip is not visualized, one cannot conclude that the appendix is normal because the inflammatory process of appendicitis may be entirely confined to the distal appendix.[23] On rare occasions, a mildly dilated fallopian tube may be misconstrued as the appendix. Secondary thickening of the ap-

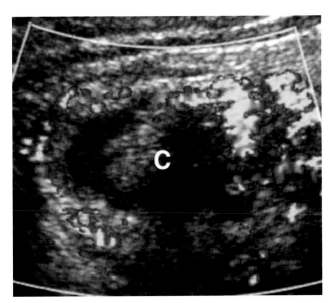

Figure 8–11 Pseudomembranous colitis of right colon. Transverse color Doppler sonogram of cecum (C) demonstrates marked mural thickening with hyperemia.

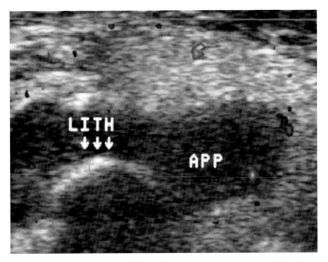

Figure 8–12 Appendicolith within gangrenous appendix. Note echogenic appendicolith (LITH) and loss of echogenic submucosal layer and prominent adjacent echogenic fat.

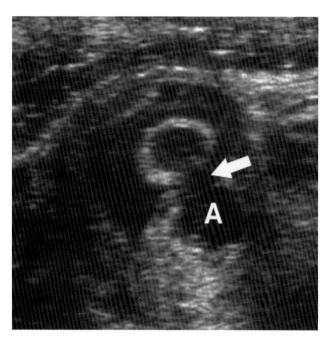

Figure 8–13 Perforated appendicitis. Transverse scan of inflamed appendix demonstrates focal loss of submucosal layer (*arrow*) and adjacent hypoechoic abscess (A).

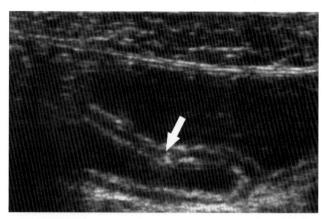

Figure 8–14 Abortive appendicitis. Mildly dilated appendix (6.5 mm) (*arrow*) is demonstrated, consistent with appendicitis. Patient's pain resolved spontaneously and no surgery was performed.

pendix may be due to extrinsic periappendiceal inflammatory processes such as tubo-ovarian abscesses or Crohn's disease (**Fig. 8–9**). The diagnosis of a periappendiceal abscess can only be established with confidence if there is an associated appendicolith or if the abscess is in continuity with mural necrosis of the appendix (**Fig. 8–13**). A rare pitfall is that inspissated stool in the right colon may cause acoustic shadowing and can be misconstrued as an appendicolith.

Spontaneous resolution of acute appendicitis may be observed in a small subset of patients (abortive appendicitis).[30] These patients may have imaging criteria for acute appendicitis in the absence of abdominal pain. This underscores the importance of always interpreting the imaging abnormalities in light of the clinical setting.

Benefits of Sonography in Diagnosing Appendicitis

Despite the fact that appendiceal sonography may be technically challenging, it has several clear imaging advantages.[31–34] Sonography is readily available, inexpensive to perform, and has no ionizing radiation. Unlike CT, it is a real-time, interactive study. Sonographic findings are relatively easy to correlate with the patient's anatomical site of maximal pain and tenderness. In addition, sonography can display bowel peristalsis and identify the discrete anatomical layers of the bowel wall, such as the echogenic submucosa. In the past several years, there have been substantial improvements in color Doppler sensitivity to enable visualization of blood flow to bowel without the use

of contrast agents.[35,36] Hyperemia, which is characteristic of acute inflammation, can thus be differentiated from ischemic disorders that cause decreased flow to the bowel. As with CT, sonography can effectively survey the remainder of the abdomen and pelvis if the appendix is normal.[37] With the use of endovaginal probes, sonography excels at diagnosing gynecologic disorders. Sonography may also be useful in identifying mesenteric adenitis, inflammatory bowel disease, pyosalpinx, small bowel obstruction (**Fig. 8–14**), and ovarian torsion.[37]

Numerous reports have established the sensitivity of sonography in the range of 76 to 89%.[20,21,34] Sonography is an operator-dependent technique that requires a dedicated sonologist willing to spend the time and effort to master the graded compression technique. Some institutions have much greater experience with CT diagnosis of appendicitis and have relegated sonography to a second-line imaging study.

Comparison of Ultrasonography and Computed Tomography for Diagnosing Appendicitis

In addition to graded compression sonography, a variety of CT techniques have been developed that are extremely valuable in the evaluation of patients with suspected appendicitis.[38–41] The differences in CT methodology relate to whether there is administration of oral, intravenous, or rectal contrast. In patients with ample intraperitoneal fat, unenhanced CT (no oral and no intravenous contrast) is an accurate technique.[39,40] It is important to note, however, that patient selection is key to the success of noncontrast CT for appendicitis. One significant limitation of noncontrast scans is that, in very thin patients with appendiceal perforation, it may be difficult to distinguish liquefied pus from indurated soft tissue inflammation. Intravenous contrast is thus routinely administered in such studies at many institutions and is particularly useful in patients

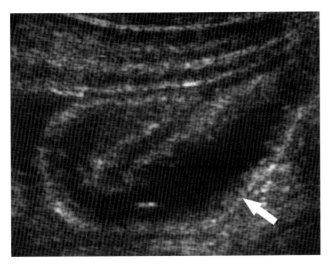

Figure 8–15 Small bowel obstruction. Dilated loop of small bowel (*arrow*) is noted in U-shaped configuration from closed loop obstruction.

with suspected appendiceal perforation (**Fig. 8–15**). Another limitation is that in very thin patients without ample intraperitoneal fat, edema of the mesoappendix, which is an important diagnostic criterion, may not be evident. Therefore, in thin patients, oral and intravenous contrast may be of significant value.

Scans performed with rectal contrast only have been shown to be highly accurate for the diagnosis of appendicitis.[40] This technique clearly identifies the cecal tip, therefore making it easier to visualize the abnormal appendix. In general, the CT criteria for acute appendicitis include identification of an appendix 7 mm or greater in diameter with adjacent edema of the mesoappendix. Secondary findings include appendicoliths and adjacent abscesses.

Graded compression sonography is often quite difficult to perform in either obese patients or in those with severe abdominal pain. It may be difficult in patients with perforation to adequately compress the cecal tip. Obese patients and patients with perforated appendicitis, however, are ideal candidates for CT. Multiple studies have demonstrated the superior sensitivity and specificity of CT compared with sonography for the evaluation of appendicitis.[42–44] Nevertheless, sonography still maintains an important role in the imaging evaluation for specific groups of patients. In particular, because of the lack of ionizing radiation, sonography should be the first-line imaging study for evaluating patients with possible appendicitis requiring imaging who are pregnant, women of child-bearing age, children, or those of slender body habitus. CT, on the other hand, excels in patients with greater mesenteric fat and should be the first-line study in patients of larger body habitus. These recommendations are supported by the most recent American College of Radiology Appropriateness Criteria.[45]

Summary

Sonography and CT play an increasingly important role in reducing the number of negative surgical explorations for acute appendicitis. Although at times technically challenging, sonography has several distinct advantages in imaging patients with right lower quadrant pain. At our institution sonography is the method of choice for imaging pediatric patients, women of reproductive age, and thin male patients. CT is complementary to sonography and excels in imaging patients who are poor candidates for sonography; namely, obese patients or patients with appendiceal perforation.

References

1. Schrock TR. Acute appendicitis. In: Sleisenger MH, Fordtran JS, eds. Gastrointestinal Disease: Pathophysiology, Diagnosis, Management. 4th ed. Philadelphia: Saunders; 1989:1382–1389
2. Telford GL, Condon RE. Appendix. In: Zuidema GD, ed. Shackelford's Surgery of the Alimentary Tract. 3rd ed. Philadelphia: Saunders; 1991:133–141
3. Velanovich V, Satava R. Balancing the normal appendectomy rate with the perforated appendicitis rate: implications for quality assurance. Am Surg 1992;58:246–269
4. Lewis FR, Holcroft JH, Boey J, et al. Appendicitis: a critical review of diagnosis and treatment in 1,000 cases. Arch Surg 1975;110:677–684
5. Sakover RP, Del Fava RL. Frequency of visualization of the normal appendix with the barium enema examination. AJR Am J Roentgenol Radium Ther Nucl Med 1974;121:312–317
6. Olutola PS. Plain film radiographic diagnosis of acute appendicitis: an evaluation of the signs. Can Assoc Radiol J 1988;39:254–256
7. Condon RE. Appendicitis. In: Sabiston DC, ed. Textbook of Surgery. 13th ed. Philadelphia: Saunders; 1986:967–982
8. Balthazar EJ, Megibow AJ, Siegel SE, Birnbaum BA. Appendicitis: prospective evaluation with high-resolution CT. Radiology 1991;180:21–24
9. Puylaert JB. Acute appendicitis: US evaluation using graded compression. Radiology 1986;158:355–360
10. Andersen M, Lilja T, Lundell L, et al. Clinical and laboratory findings in patients subjected to laparotomy for suspected acute appendicitis. Acta Chir Scand 1980;146:55–63
11. Pieper R, Kager L, Nasman P. Acute appendicitis: a clinical study of 1018 cases of emergency appendectomy. Acta Chir Scand 1982;148:51–62
12. Dunn EL, Moore EE, Elderling SC, et al. The unnecessary laparotomy for appendicitis: can it be decreased? Am Surg 1982;48:320–323
13. Cope Z. Cope's Early Diagnosis of the Acute Abdomen. New York: Oxford University Press; 1987
14. Sumpio BE, Ballantyne GH, Zdon MJ, Modlin IM. Perforated appendicitis and obstructing colonic carcinoma in the elderly. Dis Colon Rectum 1986;29:668–670
15. Dueholm S, Bagi P, Bud M. Laboratory aid in the diagnosis of acute appendicitis: a blinded, prospective trial concerning diagnostic value of leukocyte count, neutrophil differential count, and C-reactive protein. Dis Colon Rectum 1989;32:855–859
16. Bendeck SE, Nino-Murcia M, Berry GJ, et al. Imaging for suspected appendicitis: negative appendectomy and perforation rates. Radiology 2002;225:131–136

17. Rao PM, Rhea JT, Novelline RA, Mostafavi AA, McCabe CJ. Effect of computed tomography of the appendix on treatment of patients and use of hospital resources. N Engl J Med 1998;338:141–146

18. Caspi B, Zbar AP, Mavor E, et al. The contribution of transvaginal ultrasound in the diagnosis of acute appendicitis: an observational study. Ultrasound Obstet Gynecol 2003;21:273–276

19. Rioux M. Sonographic detection of the normal and abnormal appendix. AJR Am J Roentgenol 1992;158:773–778

20. Jeffrey RB Jr, Laing FC, Townsend RR. Acute appendicitis: sonographic criteria based on 250 cases. Radiology 1988;167:327–329

21. Jeffrey RB Jr, Jain KA, Nghiem HV. Sonographic diagnosis of acute appendicitis: interpretive pitfalls. AJR Am J Roentgenol 1994;162:55–59

22. Lim HK, Lee WJ, Kim TH, et al. Appendicitis: usefulness of color Doppler US. Radiology 1996;201:221–225

23. Lim HK, Lee WJ, Lee SJ, et al. Focal appendicitis confined to the tip: diagnosis at US. Radiology 1996;200:799–801

24. Kessler N, Cyteval C, Gallix B, et al. Appendicitis: evaluation of sensitivity, specificity, and predictive values of US, Doppler US, and laboratory findings. Radiology 2004;230:472–478

25. Incesu L, Yazicioglu AK, Selcuk MB, et al. Contrast-enhanced power Doppler US in the diagnosis of acute appendicitis. Eur J Radiol 2004;50:201–209

26. Sivit CJ. Diagnosis of acute appendicitis in children: spectrum of sonographic findings. AJR Am J Roentgenol 1993;161:147–152

27. Noguchi T, Hoshimitsu K, et al. Periappendiceal hyperechoic structure on sonography: a sign of severe appendicitis. J Ultrasound Med 2005;24:323–327; quiz 328–330

28. Rao PM. Presence or absence of gas in the appendix: additional criteria to rule out or confirm acute appendicitis-evaluation with US. Radiology 2000;217:599–600

29. Rettenbacher T, Hollerweger A, Macheiner P, et al. Presence or absence of gas in the appendix: additional criteria to rule out or confirm acute appendicitis-evaluation with US. Radiology 2000;214:183–187

30. Cobben LP, de Van Otterloo AM, Puylaert JB. Spontaneously resolving appendicitis: frequency and natural history in 60 patients. Radiology 2000;215:349–352

31. Jeffrey RB Jr, Ralls PW. CT and Sonography of the Acute Abdomen. 2nd ed. Philadelphia: Lippincott-Raven; 1995:289–295

32. Brown JJ. Acute appendicitis: the radiologist's role [editorial]. Radiology 1991;180:13–14

33. Schwerk WB, Wichtrup B, Ruschoff J, Rothmund M. Acute and perforated appendicitis: current experience with ultrasound-aided diagnosis. World J Surg 1990;14:271–276

34. Puylaert JB, Rutgers PH, Lalisang RI, et al. A prospective study of ultrasonography in the diagnosis of appendicitis. N Engl J Med 1987;317:666–669

35. Jeffrey RB Jr, Sommer FG, Debatin JF. Color Doppler sonography of focal gastrointestinal lesions: initial clinical experience. J Ultrasound Med 1994;13:473–478

36. Clautice-Engle T, Jeffrey RB Jr, Li KCP, Barth RA. Power Doppler imaging of focal lesions of the gastrointestinal tract: comparison with conventional color Doppler imaging. J Ultrasound Med 1996;15:63–66

37. Gaensler EH, Jeffrey RB Jr, Laing FC, Townsend RR. Sonography in patients with suspected acute appendicitis: value in establishing alternative diagnoses. AJR Am J Roentgenol 1989;152:49–51

38. Balthazar EJ, Birnbaum BA, Yee J, et al. Acute appendicitis: CT and US correlation in 100 patients. Radiology 1994;190:31–35

39. Malone AJ Jr, Wolf CR, Malmed AS, Melliere BJ. Diagnosis of acute appendicitis: value of unenhanced CT. AJR Am J Roentgenol 1993;160:763–766

40. Lane MJ, Katz DS, Ross BA, et al. Unenhanced helical CT for suspected acute appendicitis. AJR Am J Roentgenol 1997;168:405–409

41. Rao PM, Rhea JT, Novelline RA, et al. Helical CT technique for the diagnosis of appendicitis: prospective evaluation of a focused appendix CT examination. Radiology 1997;202:139–144

42. Sivit CJ, Applegate KE, Berlin SC, et al. Imaging evaluation of suspected appendicitis in a pediatric population: effectiveness of sonography versus CT. AJR Am J Roentgenol 2000;175:977–980

43. Wise SW, Labuski MR, Kasales CJ, et al. Comparative assessment of CT and sonographic techniques for appendiceal imaging. AJR Am J Roentgenol 2001;176:933–941

44. Terasawa T, Blackmore CC, Bent S, et al. Systematic review: computed tomography and ultrasonography to detect acute appendicitis in adults and adolescents. Ann Intern Med 2004;141:537–546

45. Ralls PW, Balfe DM, et al. ACR Appropriateness Criteria: Acute Right Lower Quadrant Pain. American College of Radiology; 1999

Hypertension and Bruit

Laurence Needleman

The vast majority of patients with hypertension have essential hypertension; only a minority has renovascular hypertension (RVH). Despite this fact, the impetus to identify this minority exists because there is a possibility of curing their disease.

It is impractical to screen all hypertensive patients; therefore, it is important to identify the subset of patients who are at higher risk for RVH and might benefit from screening. It is equally important to identify the imaging tests that can be applied consistently and safely to this group.

Renal artery stenosis (RAS) is the most common cause of RVH. RAS is also associated with renal insufficiency.[1-4] Interest in applying diagnostic tests and therapeutic interventions to this risk group is growing.[5] It is clear that renal artery stenosis is associated with excess morbidity and mortality. Those with renal artery stenosis are at high risk for cardiovascular death; it is less established that renal interventions provide long-term benefit.[6]

Differential Diagnosis

Goldblatt and coworkers[7] were the first to prove that a renal lesion could cause hypertension by showing that renal artery constriction in a dog was followed by hypertension and renal atrophy. In the years that followed, understanding of the renin–angiotensin system has led to an understanding of RVH. Although RAS produces RVH, the two entities are not equivalent. RAS may not produce hypertension or it may coexist with essential hypertension. Processes other than RAS, such as Page kidney or dissecting aneurysm of the renal artery may also produce RVH. Other etiologies of secondary hypertension include renal disease, hyperaldosteronism, pheochromocytoma, Cushing's syndrome, sleep apnea syndrome, and coarctation of the aorta. Renal aneurysms may be associated with hypertension.[8]

The diagnosis of RVH is established retrospectively after the patient undergoes treatment: those whose hypertension responds to revascularization of RAS have RVH. The absence of a response to revascularization may be due to a variety of factors: technical failure of the intervention, incidental RAS in a patient with essential hypertension, or irreversible renal disease superimposed on RAS or RVH. There may be no way to distinguish these groups, so it may not be possible to find a gold standard that establishes the presence or absence of RVH.

Most tests used to evaluate the hypertensive patient are anatomical—they detect RAS. A physiological test for RVH is one that bases its diagnosis on the determination of whether the renal blood flow is abnormal. Physiological tests are theoretically more likely to predict the response to therapy, and therefore, RVH.

The prevalence of RVH is quite variable, but only represents around 0.5 to 5% of the hypertensive population.[9,10] Suggestive clinical clues may raise the likelihood of RVH to 5 to 15%.[9] Certain groups will have even greater incidence of RVH. For example, 31% of patients with accelerated hypertension may have RVH.[9]

The Cooperative Study of Renovascular Hypertension evaluated clinical features that might distinguish RVH from essential hypertension. The study compared 175 patients with RVH (91 cases of arteriosclerotic stenosis and 84 cases of fibromuscular dysplasia) that had been cured by surgery to 339 patients with essential hypertension.[11] Fibromuscular dysplasia was shown to be a disease of younger, predominantly female patients with no family history of hypertension. Arteriosclerotic patients were profiled as older, with higher systolic blood pressure, and often showed evidence of arterial disease at sites other than the kidney.

Although this study showed differences between the groups, no criteria were sufficiently sensitive or specific to distinguish the groups completely (**Table 9–1**). For instance, although a bruit was more often associated with RVH, a bruit is heard as frequently in essential hypertension. This is true because, although a lower percentage of patients with essential hypertension have bruits, essential hypertension is much more common than RVH. Still, this and other studies do point out some characteristics of patients that suggest RVH.

Mann and Pickering produced indexes of clinical suspicion that can guide the evaluation of patients with hypertension.[9] Those with borderline, low, or moderate hypertension and no clinical clues have a low index of suspicion and do not require a workup. For patients with a high index of suspicion, diagnostic testing is indicated. Angiography may be the appropriate first diagnostic imaging test. They identified patients at high risk, including those with (1) severe hypertension and either progressive renal insufficiency or lack of response to therapy, (2) accelerated or malignant hypertension, (3) grade 3 or 4 retinopathy, (4) hypertension with recent unexplained elevation of serum creatinine, (5) hypertension with elevation of serum creatinine reversibly induced by angiotensin-converting en-

Table 9–1   Clinical Characteristics of 131 Matched Cases of Essential and Renovascular Hypertension

	Hypertension	
	Essential (%)	Renovascular (%)
Duration of hypertension		
Less than 1 year	12	24
Greater than 10 years	15	6
Age of onset > 50	9	15
Family history of hypertension	71	46
Grade 3 or 4 fundi	7	46
Bruit		
Abdomen	9	46
Flank	1	12
Both	9	48
BUN > 20 mg/100 mL	8	15
Serum K < 3.4 mEq/L	8	15
Serum CO_2 > 30 mEq/L	8	16
Urinary casts	9	20
Proteinuria (a trace or more)	32	46

Note: 131 cases in each group matched by age, sex, race, and blood pressure. Only statistically significant differences are noted. (From Detection, evaluation, and treatment of renovascular hypertension: final report of the working group on renovascular hypertension. Arch Intern Med 1987;147:820–829. Reprinted with permission.)

zyme inhibitor, or (6) moderate or severe hypertension with asymmetrical renal size.

The workup of those with moderate risk such as those with refractory hypertension or moderate hypertension with a bruit or occlusive vascular disease elsewhere may require additional testing. Noninvasive tests may be helpful in this group if they identify patients for angiography.

The Dutch Renal Stenosis Intervention Cooperative (DRASTIC) study is a large multicenter Dutch study looking at RVH.[12] Angiography was performed in those who did not respond to two-drug therapy in 2 months. Up to 25% of persistently hypertensive patients had RAS.[13] The investigators concluded that drug resistance is a simple and useful clinical criterion to identify patients for angiography. A more recent multicenter trial that used the DRASTIC model showed that those with abdominal bruit, atherosclerotic disease, body mass index < 25 kg/m[2], renal function < 60 mL/min, and age greater than 58 years were significantly linked to RAS.[14] In this study no variable or combination of variables predicted RAS, but the absence of all five variables excluded RAS with a probability of 98%.

Although clinical criteria may determine some characteristics that suggest RVH, using a noninvasive screening test (such as imaging) to identify a subgroup with an even higher likelihood of a positive angiogram is another widely utilized strategy. Noninvasive tests must be applied to a

subset of hypertensives with a greater likelihood of RVH. No matter how accurate the noninvasive screening test is, it will be ineffective if it is used on an unselected population of hypertensives. For example, suppose a test is quite accurate—100% sensitive and 95% specific. If this is applied to all hypertensives (3% incidence of RVH), the predictive value for RVH is only 6%. Only six of 100 angiograms will demonstrate RAS. If the population is preselected to have more RVH, the predictive value is higher. If applied to a population with 25% RVH, the test will have a predictive value of 87%; this will increase to 93% if 40% of patients have RVH. Indices of clinical suspicion are necessary to define a population that would reasonably benefit from screening.

The clinician's view about therapy also affects the workup. The results of revascularization are not entirely clear-cut in favor of subjecting patients to this treatment. In the absence of consensus, the diagnostic workup and referrals for treatment vary. The arguments made for repair of RAS cite the potential for removing or reducing a lifetime dependency on medication and for stopping or slowing the development of renal failure and other complications of hypertension. The argument against repair cites the morbidity and mortality of the procedures, the absence of long-term proven benefit, and the view that modern medical treatment may effectively treat many patients.[13,15]

Those who favor medical therapy may see no need to put patients through tests that will not alter their therapy. Those who favor revascularization are more aggressive in their efforts to detect RAS. Dean[16] has all operative candidates with diastolic blood pressure above 105 mm Hg evaluated for secondary hypertension.

Diagnostic Evaluation

Nonimaging Evaluation

Peripheral plasma renin activity and its evaluation after captopril (captopril test) are nonimaging screening tests used to determine whether hypertension is renin dependent. These tests do not localize the disease.

Vaughan's group advocates that all patients at high risk for RVH receive an ambulatory plasma renin activity level test[17] to determine the functional impact of an anatomical lesion that might be found. They find that low plasma renin activity levels are rare in untreated patients who do not have renal disease. The reported usefulness of plasma renin levels varies widely in other studies, probably due to such factors as patient preparation, medications, and assay techniques.[18,19]

Another blood test is provocative testing with captopril to elicit a hyperreninemic response. A wide range of sensitivities (34 to 100%) and specificities (72 to 95%) has been reported.[13,18,19] To perform the test correctly patients should discontinue antihypertensive medications and have an adequate amount of salt intake. Renal insufficiency, bilateral disease, and restrictive conditions make the test difficult to perform correctly. Derkx et al reported sensitivity of 84% and specificity of 93%, but the test was performed in the hospital.[13]

Renal vein determinations can be done with or without captopril stimulation. These invasive tests showed excellent results in early studies and results that are more modest on follow-up.[19]

Imaging Other than Ultrasound

Scintigraphy

Captopril renal scintigraphy (CRS) is the most widely studied noninvasive imaging test for RVH. It is used in suspected RVH, not as a general screening study. Captopril inhibits angiotensin-converting enzyme, thereby blocking angiotensin II conversion. This, in turn, prevents postglomerular efferent arteriolar vasoconstriction and decreases the glomerular filtration rate (GFR) in the stenotic kidney. The contralateral normal kidney shows an increase in GFR. This disparity in renal function can be detected by scintigraphy. Most studies have used diethylenetriamine-pentaacetic acid (DPTA), but some have also evaluated radiopharmaceuticals secreted by the tubules.

Prigent has pooled the results of several series of nuclear scans.[19] The sensitivity for RAS of these pooled data was 73%, with specificity of 85% for evaluating differences between baseline and postcaptopril scans. If only the postcaptopril scans are used, the sensitivity rises to 85% and specificity becomes 83%. The value of captopril is questioned by other investigators.[13]

Pooled data also exist on how well captopril predicts a response to revascularization, and, therefore, RVH rather than RAS. Scintigraphy has a sensitivity of 76%, with a specificity of 92%, for the prediction of a cure or improvement.[19] If only postcaptopril scans are evaluated, then the test's ability to detect kidneys that will improve rises, but specificity drops off dramatically to a disappointing 66%.

Captopril renal scintigraphy is less accurate if patients have a small kidney. In the European multicenter trial,[20] abnormal renal function markedly diminished the test's specificity and accuracy (from 93 to 55% and from 90 to 68%, respectively). When this trial removed the results of patients with small kidneys and abnormal renal function, the specificity for response to treatment rose from 82 to 100%.

Magnetic Resonance and Computed Tomographic Angiography

Magnetic resonance angiography (MRA) is being actively investigated as a means of diagnosing RAS.[21-33] A variety of tests is being evaluated, including time-of-flight and

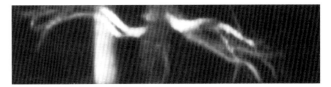

Figure 9–1 Three-dimensional reconstruction of phase-contrast magnetic resonance angiography of normal renal arteries.

phase-contrast techniques (**Fig. 9–1**). Protocols using gadolinium enhancement are also being investigated. Gadolinium has the potential to speed the examination, improve spatial resolution, and diminish artifacts. Results in the various studies have reported sensitivities from 92 to 100% with specificities of 71 to 96%[22,29,33,34] In a meta-analysis, enhanced three-dimensional MRA and computed tomographic angiography (CTA) outperformed ultrasound and other diagnostic tests, and nonenhanced MRA also outperformed ultrasound.[35] In the multicenter RADISH trial from the Netherlands, enhanced MR demonstrated less than expected sensitivity of 62% (confidence interval [CI] 54 to 71%) and specificity of 84% (CI 81 to 87%).[36]

Some of the poor results were due to inability to detect fibromuscular dysplasia (36% of the patients with RAS), but MRA for atherosclerotic RAS yielded a modestly improved sensitivity of 78% (CI 70 to 87%) and specificity of 88% (CI 86 to 91%). Raising the threshold to diagnose RAS from 50 to 70% did not change the results.

MRA misses accessory vessels and the intrarenal stenoses of fibromuscular dysplasia. In one recent study, gadolinium enhancement did allow detection of more accessory vessels, but did not improve the accuracy of the phase-contrast study for RAS detection.[22]

MR may also be used to evaluate some physiological aspects of RVH similar to nuclear scanning. Ros et al are using the passage of gadopentetate dimeglumine to determine glomerular filtration rate.[37]

CTA using multidetector CT is being evaluated for a variety of abdominal vascular diseases, including RAS.[38-41] CTA produces volumetric data that can produce three-dimensional reconstructions of arterial structures (**Fig. 9–2**). Thin-section axial scans can also be interpreted. A variety of reconstruction schemes are possible. With some thresholding techniques, stenoses may be misinterpreted.[42] The examination takes little time and the collection of data is operator-independent; however, reconstructions take additional time to create and interpret.

Studies using spiral and 16-channel multidetector CTs report high sensitivity ranging from 86 to 100%, and high specificity, ranging from 94 to 100%.[38-40,43] In the RADISH trial, CTA demonstrated less sensitivity and specificity than previous studies, 64% (CI 55 to 73%) and 92% (CI 90 to 95%).[36] Only one of six centers used a multidetector CT (four slice); nonetheless, all scanners yielded similar results. As with MRA, some of the poor results were due to inability to detect fibromuscular dysplasia. CTA for ath-

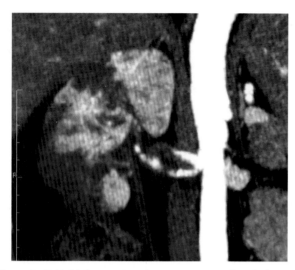

Figure 9–2 Multiplanar coronal reconstruction of multidetector computed tomographic angiogram. There is a right renal artery dissection and multiple renal infarcts. The patient has Ehlers-Danlos syndrome.

erosclerotic RAS yielded a better sensitivity of 77% (CI 67 to 86%).

Olbricht et al found some loss of accuracy when there was impaired renal function, but the numbers were too small for statistical evaluation.[40] Accessory vessels may be missed if they are outside of the acquired volume. A potential drawback to CTA is the requirement of iodinated contrast medium.

Both MRA and CTA are emerging techniques. Clinical trials with newer equipment (e.g., 16 and higher detector CT) and standardization of techniques (particularly for MR) are needed to determine their final place. For those patients whose doctor has a high clinical suspicion, angiography may still be required for a definitive diagnosis, despite a negative scan.

Ultrasound

Kidney atrophy and loss of mass over time are related to RAS.[44] In patients suspected of RVH, kidney size should be measured. In serial studies, it should be determined if there is a loss of renal mass. The demonstration of a small kidney (< 7.5 cm) is important because the shrunken kidney is unlikely to respond to revascularization.[4] Testing should concentrate on detecting a potentially curable lesion in the normal-sized kidney.

The role of Doppler ultrasound in evaluating a patient for RAS is far from clear. Although some investigators have shown superb results with Doppler ultrasound imaging, others have failed to duplicate these results. Successful groups and skeptics all agree the test is technically challenging. Investigations to diagnose Doppler examinations to diagnose RAS have fallen into two broad techniques:

those that evaluate the renal arteries directly and those that evaluate the intrarenal vasculature.

Direct Doppler Evaluation of the Renal Artery

In this test, the renal artery is insonated along its course, and spectral Doppler tracings are obtained from the origin of the vessel to their entry into the kidney. Scanning is typically directed by color Doppler scanning (**Fig. 9–3**). For examination of the renal arteries, lower frequency transducers are often preferable, especially those at 2 to 2.5 MHz. Although resolution decreases with lower frequency transducers, attenuation also decreases, and this is the more critical factor. Filter settings should be set low yet high enough to suppress peristalsis, noise, and respiratory movement.

The left renal artery is found behind the left renal vein. The right renal artery originates at a similar level, or it can be found behind the inferior vena cava. Although the vessels travel posteriorly, their origins are typically from the middle, or even the anterior third, of the aorta. In certain patients, a decubitus view is helpful to move bowel out of the way. One can detect the renal origins in a coronal plane (**Fig. 9–4**).

Localization of the site of RAS is based on the detection of a high-velocity jet at the stenosis (**Fig. 9–5**). The velocity is maximal at the site of the tightest stenosis. Distal to the jet, secondary flow disturbances may exist. These include spectral broadening, shift of the distribution of blood velocities toward the baseline and away from the envelope, and simultaneous forward and reverse flow (**Fig. 9–6**). Velocities downstream from the stenotic jet are diminished. In some patients a bruit may be seen or heard. It appears on the spectrum as a low-velocity signal that is symmetrically above and below the baseline (**Fig. 9–7, Fig. 9–8**). Color Doppler may demonstrate a bruit as random color

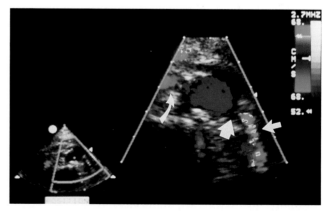

Figure 9–3 Renal color Doppler flow image of left renal artery stenosis shows marked narrowing of origin of the left renal artery (*thick straight arrow*). Red in the left renal artery, just after color is detected, represents aliasing (*thin straight arrow*). Normal right renal artery is also noted (*curved arrow*).

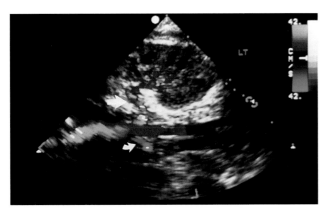

Figure 9–4 Coronal color Doppler flow image of renal artery origins. Left renal artery (*straight arrow*) can be traced in its entirety into the kidney. Proximal right renal artery (*curved arrow*) can also be seen.

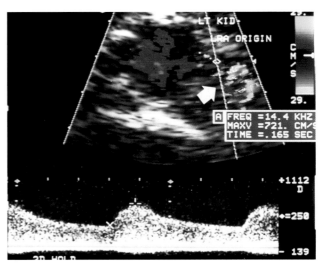

Figure 9–5 Left renal artery stenosis. Spectral color Doppler flow image shows marked narrowing of color column at origin of left renal artery. Sample volume within the narrowing yields a peak systolic velocity of 721 cm/s. Poststenotic dilatation (*arrow*) is seen distal to the narrowing. Note mosaic pattern, a mixture of colors in poststenotic regions that indicates aliasing.

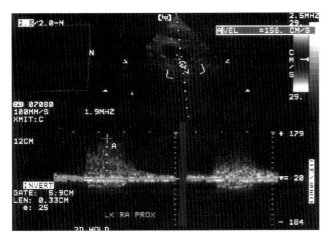

Figure 9–6 Spectral duplex Doppler image demonstrates downstream flow disturbances distal to a site of renal artery stenosis. Edge of the waveform is poorly seen. Whiter shades near the baseline indicate that more blood is moving at the lower velocities. Many different velocities are represented, which produces spectral broadening. Note simultaneous forward and reverse flow, probably the result of vortices and flow in many directions.

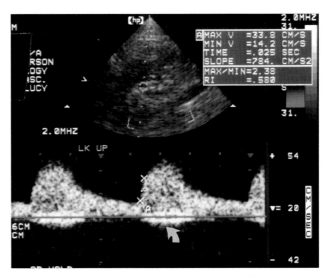

Figure 9–7 Spectral duplex Doppler intrarenal waveform with bruit. A strong, low-frequency symmetric signal above and below the baseline indicates a bruit (*arrow*). The bruit is pansystolic. Early systolic acceleration is measured as the slope in the fastest accelerating part of systole. Its value is 7.8 m/s^2. It is not measured to the peak systolic frequency, which occurs later in systole.

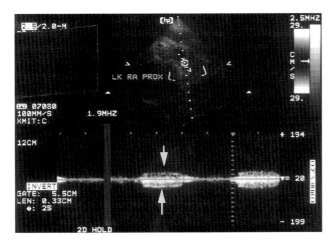

Figure 9–8 Spectral duplex Doppler image demonstrates bruit. Because bruits (*arrows*) travel through tissue, they can be detected even where no blood is flowing, as in this case. Bruits detected with Doppler imaging may not necessarily be auscultated and vice versa.

appearing in the adjacent soft tissues. Spectral or color bruits are usually detected in systole.

Color Doppler flow imaging can help detect stenoses as well as show the course of the vessels. Stenoses may be seen as narrowing of the color lumen (**Fig. 9–3, Fig. 9–5**). Poststenotic dilatation may also be appreciated (**Fig. 9–5**). The edge of the color does not exactly correspond to the edge of the flow because it may over- or underestimate the lumen, depending on the unit settings.

The high-velocity jet is seen as a change in color that reflects the change in velocity. The jet can be seen as a different intensity of the same color, but more frequently, it is seen as aliased color. Aliasing is produced by an inadequate sampling rate for the velocity that is being sampled. Color aliasing may be seen in a variety of ways: it may appear as a region where flow appears reversed (**Fig. 9–3**), as bands of color changes (an onion-skin appearance), or as a wilder "mosaic" pattern (**Fig. 9–5**).

Because the normal renal artery has no fixed velocity, many investigators have chosen to compare the velocity of the jet to that of the aorta where the renal arteries originate. The diagnosis of RAS is made when the value of the "renal:aortic ratio" (RAR) is elevated. The ratio is calculated by dividing the highest velocity obtained in the renal artery jet by the peak systolic velocity (PSV) of the aorta. A ratio over 3.5 has been correlated to RAS above 60% diameter reduction.[45–47] Other studies have looked at absolute velocities in the renal artery jet. Although earlier studies used lower values,[48] later studies used abnormal values of PSV > 180 cm/s[49,50] or > 200 cm/s with poststenotic flow disturbances to diagnose a stenosis greater than 60%.[46,51]

In an accredited laboratory, using colorflow duplex scanning, receiver operating characteristics (ROC) analysis determined that RAR and PSV had similar accuracy.[52] In this analysis, a PSV of 220 cm/s or greater yielded a sensitivity of 91% and specificity of 85%. The best RAR was 3.2, which yielded a sensitivity of 81% and a specificity of 89%. An RAR of 3.5 yielded a sensitivity of 72% with a specificity of 92%.

In an early prospective evaluation of ultrasound duplex scanning of the main renal artery, Taylor et al[45] found a sensitivity of 84%, specificity of 97%, and positive predictive value of 94%; 12% of scans were technically inadequate.

Olin et al[46] reported detection of 98% of stenoses and occlusions (31/32 cases with stenoses of 60 to 79%, 67/69 cases with stenoses of 80 to 99%, and 22/23 cases with occlusions). Specificity was 99%. One hour was allowed for the studies, which were performed by vascular technologists. Because only main renal arteries were reported, the analysis did not evaluate any accessory renal vessels.

Hoffman et al[49] had a 10% failure rate. In this study sensitivity was 92% (44/48 cases with stenoses) but the specificity was only 62% for 60% stenoses. Ten of 11 patients with occlusions were correctly identified.

Hansen, et al[53] showed excellent results for cases where there was one renal artery (sensitivity 93%, specificity 98%). However, only 49% of accessory vessels were detected. When all kidneys were considered, the resultant sensitivity was 88%.

Halpern et al[54] used similar techniques and employed experienced vascular technologists, taking as long as necessary to produce an examination. The sensitivity for the RAR was 71% with a specificity of 91%. This is also identical to the results of Krumme et al,[55] who showed 71% sensitivity and 96% specificity for abnormal PSV greater than 200 cm/s.

Spies et al[56] evaluated 135 consecutive patients using color duplex sonography. Although they had trouble identifying all segments of the renal arteries, in those with adequate scans (75% of patients, 195 arteries), the sensitivity was 93% and specificity 92%. All 12 stenosis above 75% were detected, although one was considered a 50 to 74% stenosis.

A more recent report utilized colorflow and tissue harmonic imaging.[49] Despite these technical advances, bowel gas made arteries in 9% of patients unevaluable and accessory arteries were not seen in 16 of the 19 present. All patients had atherosclerotic RAS. Doppler detected 91% (CI 89 to 93%) of stenoses and had a specificity of 97% (CI 92 to 96%).

Scanning the main renal artery is time consuming and does not reliably detect accessory vessels. Technical failure continues to be a problem because bowel gas can obscure the vessels. An overnight fast and bowel prep can help minimize this.[50,53]

Van der Hulst et al[57] validated the use of PSV and renal artery ratios for RAS. Using a Doppler guidewire, this group compared the renal artery parameters to hemodynamically significant RAS as determined by transstenotic pressure gradients in 30 vessels. This group determined that PSV and velocity ratios did correlate with RAS. Furthermore, the ROC curves produced by absolute velocity measurements were equal to those generated by digital subtraction angiography.

Intrarenal Artery Evaluation

Handa et al[58,59] described abnormal waveforms in vessels downstream from renal stenoses. Handa's group described a series of indices using frequency: the acceleration index, acceleration time, and a comparison of acceleration time in the renal artery compared with the aorta. Several years later Martin et al[60] described successful results with a flank rather than translumbar approach. This Australian group described the initial systolic (the so-called compliance) peak but did not use its appearance to make a diagnosis. The work of Stavros et al[61] resulted in more widespread interest in the technique in the United States. Several European groups were also pursuing intrarenal evaluation at that time.[62–64]

Normal intrarenal signals show a rapid rise during early systole and continuous flow through diastole (**Fig. 9–9, Fig. 9–10**). To be accurate when one measures intrarenal waveforms, the scale should be diminished so the waveform fills the spectrum. The sweep rate should be fast so only one or two waveforms are in the image. Measurement errors are reduced if the size of the spectral display is larger. The highest frequency transducer that can give an adequate signal is used, preferably 3 to 5 MHz. Position and Doppler settings should be optimized to maximize signal to noise. The Doppler angle should be minimized. Doppler parameters such as acceleration are angle-dependent because they re-

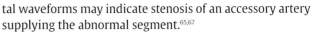

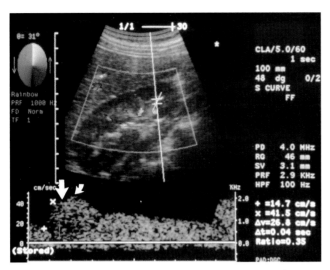

Figure 9–9 Normal intrarenal spectral Doppler waveform. The spectrum has been optimized so that one waveform fills the whole spectrum. Sweep speed is rapid so only one complete cardiac cycle is displayed. Doppler angle is determined by direction of blood flow on the color image. The angle of 31 degrees is acceptably low. Early systolic acceleration is the slope from the + marker to the x marker. In early systole, the fast-moving flow hesitates (*straight arrow*), slows down, then speeds up to peak systole (*curved arrow*). The acute angle at the hesitation marks the early systolic compliance peak/reflective wave complex.

quire velocity measurements. One should attempt measurement along the plane of the intrarenal arteries, and angles should be routinely less than 30 degrees.

Intrarenal waveforms are taken from the hilus and from segmental waveforms from the upper, middle, and lower kidney (**Fig. 9–9**). Interlobar or interlobular arteries can be used,[65] although it is not known if the same normal values will apply because waveform shapes can vary along the vessels.[66] Differences in the appearance between segmen-

tal waveforms may indicate stenosis of an accessory artery supplying the abnormal segment.[65,67]

In distinction to the main renal artery test, which may take an hour or more, intrarenal scanning usually takes around 20 minutes. Technical failures rarely occur because the kidney can usually be insonated. Martin et al[60] reported a failure rate of 1.5%, although a recent investigation had a 16% failure rate.[68] Patients' inability to hold their breath is the most common cause of technical difficulties. A small kidney or poor flow caused by severe occlusive disease are other causes.

In stenosis, there is a slow rise to the peak velocity distal to the stenosis, the so-called pulsus tardus. The slope (which is the systolic acceleration) of the systolic rise is diminished and the time to the first peak velocity is lengthened (diminished acceleration time) (**Fig. 9–10, Fig. 9–11**). The arterial stenosis "filters" the normally complex arterial pulse. In early systole, this filtering accounts for diminished acceleration. The stenosis evens out the changes between systole and diastole and produces diminished pulsatility. In extreme cases, pulsatility is so diminished that the artery may resemble a vein (**Fig. 9–12**).

Martin et al and others[60,61] have described a normal early systolic compliance peak (ESP), which is an acute angle formed after the early systolic rise (**Fig. 9–9, Fig. 9–10**). ESP was associated with normal upstream vessels and was lost if there was proximal RAS. Halpern et al evaluated this phenomenon with a phantom.[66] Their results suggest the early peak is caused by transmitted systole. Following this the blood slows and may speed up again. It is this region, in the later part of systole, which is the produced by compliance. Furthermore, phantom studies suggested that changes in compliance could significantly affect the appearance of renal waveforms.[66,69]

In Martin et al's study, acceleration time and acceleration index were 87% sensitive and 98% specific.[60] Stavros et

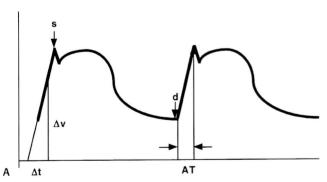

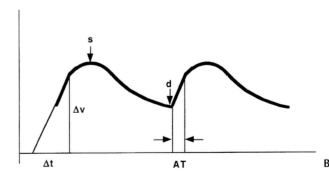

Figure 9–10 Intrarenal waveform parameters in (**A**) a normal and (**B**) abnormal waveform. Early systolic acceleration is the slope of the fastest-moving portion of the systolic component (v/t). It is not the slope of the waveform to peak systole (s) unless there is one continuous straight line to peak systole [as is the case in waveform (**B**) but not waveform (**A**)]. Acceleration time (AT) is the time it takes to get to the first inflection of the waveform (between two arrows). In the normal case (**A**) this is the time to peak systole. In the abnormal waveform (**B**)

this is the time to the first inflection, which occurs earlier than peak systole. The early systolic compliance peak/reflective wave complex (ESP) is identified in waveform (**A**) at the acute angle in the waveform just after the first peak (s). The ESP is not present in waveform (**B**). Resistance index is calculated by the (peak systolic velocity − end diastolic velocity)/peak systolic velocity or (s − d)/s. The pulsatility index uses the mean velocity (not shown) as the denominator.

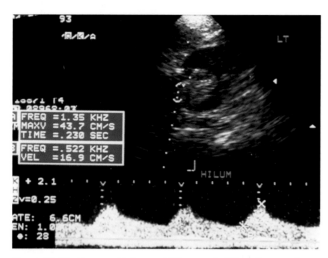

Figure 9–11 Abnormal intrarenal hilar spectral Doppler waveform. The slope of systolic acceleration is diminished, and the time to peak systole is prolonged (0.23 s), indicating proximal stenosis.

al[61] found the acceleration time to be only 78% sensitive and 94% specific, and the acceleration index to be 89% sensitive and 83% specific. Kliewer et al[70] found that the acceleration time and index distinguished normal from abnormal vessels only when the stenosis was severe (80 to 95%), but not when all the stenoses above 50% were considered. The result is not entirely unexpected because 50% diameter-reducing lesions are not hemodynamically significant in the kidneys. Higher-grade lesions of 60 to 75% may actually be necessary to produce downstream changes.[65,71,72] Indirect measures are generally less sensi-

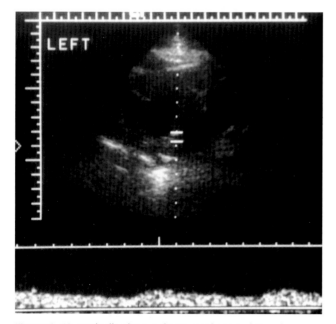

Figure 9–12 Markedly abnormal intrarenal spectral Doppler waveform shows greatly diminished systolic acceleration. Pulsatility is markedly low, to the extent that the artery might be mistaken for a vein. Note loss of the early systolic compliance peak.

tive; Motew et al demonstrated only a sensitivity of 58% using acceleration time for stenoses greater than 60%.[51]

Halpern et al[54] found the best intrarenal test to be early systolic acceleration, which is the slope of the fastest moving part of the early waveform. Early systolic acceleration is not always the slope to the PSV (**Fig. 9–7, Fig. 9–10**). Values of less than 3 m/s^2 were considered abnormal. Minimum early systolic acceleration had 86% sensitivity and 91% specificity. Halpern et al[54] concluded that a slope was better than acceleration time because the onset of acceleration is not precisely defined. Gottlieb et al[73] also determined that difficulty determining the onset of systole was the largest source of error in intrarenal measurements.

Stavros et al[61] found that a visual estimate of an abnormal waveform, as determined by the loss of the ESP, was better than any calculated measure. This loss had a sensitivity of 95% and a specificity of 97%. Because recognition of ESP is a visual parameter that describes the waveform shape, it does not require any calculation. Visual estimates of waveform shape were unsuccessful in the study by Halpern et al,[54] with the exception of a truly blunted waveform, which had a specificity of 100%. Kliewer et al[74] also found the interpretation of waveform morphology to be unsuccessful in predicting the presence or severity of RAS. However, in another study using pattern recognition before and after captopril, Rene et al[75] found this technique useful after captopril. Pattern recognition was only 68% sensitive at baseline, but rose to 100% after captopril.

Accessory vessels were identified as contributing to the misses in several of the studies.[60,70,76] Increased pulsatility in renal vessels is also associated with missed diagnosis,[60,65,77] which may be due to diminished compliance or elevated resistance.[69]

Pulsatility parameters evaluate the shape of a Doppler waveform by evaluating the relationship between peak systolic velocity and end diastolic velocity. Two common indices are the pulsatility index (PI), which is (peak systolic velocity − end diastolic velocity)/mean velocity, and the resistance index (RI), which is (peak systolic velocity − end diastolic velocity)/end diastolic velocity.

Soulen et al[78] showed that the intrarenal RI changed significantly from baseline following angioplasty. Ozbek et al[64] showed there were significant differences in PI and RI between normal kidneys and those with RAS. Bardelli et al[62] used side-to-side PI differences to diagnose unilateral RAS. In initial trials, Schwerk et al[79] determined that a difference of the RI of greater than 5% between the kidneys was 82% sensitive and 92% specific for RAS, while greater than 50% and 100% sensitive and 94% specific for stenoses with greater than 60% diameter reduction. The group conceded the test might not be as good for bilateral stenoses, and they recommended considering bilaterally low indices as suggesting bilateral RAS.

Subsequent studies using pulsatility have not been as encouraging. Burdick et al[80] evaluated acceleration, acceleration time, PI, RI, and side-to-side differences of PI and RI.

This group found acceleration and acceleration time to be superior to any of the pulsatility parameters. Side to side RI differences were only 73% sensitive and 86% specific. Bilateral disease accounted for some of the errors in using RI or PI. Acceleration time was significantly correlated with the degree of narrowing, whereas RI and PI correlated with age rather than RAS. Both acceleration time and pulsatility worked better in those with fibromuscular dysplasia than atherosclerosis. The authors postulated that changes in pulsatility due to age and atherosclerosis reduced the accuracy of the pulsatility parameters. This was probably due to resistance and compliance differences in the older, stiffer vessels. Pedersen et al[81] found a kidney length difference of 1 cm or a PI difference of greater than 0.1 to be only 75% sensitive and 76% specific for stenoses above 50%, and 84% sensitive and 73% specific for stenoses above 70%. Krumme et al[55] had a sensitivity of only 51% for bilateral stenosis.

Doppler to Predict Response to Revascularization

Preprocedural Doppler parameters have shown conflicting results to predict blood pressure or renal function response after revascularization. Pulsatility parameters change after successful revascularization for RVH.[64,65,78] Although Frauchiger et al[82] showed intervention was less successful if diastole was less than 30% of systole, Hansen et al[53] did not find a relationship between end diastolic values and the response of blood pressure or renal function to revascularization. Krumme et al[55] were also unable to show a relationship between preoperative side-to-side differences of RI and blood pressure response after successful treatment.

A prospective trial by Radermacher et al of 131 patients suggested that those with resistive indices above 0.80 were unlikely to improve their hypertension or renal function after balloon angioplasty.[83] More recently, authors have questioned this after revascularization with stents demonstrated better results despite nephrosclerosis.[84] A Doppler study by Garcia-Criado et al also does not support an upper limit of the pulsatility index to withhold revascularization.[85] Their prospective evaluation in 36 patients followed for 23 ± 15 months demonstrated improvement in blood pressure and renal function for some patients with an RI greater than 0.80. More patients showed benefit if the RI was lower, but blood pressure improved in both groups (85% for those with low RI compared with 50% in the high RI group, a significant difference), as did renal function (45% vs 28.5%, not significant). A decline in renal function occurred in 18% of the low RI group compared with 35% in the high RI group ($P = .407$). Larger studies will be necessary to determine if Doppler indices can be used to predict who may or may not benefit from revascularization.[76]

Renal Artery or Intrarenal Evaluation

Van der Hulst et al[57] seriously challenged the validity of all the intrarenal Doppler analyses. In this study using pressure gradients as a gold standard, no intrarenal parameter (acceleration time, acceleration, RI, PI, or loss of ESP) correlated with the presence of RAS. The group also found that the ROC curve of PSV is equal to angiography. This indicates that the direct renal artery study is potentially as accurate as an angiogram. However, in the real world, transabdominal scanning is not as accurate as the Doppler guidewire. The changing Doppler angle, bowel gas, deep position, and diminished signal from flow-reducing lesions all contribute to transabdominal inaccuracies and technical failures.

It is the technical difficulties encountered in certain patients rather than the interpretation of the test that makes direct renal artery duplex difficult. The criteria of an RAR above 3.5 or a PSV of greater than 180 to 200 cm/s is reproducible. In technically adequate examinations, renal artery duplex scanning can reliably detect and exclude main renal artery stenosis. An adequate amount of time must be allowed to perform the study. The experience of the sonographer or vascular technologist is crucial; the more experienced sonographer will make fewer mistakes and produce fewer inadequate examinations. An experienced examiner will also be able to determine if the study is reliable or limited. When color or spectral Doppler evaluation does not demonstrate substantial portions of the renal arteries, the results should be reported as less reliable unless there is unequivocal evidence for RAS in the region seen. Those with limited examinations may need additional testing with another modality.

Intrarenal Doppler parameters are easier to produce, but their significance is more difficult to interpret. The degree of stenosis,[71] etiology of the lesion,[55] resistance and compliance,[66,69] age of the patient, presence of parenchymal disease,[66] and arterial pressure[63]—all affect the final waveform shape. It is unknown if medical therapy itself affects waveform shape. Severe stenoses are correlated with the intrarenal indices, but less severe stenoses are not. Some investigators feel this is because those lesser stenoses are not hemodynamically significant based on some experimental data.[65] The results of van der Hulst et al, appear to refute this concept.[57]

The slope of the early systolic acceleration is more reproducible than acceleration time.[54,73] Acceleration and acceleration time are less accurate in pulsatile renal arteries, presumably due to intrinsic renal disease. Determining if there is loss of ESP is operator dependent[65] and not reproducible.[54,70,74,86] Pulsatility parameters are not accurate enough and miss many bilateral stenoses.

A very blunted waveform[54] or a very long acceleration time (above 0.12 s[68]) have a high predictive value for RAS. Normal intrarenal waveforms and mildly abnormal measurements are less reliable. Direct renal artery evaluation should always be performed if there are normal or equivocal intrarenal results. This is particularly true if there is diminished diastolic flow.

Future research efforts should be made to make direct renal evaluation simpler and to diminish the number of inadequate studies. It is hoped that by increasing the signal from the blood, intravenous microbubble contrast agents can improve the accuracy of renal Doppler. In two initial studies of direct renal artery evaluation,[87] and intrarenal evaluation,[77] contrast enhancement improved the results and shortened the examination time. In a multicenter trial, the number of inadequate scans decreased with contrast, but neither the sensitivity nor the specificity improved.[88]

The etiology of suspected RAS helps determine if Doppler should be performed and how it should be interpreted. Direct renal artery duplex scanning detects RAS in large, typically main vessels. Accessory vessels are routinely missed.[31,48,53,56,89,90] This may be less important in atherosclerotic patients because some investigators feel renal artery stenosis in small accessory vessels rarely causes hypertension in this group.[89] Fibromuscular dysplasia is different—patients may have RVH from main or intrarenal stenoses. In those suspected of fibromuscular dysplasia, the significance of a normal Doppler study is not reassuring because accessory and branch disease may be missed. Patients with suspected fibromuscular dysplasia might require angiography because angiography is currently the only examination that has the resolution to evaluate intrarenal stenoses well.

Other Causes of Abdominal Bruit

Significant stenoses in any vessel may produce a bruit. In the abdomen, common locations for occlusive disease are the celiac axis and superior mesenteric artery. In patients who present with a bruit, and in whom the renal arteries are not stenotic, evaluating the celiac axis and superior mesenteric artery may be worthwhile to determine if they are stenosed (**Fig. 9–13**). Bruits from stenoses in the iliac artery are heard lower in the abdomen than the bruit from upper abdominal vessels. Bruits from arteriovenous fistulas usually have a continuous quality. Epigastric bruits are more common from the celiac axis or superior mesenteric artery, whereas flank bruits are more typical for a renal origin.

Renal arteriovenous fistulas (**Fig. 9–14**) are associated with bruits.[8] They often appear as a cystic mass, typically in a hilar location. Color flow imaging demonstrates flow in these lesions. Arteriovenous fistulas have a typical high-velocity spectral waveform with low pulsatility. Fistulas are often congenital, although they are found in renal car-

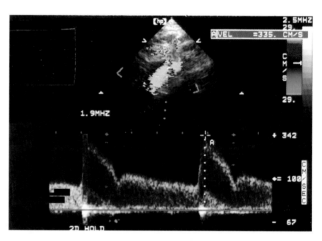

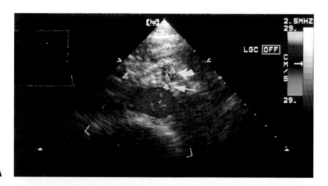

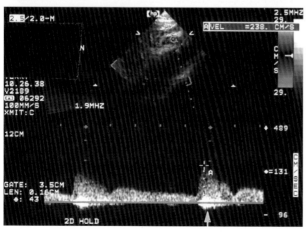

Figure 9–13 Celiac axis stenosis producing abdominal bruit. Patient had a bruit, and a diagnosis of renal artery stenosis had been ruled out. **(A)** Color Doppler flow image shows celiac stenosis with narrowing of color column immediately after the celiac origin (*straight arrow*). Distal to the stenosis, a mosaic pattern of color can be seen (*curved arrow*), which represents aliasing. **(B)** Spectral Doppler image shows celiac stenosis with high-velocity jet (335 cm/s) at origin of the celiac axis. Jet has a well-defined envelope and no spectral broadening because jets have laminar flow. A second, smaller waveform, superimposed on the celiac waveform, is the aortic signal, which is partially in the sample volume. **(C)** Spectral Doppler image shows celiac stenosis with bruit. Downstream from the jet, the velocity diminishes (238 cm/s). Note the spectral broadening. Systolic bruit is shown (*arrow*) as a symmetrical, low-velocity waveform above and below the baseline.

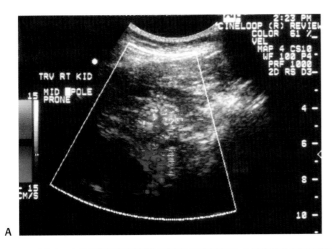

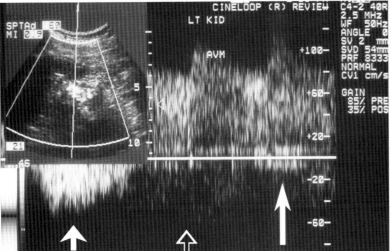

Figure 9–14 Renal arteriovenous fistula. **(A)** Transverse color Doppler flow image of the right renal hilum shows a large area of color not conforming to normal vessels indicating a vascular malformation. **(B)** Spectral Doppler image shows an increased velocity and markedly increased diastolic velocity indicating diminished pulsatility from arteriovenous shunting. Systolic acceleration is normal and there is spectral broadening. A continuous bruit can be seen as a symmetrical, low-velocity waveform above and below the baseline (*arrow*). Flow below the baseline is renal vein in the early portion of the spectrum (*from a short arrow*) and disturbed flow in the later portion (*open arrow*). (Case courtesy of Beatrice Madrazo, M.D., William Beaumont Hospital, Royal Oak, MI)

cinoma and after trauma. Parenchymal arteriovenous fistulas may be seen after kidney biopsy.

Midaortic syndrome may cause hypertension and bruit. In this case, the aorta is narrowed, possibly affecting the renal, celiac, or superior mesenteric arteries. More commonly, the aorta alone is narrowed. Because the renal arteries are downstream from the stenosis, their waveforms are abnormal, showing diminished pulsatility and systolic upstroke. A jet may be identified in the aorta at the site of the narrowing. Distal flow disturbances such as spectral broadening can be identified in the aorta beyond the narrowing.

Summary

Although clinicians can identify some patients at greater risk for RVH, there is no consensus on who should be tested. A noninvasive test cannot be applied to all hypertensive patients. Clinical criteria are needed to establish a subgroup of patients with a high prevalence of RVH. Part of the reluctance to study patients results from the lack of well-defined criteria for defining who will benefit from

revascularization, and from the lack of a clearly effective screening test. Angiography is the standard, but it is invasive and carries some risk. Nuclear scanning after captopril has some appeal because it reflects the pathophysiology of RAS. However, the ability of scintigraphy to predict the outcome after revascularization is not as good as might be expected. Nuclear scanning is not warranted if there is renal insufficiency or a small kidney.

Ultrasound studies show wide variations. Although there are technical failures, direct evaluation is generally accurate if the technical quality of the study is adequate. Intrarenal waveform analysis has not been the panacea it was hoped to be. The use of renal pulsatility indices to predict the results of catheter-based treatments has shown variable results and awaits further study.

MRA and CTA are more accurate than nuclear medicine or ultrasound; however, not all patients are candidates for these tests for reasons such as renal insufficiency, claustrophobia, or allergy. Technical failures also occur with these tests, which are far more expensive than ultrasound.

Outcome analyses incorporating the accuracy, cost, technical success, and complication rates are not available and need to be performed. Various diagnostic pathways should be evaluated, including proceeding straight to angiography, directly to CT or MRA, and using ultrasound. Decision analyses should not simply use positive and negative results but should evaluate technically limited studies to determine how they might be handled.

In high-risk groups, it may not be appropriate to use a screening test. In some patients (for instance, those with suspected fibromuscular dysplasia and normal renal function), it is appropriate to go directly to angiography.

References

1. Schreiber MJ, Pohl MA, Novick AC. The natural history of atherosclerotic and fibrous renal artery disease. Urol Clin North Am 1984; 11:383–392
2. Meyrier A. Renal vascular lesions in the elderly: nephrosclerosis or atheromatous renal disease? Nephrol Dial Transplant 1996;11 (Suppl 9):45–52
3. O'Neil EA, Hansen KJ, Canzanello VJ, Pennell TC, Dean RH. Prevalence of ischemic nephropathy in patients with renal insufficiency. Am Surg 1992;58:485–490
4. Textor SC, Wilcox CS. Renal artery stenosis: a common, treatable cause of renal failure? Annu Rev Med 2001;52:421–442
5. Palmaz JC. The current status of vascular intervention in ischemic nephropathy. J Vasc Interv Radiol 1998;9:539–543
6. Weinrauch LA, D'Elia JA. Renal artery stenosis: "fortuitous diagnosis," problematic therapy. J Am Coll Cardiol 2004;43:1614–1616
7. Goldblatt H, Lynch J, Hanzal RF, Summerville WW. Studies on experimental hypertension, I: The production of persistent elevation of systolic blood pressure by means of renal ischemia. J Exp Med 1934;59:347–378
8. Van Way CW. Renal artery aneurysms and arteriovenous fistulas. In: Rutherford RB, ed. Vascular Surgery. 4th ed. Philadelphia: WB Saunders; 1995:1274–1286
9. Mann S, Pickering T. Detection of renovascular hypertension: state of the art: 1992. Ann Intern Med 1992;117:845–853
10. Detection, evaluation, and treatment of renovascular hypertension: final report of the working group on renovascular hypertension. Arch Intern Med 1987;147:820–829
11. Simon N, Franklin SS, Bleifer KH, Maxwell MH. Clinical characteristics of renovascular hypertension. JAMA 1972;220:1209–1218
12. van Jaarsveld BC, Derkx FH, Krijnen P, et al. Hypertension resistant to two-drug treatment is a useful criterion to select patients for angiography: the Dutch Renal Artery Stenosis Intervention Cooperative (DRASTIC) study. Contrib Nephrol 1996;119:54–58
13. Derkx FH, van Jaarsveld BC, Krijnen P, et al. Renal artery stenosis towards the year 2000. J Hypertens Suppl 1996;14:S167–S172
14. Ducher M, Cerutti C, Marquand A, et al. How to limit screening of patients for atheromatous renal artery stenosis in two-drug resistant hypertension? J Nephrol 2005;18:161–165
15. Textor SC. Pitfalls in imaging for renal artery stenosis. Ann Intern Med 2004;141:730–731
16. Dean RH. Renovascular hypertension: an overview. In: Rutherford RB, ed. Vascular Surgery. 4th ed. Philadelphia: WB Saunders; 1995: 1371–1377
17. Vaughan ED. Pathophysiology of renovascular hypertension. In: Rutherford RB, ed. Vascular Surgery. 4th ed. Philadelphia: WB Saunders; 1995:1377–1390
18. Nally JV. Provocative captopril testing in the diagnosis of renovascular hypertension. Urol Clin North Am 1994;21:227–234
19. Prigent A. The diagnosis of renovascular hypertension: the role of captopril renal scintigraphy and related issues. [see comments] Eur J Nucl Med 1993;20:625–644
20. Fommei E, Ghione S, Hilson AJ, et al. Captopril radionuclide test in renovascular hypertension: a European multicentre study. European Multicentre Study Group. Eur J Nucl Med 1993;20: 617–623
21. Borrello JA, Li D, Vesely TM, et al. Renal arteries: clinical comparison of three-dimensional time-of-flight MR angiographic sequences and radiographic angiography. Radiology 1995;197:793–799
22. De Cobelli F, Mellone R, Salvioni M, et al. Renal artery stenosis: value of screening with three-dimensional phase-contrast MR angiography with a phased-array multicoil. Radiology 1996;201: 697–703
23. Debatin JF, Spritzer CE, Grist TM, et al. Imaging of the renal arteries: value of MR angiography. AJR Am J Roentgenol. 1991;157:981–990
24. Gedroyc WM, Neerhut P, Negus R, et al. Magnetic resonance angiography of renal artery stenosis. Clin Radiol 1995;50:436–439
25. Loubeyre P, Revel D, Garcia P, et al. Screening patients for renal artery stenosis: value of three-dimensional time-of-flight MR angiography. AJR Am J Roentgenol 1994;162:847–852
26. Kim D, Edelman RR, Kent KC, Porter DH, Skillman JJ. Abdominal aorta and renal artery stenosis: evaluation with MR angiography. Radiology 1990;174:727–731
27. Kent KC, Edelman RR, Kim D, et al. Magnetic resonance imaging: a reliable test for the evaluation of proximal atherosclerotic renal arterial stenosis. J Vasc Surg 1991;13:311–318
28. Postma CT, Hartog O, Rosenbusch G, Thien T. Magnetic resonance angiography in the diagnosis of renal artery stenosis. J Hypertens 1993;11(Suppl):S204–S205
29. Rieumont MJ, Kaufman JA, Geller SC, et al. Evaluation of renal artery stenosis with dynamic gadolinium-enhanced MR angiography. AJR Am J Roentgenol 1997;169:39–44
30. Servois V, Laissy JP, Feger C, et al. Two-dimensional time-of-flight magnetic resonance angiography of renal arteries without maximum intensity projection: a prospective comparison with angiography in 21 patients screened for renovascular hypertension. Cardiovasc Intervent Radiol 1994;17:138–142
31. Strotzer M, Fellner CM, Geissler A, et al. Noninvasive assessment of renal artery stenosis: a comparison of MR angiography, color Doppler sonography, and intraarterial angiography. Acta Radiol 1995;36:243–247
32. Yucel EK, Kaufman JA, Prince M, et al. Time of flight renal MR angiography: utility in patients with renal insufficiency. Magn Reson Imaging 1993;11:925–930
33. Bakker J, Beek FJ, Beutler JJ, et al. Renal artery stenosis and accessory renal arteries: accuracy of detection and visualization with gadolinium-enhanced breath-hold MR angiography. Radiology 1998;207:497–504
34. Postma CT, Joosten FB, Rosenbusch G, Thien T. Magnetic resonance angiography has a high reliability in the detection of renal artery stenosis. Am J Hypertens 1997;10(9 Pt 1):957–963
35. Vasbinder GB, Nelemans PJ, Kessels AG, Kroon AA, De Leeuw PW, Van Engelshoven JM. Diagnostic tests for renal artery stenosis in patients suspected of having renovascular hypertension: a meta-analysis. Ann Intern Med 2001;135:401–411
36. Vasbinder GB, Nelemans PJ, Kessels AG, et al, Renal Artery Diagnostic Imaging Study in Hypertension (RADros Inf ServH) Study Group. Accuracy of computed tomographic angiography and magnetic res-

onance angiography for diagnosing renal artery stenosis. Ann Intern Med 2004;141:674–684; discussion 682

37. Ros PR, Gauger J, Stoupis C, et al. Diagnosis of renal artery stenosis: feasibility of combining MR angiography, MR renography, and gadopentetate-based measurements of glomerular filtration rate. AJR Am J Roentgenol 1995;165:1447–1451

38. Kaatee R, Beek FJA, de Lange EE, et al. Renal artery stenosis: detection and quantification with spiral CT angiography versus optimized digital subtraction angiography. Radiology 1997;205:121–127

39. Elkohen M, Beregi JP, Deklunder G, et al. A prospective study of helical computed tomography angiography versus angiography for the detection of renal artery stenoses in hypertensive patients. J Hypertens 1996;14:525–528

40. Olbricht CJ, Paul K, Prokop M, et al. Minimally invasive diagnosis of renal artery stenosis by spiral computed tomography angiography. Kidney Int 1995;48:1332–1337

41. Zeman RK, Fox SH, Silverman PM, et al. Helical (spiral) CT of the abdomen. AJR Am J Roentgenol 1993;160:719–725

42. Halpern EJ, Wechsler RJ, DiCampli D. Threshold selection for CT angiography shaded surface display of the renal arteries. J Digit Imaging 1995;8:142–147

43. Willmann JK, Wildermuth S, Pfammatter T, et al. Aortoiliac and renal arteries: prospective intraindividual comparison of contrast-enhanced three-dimensional MR angiography and multi-detector row CT angiography. Radiology 2003;226:798–811

44. Guzman RP, Zierler RE, Isaacson JA, Bergelin RO, Strandness DJ. Renal atrophy and arterial stenosis: a prospective study with duplex ultrasound. Hypertension 1994;23:346–350

45. Taylor DC, Kettler MD, Moneta GL, et al. Duplex ultrasound scanning in the diagnosis of renal artery stenosis: a prospective evaluation. J Vasc Surg 1988;7:363–369

46. Olin JW, Piedmonte MR, Young JR, et al. The utility of duplex ultrasound scanning of the renal arteries for diagnosing significant renal artery stenosis. Ann Intern Med 1995;122:833–838

47. Kohler TR, Zierler RE, Martin RL, et al. Noninvasive diagnosis of renal artery stenosis by ultrasonic duplex scanning. J Vasc Surg 1986;4:450–456

48. Desberg AL, Paushter DM, Lammert GK, et al. Renal artery stenosis: evaluation with color Doppler flow imaging. Radiology 1990;177:749–753

49. Hoffmann U, Edwards JM, Carter S, et al. Role of duplex scanning for the detection of atherosclerotic renal artery disease. Kidney Int 1991;39:1232–1239

50. Nchimi A, Biquet JF, Brisbois D, et al. Duplex ultrasound as first-line screening test for patients suspected of renal artery stenosis: prospective evaluation in high risk group. Eur Radiol 2003;13:1413–1419

51. Motew SJ, Cherr GS, Craven TE, et al. Renal duplex sonography: main renal artery versus hilar analysis. J Vasc Surg 2000;32:462–469;462–471

52. Hua HT, Hood DB, Jensen CC, Hanks SE, Weaver FA. The use of colorflow duplex scanning to detect significant renal artery stenosis. Ann Vasc Surg 2000;14:118–124

53. Hansen KJ, Tribble RW, Reavis SW, et al. Renal duplex sonography: evaluation of clinical utility. J Vasc Surg 1990;12:227–236

54. Halpern EJ, Needleman L, Nack TL, East SA. Renal artery stenosis: should we study the main renal artery or segmental vessels? Radiology 1995;195:799–804

55. Krumme B, Blum U, Schwertfeger E, et al. Diagnosis of renovascular disease by intra- and extrarenal Doppler scanning. Kidney Int 1996;50:1288–1292

56. Spies KP, Fobbe F, El-Bedewi M, et al. Color-coded duplex sonography for noninvasive diagnosis and grading of renal artery stenosis. Am J Hypertens 1995;8(12 Pt 1):1222–1231

57. van der Hulst VP, van Baalen J, Kool LS, et al. Renal artery stenosis: endovascular flow wire study for validation of Doppler US. [see comments] Radiology 1996;200:165–168

58. Handa N, Fukanaga R, Etani H, et al. Efficacy of echo-Doppler examination for the evaluation of renovascular disease. Ultrasound Med Biol 1988;14:1–15

59. Handa N, Fukanaga R, Uehara A, et al. Echo-Doppler velocimeter in the diagnosis of hypertensive patients: the renal artery Doppler technique. Ultrasound Med Biol 1986;12:945–952

60. Martin RL, Nanra RS, Wlodarczyk J, DeSilva A, Bray AE. Renal hilar Doppler analysis in the detection of renal artery stenosis. J Vasc Tech 1991;15:173–180

61. Stavros AT, Parker SH, Yakes WF, et al. Segmental stenosis of the renal artery: pattern recognition of tardus and parvus abnormalities with duplex sonography. [see comments] Radiology 1992;184:487–492

62. Bardelli M, Jensen G, Volkmann R, Aurell M. Noninvasive ultrasound assessment of renal artery stenosis by means of the Gosling pulsatility index. J Hypertens 1992;10:985–989

63. Veglio F, Provera E, Pinna G, et al. Renal resistive index after captopril test by echo-Doppler in essential hypertension. [see comments] Am J Hypertens 1992;5:431–436

64. Ozbek SS, Aytac SK, Erden MI, Sanlidilek NU. Intrarenal Doppler findings of upstream renal artery stenosis: a preliminary report. Ultrasound Med Biol 1993;19:3–12

65. Stavros T, Harshfield D. Renal Doppler: renal artery stenosis, and renovascular hypertension: direct and indirect duplex sonographic abnormalities in patients with renal artery stenosis. Ultrasound Q 1994;12:217–263

66. Halpern EJ, Deane CR, Needleman L, Merton DA, East SA. Normal renal artery spectral Doppler waveform: a closer look. Radiology 1995;196:667–673

67. Hall NJ, Thorpe RJ, MacKechnie SG. Stenosis of the accessory renal artery: Doppler ultrasound findings. Australas Radiol 1995;39:73–77

68. Baxter GM, Aitchison F, Sheppard D, et al. Colour Doppler ultrasound in renal artery stenosis: intrarenal waveform analysis. Br J Radiol 1996;69:810–815

69. Bude RO, Rubin JM, Platt JF, Fechner KP, Adler RS. Pulsus tardus: its cause and potential limitations in detection of arterial stenosis. Radiology 1994;190:779–784

70. Kliewer MA, Tupler RH, Carroll BA, et al. Renal artery stenosis: analysis of Doppler waveform parameters and tardus-parvus pattern. Radiology 1993;189:779–787

71. Lafortune M, Patriquin H, Demeule E, et al. Renal arterial stenosis: slowed systole in the downstream circulation: experimental study in dogs. Radiology 1992;184:475–478

72. Strandness DE Jr. Duplex imaging for the detection of renal artery stenosis. Am J Kidney Dis 1994;24:674–678

73. Gottlieb RH, Snitzer EL, Hartley DF, Fultz PJ, Rubens DJ. Interobserver and intraobserver variation in determining intrarenal parameters by Doppler sonography. AJR Am J Roentgenol 1997;168:627–631

74. Kliewer MA, Tupler RH, Hertzberg BS, et al. Doppler evaluation of renal artery stenosis: interobserver agreement in the interpretation of waveform morphology. AJR Am J Roentgenol 1994;162:1371–1376

75. Rene PC, Oliva VL, Bui BT, et al. Renal artery stenosis: evaluation of Doppler US after inhibition of angiotensin-converting enzyme with captopril. [see comments] Radiology 1995;196:675–679

76. Nazzal MMS, Hoballah JJ, Miller EV, et al. Renal hilar Doppler analysis is of value in the management of patients with renovascular disease. Am J Surg 1997;174:164–168

77. Missouris CG, Allen CM, Balen FG, et al. Noninvasive screening for renal artery stenosis with ultrasound contrast enhancement. J Hypertens 1996;14:519–524

78. Soulen MC, Benenati JF, Sheth S, Merton D, Rothgeb J. Changes in renal artery Doppler indexes following renal angioplasty. J Vasc Interv Radiol 1991;2:457–461

79. Schwerk WB, Restrepo IK, Stellwaag M, Klose KJ, Schade-Brittinger C. Renal artery stenosis: grading with image-directed Doppler US evaluation of renal resistive index. [see comments] Radiology 1994;190: 785–790

80. Burdick L, Airoldi F, Marana I, et al. Superiority of acceleration and acceleration time over pulsatility and resistance indices as screening tests for renal artery stenosis. J Hypertens 1996;14:1229–1235

81. Pedersen EB, Egeblad M, Jorgensen J, et al. Diagnosing renal artery stenosis: a comparison between conventional renography, captopril renography and ultrasound Doppler in a large consecutive series of patients with arterial hypertension. Blood Press 1996;5:342–348

82. Frauchiger B, Zierler R, Bergelin RO, Isaacson JA, Strandness DE Jr. Prognostic significance of intrarenal resistance indices in patients with renal artery interventions: a preliminary duplex sonographic study. Cardiovasc Surg 1996;4:324–330

83. Radermacher J Chavan A, Bleck J, et al. Use of Doppler ultrasonography to predict the outcome of therapy for renal-artery stenosis. N Engl J Med 2001;344:410–417

84. Zeller T, Frank U, Muller C, et al. Predictors of improved renal function after percutaneous stent-supported angioplasty of severe atherosclerotic ostial renal artery stenosis. Circulation 2003;108: 2244–2249

85. Garcia-Criado A, Gilabert R, Nicolau C, et al. Value of Doppler sonography for predicting clinical outcome after renal artery revascularization in atherosclerotic renal artery stenosis. J Ultrasound Med 2005;24:1641–1647

86. Postma CT, Bijlstra PJ, Rosenbusch G, Thien T. Pattern recognition of loss of early systolic peak by Doppler ultrasound has a low sensitivity for the detection of renal artery stenosis. J Hum Hypertens 1996;10:181–184

87. Melany ML, Grant EG, Duerinckx AJ, Watts TM, Levine BS. Ability of a phase shift US contrast agent to improve imaging of the main renal arteries. Radiology 1997;205:147–152

88. Claudon M, Plouin PF, Baxter GM, et al. Renal arteries in patients at risk of renal arterial stenosis: multicenter evaluation of the echo-enhancer SH U 508A at color and spectral Doppler US. Levovist Renal Artery Stenosis Study Group. Radiology 2000;214: 739–746

89. Miralles M, Cairols M, Cotillas J, Gimenez A, Santiso A. Value of Doppler parameters in the diagnosis of renal artery stenosis. J Vasc Surg 1996;23(3):428–435

90. Antonica G, Sabba C, Berardi E, et al. Accuracy of echo-Doppler flowmetry for renal artery stenosis. J Hypertens Suppl 1991;9: S240–S241

10 Elevated PSA and/or Abnormal Prostate Physical Examinations: Diagnosing Prostate Cancer

Ulrike Hamper

Carcinoma of the prostate is the most common malignancy in Western men and the second leading cause of cancer death among men in the United States. It is estimated that 234,460 new cases were diagnosed in the United States during 2006. An estimated 27,350 men died from the disease during the same year.

Prostate cancer and incidence rates vary among ethnic and racial groups. Prostate cancer incidence rates are 37% higher for black than for white men, and mortality rates are more than two times higher for black than for white men. The disease is common in North America and northwestern Europe and rare in Asia, Africa, and South America. According to recent genetic studies, an inherited predisposition may account for 5 to 10% of prostate cancers. In addition, international studies suggest that dietary fat and high plasma testosterone levels may also be a factor.

The incidence of prostate cancer increases with age, and ~80% of all prostate cancers are diagnosed in men over the age of 65. Between 1988 and 1992 the prostate cancer incidence rate increased by 65%, mostly due to improved detection. A decline in prostate cancer incidence began in 1992 for white men, and in 1993 for African Americans.[1] This trend is likely related to the effects of prostate-specific antigen (PSA) screening. Prostate cancer incidence rates are expected to continue to decline and stabilize at rates that were in effect prior to the widespread use of PSA screening.[1]

To detect prostate cancer early, every man aged 40 and older should undergo a digital rectal examination (DRE) as part of his annual physical checkup. In addition, the American Cancer Society recommends that all men aged 50 or over should have an annual PSA blood test. Earlier screening is recommended for men at increased risk for prostate cancer, such as men with a positive family history or African Americans. These patients should undergo annual DRE and PSA screening starting at age 40. If either one of these test results appears suspicious, further evaluation with a transrectal ultrasound (TRUS) should be performed.[1]

Differential Diagnosis

Both prostate cancer and benign processes such as benign prostate hyperplasia (BPH) or prostatitis may cause elevation of serum PSA levels and can cause an abnormal DRE.

The most troublesome differentiation is between cancer and BPH. Elevated PSA levels are found in 16 to 86% of men with BPH (average one third of men with BPH) and in 60 to 70% of patients with prostate cancer. Multiple studies have shown that the measurement of PSA serum concentration is well established in the diagnosis and follow-up of patients with prostate cancer and may better identify patients with organ-confined, potentially curable disease.[2-6]

Over 30% of men over the age of 50 will have small cancers in their gland, which remain clinically insignificant and may never require treatment.[5,8] Therefore, skeptics of PSA testing have raised the issue of increased detection of biologically insignificant tumors.[9] Often prostate cancers are detected when the patient has symptoms of bladder outlet obstruction or when routine DRE or PSA tests detect abnormalities.[6] Systemic symptoms such as weakness, bone pain, or azotemia may be the presenting features; however, most of the time patients presenting with these symptoms have more advanced and usually metastatic disease. In general, survival of the disease has an inverse relationship with the stage of the cancer at time of detection. Survival rates also vary with race and ethnicity, with African American men having a lower 5-year survival rate compared with white men.[1] To decrease the mortality rate from prostate cancer it will be necessary to (1) detect cancers that are still organ confined and, therefore, potentially curable, and (2) initiate definitive therapy, either radical prostatectomy or radiation therapy.

Diagnostic Evaluation

Nonimaging Tests

Prostate-Specific Antigen Testing

Serum PSA testing has become a valuable tool in the diagnosis of prostate cancer, emerging as the best single test for early detection of prostate cancer, and its routine use results in a higher percentage of patients with pathologically organ-confined disease at diagnosis.[2,4,9-11] PSA is an objective measurement, unlike DRE or TRUS, which are operator-dependent and subjective examination techniques.

Prostate-specific antigen is a serum protease originally isolated from prostate tissue by Wang et al in 1979.[12] PSA levels of 4.0 ng/mL or less, are considered normal.[5]

The synthesis of PSA is restricted to prostatic epithelium. Elevated serum PSA protein levels can be found in both benign and malignant diseases of the prostate, and are caused not only by prostate cancer, but also by BPH, bacterial prostatitis, prostatic intraepithelial neoplasia (PIN), and prostatic infarction, as well as by selective manipulations (e.g., TRUS, prostate massage, prostate biopsy, catheterization, and cystoscopy).[13,14] In benign glands, the factors that affect PSA levels most are prostatic volume and patient's age. It has been estimated that 1 g of prostatic hyperplastic tissue will elevate the PSA level by 0.3 ng/mL, whereas cancer will cause an increase of about 10-fold (3.5 ng/mL) compared with BPH.

Limitation of PSA sensitivity includes the fact that not all patients with prostate cancer have elevated PSA concentrations. In earlier series, 14 to 27% of patients with organ-confined cancer had elevated PSA levels.[15] Likewise, nearly 33% of cancers are detected in men who had PSA levels in the normal range.[16] A large study by Catalona et al[10] evaluated 1653 men over age 50 without cancer or prostatitis with PSA levels in the 4 to 10 ng/mL range with DRE and TRUS, followed by TRUS-guided biopsy if an abnormality was found. Twenty-two percent of patients with midrange PSA values (4 to 10 ng/mL) had cancer on their biopsy, compared with 67% with PSA levels (>10 ng/mL). DRE alone would have missed 32% and TRUS alone 43% of cancers in this series. Therefore, elevated PSA levels > 10 ng/mL warrant a prostate biopsy regardless of the findings on DRE.[3,10]

A study by Rietbergen et al[11] concluded that if PSA levels had not been used as part of the screening regimen, DRE would have missed 52.9% of cancers and TRUS would have missed 54.7%. The most recent results from the Prostate Cancer Prevention Trial showed that the prevalence of high-grade cancer increased from 12.5% of cancers with a PSA level of ≤ 0.5 ng/mL to 25% of cancers associated with a PSA level of 3.1 to 4.0 ng/mL.[17] Another controversial aspect of PSA testing for prostate cancer detection is that over 30% of men over the age of 50 will have small cancers in their gland that remain clinically insignificant and may never require treatment. Although the serum PSA levels correlate with the extent of disease in patients with prostate cancer, it is impossible to predict occult metastatic disease accurately except in individuals with extreme serum PSA elevations.

Because a substantial overlap in serum PSA levels in men with prostate cancer and those with BPH exists, better methods of using serum PSA in the diagnosis and management of patients with prostate cancer have been explored, including but not limited to the determination of PSA density, excess PSA, PSA velocity, age-specific PSA ranges, and, most recently, the use of molecular forms of PSA.[7,18–21]

Prostate Specific Antigen Density and Excess Prostate Specific Antigen

As previously mentioned, elevated levels of PSA are not specific for prostate cancer. Therefore, attempts have been made to correct for an elevated PSA level contributed by benign prostate enlargement through the use of prostate specific antigen density (PSAD), especially in the intermediate range (4 to 10 ng/mL), where such elevations may occur in patients with BPH or prostate cancer.[18,22–28] PSAD is calculated as the quotient of the serum PSA level divided by the estimated volume of the prostate gland as measured by TRUS. This technique may be useful to determine which patients with ambiguous PSA findings should undergo prostate biopsy. For tests using monoclonal antibody to detect PSA, PSAD values of 0.10,[26] 0.12,[24] and 0.14[23] have been recommended. A PSAD of 0.12 has been shown to maximize the sensitivity of PSAD while maintaining a moderate specificity.[26,27] Some studies have advocated that a combination of PSAD and PSA values is more sensitive and specific for the detection of prostate cancer.[22–26] However, other studies showed that the combination of PSAD and PSA did not have a higher predictive value than PSA alone.[18,25–27]

Prostate Specific Antigen Velocity

A case-controlled study of 54 men showed that serial PSA measurements that followed the rate of change over time allowed a more accurate correlation between the serum PSA and the clinical status of the prostate than was possible with a single reading.[29] Because daily variations of PSA values up to 10% can occur, only PSA changes of at least 0.75 ng/mL per year are considered significant.

Age-Specific Prostate Specific Antigen

Age-related reference ranges for PSA in combination with DRE findings were introduced by Oesterling et al[30] in 1993 in an attempt to improve specificity for biopsy in older men while improving sensitivity in younger patients.

Littrup et al[27,28] have shown that minimal cost reductions are achieved with age-related PSA when combined with universal systematic biopsy; this was in contrast to potential savings achieved with tailored biopsies. The increase in PSA levels with age probably merely reflects a contribution from the increased incidence of BPH in older men.[31]

Molecular Forms of Prostate Specific Antigen (Total PSA, Free PSA, and Complexed PSA)

PSA can be detected in different molecular forms in sera of men. Although PSA is predominantly bound by α 1-antichymotrypsin (PSA-ACT), it may exist in a "free," or unbound, form or it may be bound to α 2-macroglobulin (PSA-AZM).[32–37] Current commercially used assays for PSA measure total PSA, detect free PSA, and PSA-ACT. There is evidence that PSA bound to ACT may be higher in men with prostate cancer than in men with BPH. Determining a ratio of free PSA to total PSA may help decrease the number of unnecessary biopsies in men with diagnostically vague serum PSA levels between 4.0 and 10.0 ng/mL. Extensive prospective studies are in progress to evaluate the clinical utility of these methods for early and optimal prostate cancer detection.[5,25,32-37]

Enhanced reverse transcriptase (RT) molecular polymerase chain reaction (PCR) assay for PSA (RT-PCR assay for PSA) is a molecular assay specific for the human PSA. This assay identifies PSA-synthesizing cells from reverse transcribed messenger ribonucleic acid (mRNA) and is a marker for circulating tumor cells in the blood of patients with prostate cancer.[38-40] It has been reported to be a more sensitive modality to identify patients with extracapsular extension of disease (sensitivity 86%, specificity 84%) and positive surgical margins (sensitivity 87%, specificity 84%). It is superior to the DRE, computed tomography (CT), endorectal coil magnetic resonance imaging (MRI), PSA, PSAD, or Gleason score in staging correctly apparently localized prostate cancer prior to surgery.[39,40] However, further work is needed and currently in progress to validate this method for routine use in daily clinical practice. Recent and future work is focusing on the analysis of multiple gene expression or proteins simultaneously via gene chip or proteomics technology.[21,41]

Prostate Acid Phosphatase

The determination of prostate acid phosphatase (PAP) levels, whether performed by enzymatic or radioimmune assays, has severe limitations because the levels may be normal in 57 to 73% of patients with localized prostate cancer. In addition, most patients with elevated PAP levels have

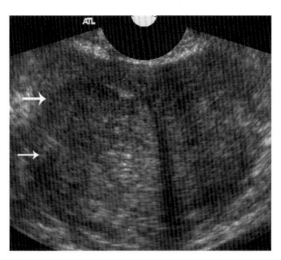

Figure 10–1 A 71-year-old man with elevated prostate specific antigen (7 ng/mL) and right-sided palpable nodule on physical examination. Coronal transrectal ultrasound shows an asymmetric nodule of benign prostatic hypertrophy (*arrows*) accounting for the abnormal digital rectal exam.

advanced disease, severely limiting its specificity.[32,33,42] Therefore, this test is no longer used in daily practice.

Digital Rectal Examination

The DRE is relatively cheap and easy to perform; however, it has significant limitations for the detection of prostate cancer because it is a very subjective and operator-dependent test with high interobserver variability. An abnormal-feeling prostate gland on DRE may be caused by prostate cancer, but also by benign processes such as asymmetric prostatic enlargement, calcifications, cystic lesions, or chronic inflammatory changes (**Fig. 10–1, Fig. 10–2,**

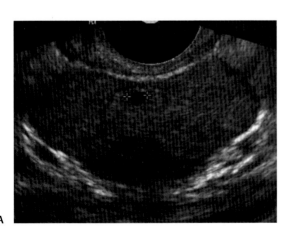

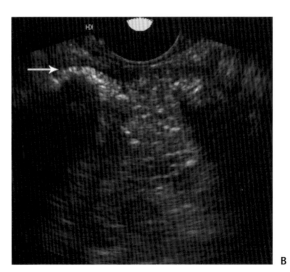

Figure 10–2 (A) A 48-year-old man with a midline mass and induration felt on physical examination. Coronal transrectal ultrasound demonstrates a cystic mass (between calipers), compatible with a small utricular cyst. **(B)** A 75-year-old man with large right-sided area of calcifications (*arrow*) accounting for the palpable abnormality on physical examination.

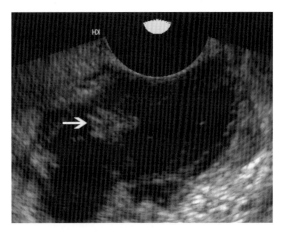

Figure 10–3 A 42-year-old man, positive for human immunodeficiency virus, with an enlarged left prostatic lobe on physical exam. Sagittal transrectal ultrasound shows an ill-defined hypoechoic mass in the left central gland, with fluid-filled components and internal echoes (*arrow*). This mass aspirated transrectally and proved to be a prostatic abscess.

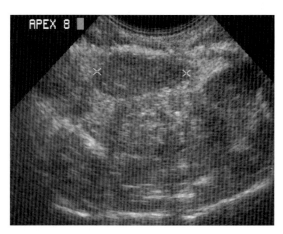

Figure 10–4 A 78-year-old man with an elevated prostate specific antigen level (5.4 ng/mL) and a left apical nodule felt on physical exam. Sagittal transrectal ultrasound (TRUS) demonstrates a well-defined, hypoechoic nodule in the left apex (between calipers). TRUS-guided biopsy of this nodule showed benign prostatic tissue with caseating and noncaseating granulomas, compatible with prior Bacille Calmette–Guerin therapy for bladder tumor.

Fig. 10–3, Fig. 10–4). The detection rate for prostate cancer by DRE has been reported to be only ~50% in several studies.[11,13,37,43]

Tumors occurring anterior to midline, which constitute ~40 to 50% of prostate cancer, are usually not detected by DRE, which predominantly allows palpation of the posterolateral aspects of the gland. Lesion size is an important factor for detection by DRE. For lesions less than 1.5 cm, the sensitivity of DRE has been reported to be only 41%.[44] The discrepancy between the clinical and surgical stage in several series[4-6] illustrates the limitations of DRE. Studies by Catalona et al[2,3,10] showed that DRE alone would have missed 32% of biopsy-proven cancers. In the large European series by Rietbergen et al, DRE alone would have missed ~53% of cancers.[11] Screening with DRE alone also fails to increase the proportion of pathologically organ-confined cancers detected, and clinical staging of prostate cancer has resulted in a 30 to 70% understaging of stage B disease.[4]

Imaging Tests Other than Ultrasound

CT and MRI with a body coil have not proven to be valuable for detecting and staging prostate cancer and are not recommended for the initial evaluation of patients with a prostate problem.[45] In terms of detection and localization of cancerous lesions larger than 5 mm, MRI only identified 60% of the tumors in one older series. The staging accuracy of body coil MRI in this series was 57% for localized and 77% for advanced disease.[45] MRI with endorectal coils, however, seems to be superior to other imaging techniques in the preoperative assessment of local tumor stage, particularly for prediction of extracapsular extension in patients with prostate cancer.[46,47]

Achieving high accuracies is directly related to the technique used and the experience of the reader.[41] Nuclear medicine bone scans, positron emission tomography (PET), CT, and/or body coil MRI are used as staging radiographic studies for metastatic disease prior to the implementation of therapy. A study by Huncharek and Muscat[48] questioned the need for staging bone scans in asymptomatic patients with newly diagnosed prostate cancer and PSA levels of less than 10 ng/mL and staging CT/MRI with PSA levels of less than 20 ng/mL. There would be significant economic savings if the scans were not done.

New developments in the field of nuclear medicine, such as hormone receptor scintigraphy or PET, are emerging. These techniques allow in vivo characterization of tumors, which may have important implications for the diagnosis of prostate cancer in the future. Although the role of PET imaging is evolving, it currently seems to be most important in the determination of the early spread of disease in patients with aggressive tumors, and in monitoring the response to therapy in more advanced patients.[49,50] Diffusion-weighted MRI remains untested clinically and a work in progress for future research.[49]

Ultrasound Imaging

TRUS with high-frequency (6 to 9 MHz) transducers is a valuable diagnostic tool for the workup of patients with a prostate problem. TRUS is performed in sagittal and transverse or coronal planes to evaluate glandular changes, delineate and measure focal lesions, and primarily guide biopsies. It is used to calculate the size of the prostate gland and can accurately assess prostate volume in glands less than 50 g. Gland volume is important for PSAD analyses, which can be used to select patients for a TRUS-guided

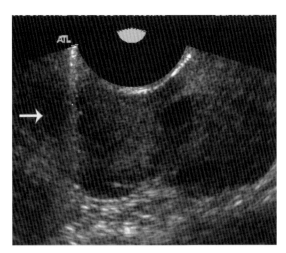

Figure 10–5 An 82-year-old man with rising prostate-specific antigen up to 7 ng/mL and left-sided firmness noted on physical exam. Transrectal ultrasound–guided biopsy of a hypoechoic lesion in the right base (*arrow*) yielded adenocarcinoma, Gleason score 4 + 3 = 7.

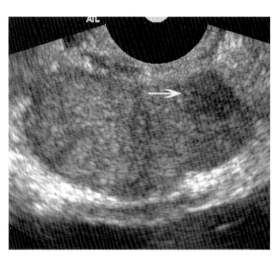

Figure 10–7 A 64-year-old man with elevated prostrate specific antigen (8.6 ng/mL). No palpable abnormality. Coronal transrectal ultrasound demonstrates an irregularly shaped hypoechoic nodule in the left peripheral zone (*arrow*).

biopsy. Furthermore, TRUS in patients with an abnormal DRE can identify mimics of carcinoma, such as prostatic calculi, cysts, or other benign processes (**Fig. 10–1, Fig. 10–2, Fig. 10–3, Fig. 10–4**) or clarify equivocal findings on DRE, especially when the physical examination was not performed by an experienced urologist or practitioner. In addition, TRUS has become the modality for routine guidance of a prostate biopsy, prostate brachytherapy, and experimental gene therapy.[51]

Abnormal PSA levels and/or an abnormal DRE usually initiate the performance of a TRUS-guided biopsy, which is

simple, safe, and can be accurately performed with automatically triggered core biopsy devices (**Fig. 10–5**). Because cancers detected before they spread beyond the confines of the prostate gland have an excellent cure rate, many authorities believe that any patient with an elevated serum PSA, especially when the DRE is also abnormal, should undergo a biopsy.[52]

Focal lesions are targeted, followed by systematic, usually sextant, octant, or even more biopsies of the remainder of the gland.[53] Some series have shown that 61% of cancers would have been missed if only the site of palpable induration had been biopsied, and 40 to 52% if only the site of a hypoechoic lesion had been biopsied.[3] Some authors recommend tailored sextant biopsies or targeting areas of increased flow in the absence of focal

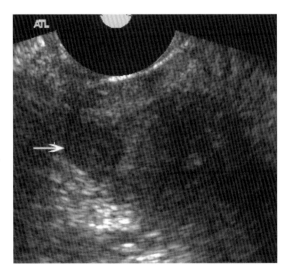

Figure 10–6 An 82-year-old man with rising prostrate-specific antigen up to 7 ng/mL and left-sided firmness noted on physical exam. No palpable abnormality in the right gland. Coronal transrectal ultrasound shows a hypoechoic lesion in the right base (*arrow*). Biopsy of this lesion yielded adenocarcinoma of the prostate, Gleason score 4 + 3 = 7 (same patient as **Fig. 10–5**).

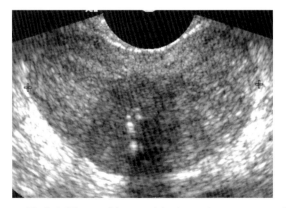

Figure 10–8 A 68-year-old man with elevated prostrate-specific antigen (7 ng/mL). No palpable abnormality. Coronal transrectal ultrasound demonstrates no focal abnormality in either peripheral zone. Systematic octant biopsy of the gland revealed extensive bilateral adenocarcinoma, Gleason score 3 + 3 = 6.

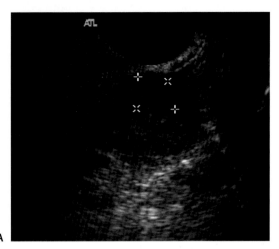

Figure 10–9 (A) A 72-year-old man with elevated prostrate specific antigen (PSA) (27 ng/mL). Transrectal ultrasound (TRUS) shows a hypoechoic lesion in the left peripheral zone with small echogenic foci (between calipers). TRUS- guided biopsy yielded adenocarcinoma, Gleason score 4 + 4 = 8. **(B)** A 71-year-old man with elevated PSA (7 ng/mL). TRUS demonstrated an acrogenic nodule (between calipers) in the right central gland. TRUS-guided biopsy of the lesion showed adenocarcinoma, Gleason score 3 + 3 = 6.

hypoechoic lesions.[27,28,54–56] In addition, staging biopsies of the seminal vesicles, ejaculatory ducts, and apex can be performed.

At some institutions, patients with PSA between 4.0 and 10.0 ng/mL undergo DRE plus TRUS-guided biopsy. Others use PSAD to determine who should undergo biopsy. Patients with PSA levels of greater than 10 ng/mL should definitely be biopsied.[18] If the biopsy shows insignificant tumor, defined as cancer cells found only in one or two needle cores with tumor present in less than half of these cores, a Gleason score of 6 or lower, and a PSAD of less than 0.1 to 0.15, then it has been advocated that the patient be followed by "watchful-waiting," serial PSA testing, and repeat prostate biopsies.[57,58] In addition, patients with an initially negative biopsy but increasing PSA velocity usually undergo repeat biopsy. Some studies have shown an incremental increase in detection rate of cancers on second and even third biopsies.[59] Patients with early prostate carcinoma may have a good survival without therapy; however, aggressive screening should be limited by the patient's age and requires a life expectancy of at least 10 years.[60]

Accuracy of Transrectal Ultrasound

TRUS can document areas of abnormalities in the prostate gland that may be suspicious for cancer, such as focal hypoechoic lesions.[61,62] The sonographic appearance of early prostate cancer is a hypoechoic lesion in the peripheral zone (**Fig. 10–6, Fig. 10–7**). This sonographic appearance is, however, not specific because not all cancers are hypoechoic and not all hypoechoic lesions are malignant. Sonographic pathological correlation studies have shown

that ~70 to 75% of tumors are hypoechoic, whereas 25 to 30% of tumors are isoechoic and blend with the surrounding tissues[61,63] (**Fig. 10–8**). These lesions are usually not detected by TRUS. A small number of cancers are echogenic or have a heterogeneous echotexture with small echogenic foci within echogenic lesions (**Fig. 10–9**).[64] The positive predictive value (PPV) of a hypoechoic lesion to be cancer increases with the size of the lesion, a palpable nodule, and an elevated PSA.[13] Overall, the incidence of malignancy in a sonographically suspicious lesion is ~20 to 25%.[13,65]

Various benign lesions mimic the sonographic appearance of early prostate cancer, including inflammatory conditions, granulomatous prostatitis, dilated acinar glands, hyperplasia, scarring, and fibrosis from previous transurethral resection of the prostate (**Fig. 10–1**, **Fig. 10–2, Fig. 10–3, Fig. 10–4**).[66,67] Normal variants such as prominent vessels in the peripheral gland or smooth muscle near the apex and ejaculatory ducts, as well as positional "pseudolesions," may be mistaken for carcinoma.[67] Even with high-resolution equipment, many potentially clinically significant tumors are not visualized by TRUS. A large multicenter study[45] showed that up to 40% of significant cancers were missed by gray-scale ultrasound. The overall sensitivity of TRUS in detecting neurovascular bundle invasion has been reported to be 66%, with a specificity of 78%.[68] To improve lesion detection TRUS, secondary signs such as bulging and contour abnormalities, and increased flow on color Doppler ultrasound (CDUS) have been advocated, especially for isoechoic lesions (**Fig. 10–10**).[69–71]

Small tumors (< 2 mm) have been reported to have no detectable flow, whereas tumors at least 1 cm³ demonstrate

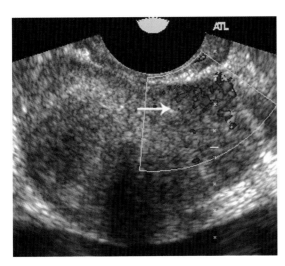

Figure 10–10 A 56-year-old man with elevated prostate-specific antigen. Coronal transrectal ultrasound (TRUS) with color Doppler ultrasound demonstrates increased flow in an isoechoic region of the left gland (*arrow*). TRUS-guided biopsy of this region showed high-grade adenocarcinoma, Gleason score 5 + 4 = 9.

vascularity.[54,72] Results of CDUS studies[58,68] are conflicting and demonstrate a problematic overlap between increased flow detected in cancers, inflammatory condition, and benign lesions (**Fig. 10–11A–C**). Also, not every cancer has sufficient flow to be detected by CDUS[70] (**Fig. 10–12**). CDUS will and should not replace gray-scale ultrasound, but CDUS findings have been advocated to initiate a TRUS-guided biopsy that otherwise may not have been performed, thus tailoring the biopsy to target isoechoic, yet hypervascular areas of the prostate gland (**Fig. 10–10**).

Some investigators have suggested that tumor vascularization may allow correlation with the biological behavior of a lesion, especially its potential for rapid growth and distant metastases.[72-74] If this holds true, CDUS may have potential for identifying an important subgroup of patients. Further research in this area is still needed. Newer color flow techniques such as power Doppler ultrasound (PDUS) may be helpful in this respect due to increased sensitivity to flow allowing visualization and demonstration of vascularity in even smaller vessels (**Fig. 10–11A,C**). A recent

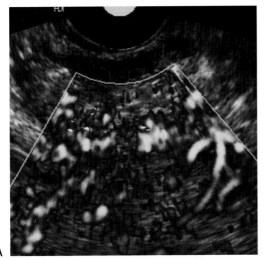

A

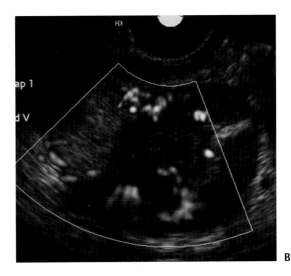

B

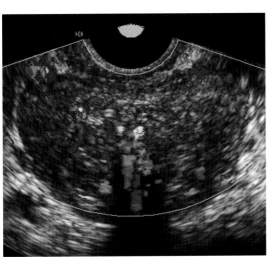

C

Figure 10–11 (A) An 80-year-old man with elevated prostate-specific antigen (PSA) and abnormal digital rectal exam. Coronal transrectal ultrasound (TRUS) with power Doppler ultrasound demonstrates diffuse increased flow in a lobulated, predominantly left-sided prostate mass. Biopsy yielded adenocarcinoma, Gleason score 4 + 4 = 8, with ductal features. **(B)** A 42-year-old man with elevated PSA and bulging prostate on physical exam. Power Doppler TRUS demonstrates diffuse increased flow to centrally hypoechoic areas, which proved to be acute prostatitis with abscess formation. **(C)** A 73-year-old man with a history of prostate carcinoma and failed radiotherapy. The patient underwent experimental TRUS-guided gene therapy. Color Doppler TRUS 3 days postprocedure demonstrates diffuse increased flow throughout the gland caused by acute prostatitis, as proven by TRUS-guided biopsy.

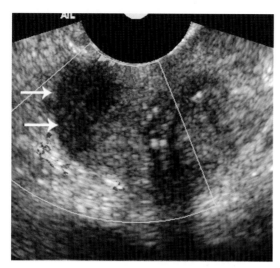

Figure 10–12 A 69-year-old man with elevated prostate-specific antigen (5.3 ng/mL) and irregular right lower lobe felt on digital rectal exam. Coronal transrectal ultrasound (TRUS) demonstrates a large hypoechoic, avascular mass in the right lobe (*arrows*). TRUS-guided biopsy showed extensive right-sided adenocarcinoma, Gleason score 3 + 3 = 6, with perineural invasion.

study by Wilson et al[55] demonstrated that PDUS signals were of value as an indicator of microvessel density, correlating with a higher Gleason score. This may ultimately predict clinical outcome in prostate cancer.

Other recent developments such as intravenous ultrasound contrast agents and harmonic imaging (**Fig. 10–13A,B**) have shown in preliminary studies a possible role for these agents and techniques to delineate subtle prostate cancers when used in combination with CDUS, PDUS, or harmonic imaging. Further research in this area, however, is needed and is under way.[75–80] In addition, preliminary reports about the use of three-dimensional TRUS have shown promise and incremental value for volume de-

terminations in patients with BPH and assessment of extracapsular spread in prostate cancer[81,82] (**Fig. 10–14A–C**).

Limitations of Ultrasound

TRUS has been shown to be too insensitive and not specific enough to be used as a screening tool in patients with either a normal DRE or a normal PSA test. The American College of Radiology (ACR), the American Urological Association (AUA), and the American Cancer Society (ACS) have made recommendations to limit TRUS to patients with either or both abnormal DRE and PSA elevation. TRUS, however, is useful to delineate possible prostate pathology in patients with abnormal PSA or DRE results. As previously mentioned, however, not all gray-scale abnormalities represent tumor, and similar hypoechoic lesions may be caused by atrophy, inflammation, infarction, and other benign processes, thus limiting the specificity of TRUS. Likewise, isoechoic lesions are usually not detected unless secondary tumor signs such as focal bulge or contour irregularity are identified. As mentioned earlier, CDUS may be useful in those patients.

Small cancers (< 5 mm) are rarely detected by TRUS, and very extensive tumors involving the entire peripheral zone are difficult to identify because comparison with normal tissue is not possible. Almost 50% of cancers are located in the anterior half of the prostate, and 20 to 30% of tumors arise from the central or transition zone and usually remain undetected by TRUS. Estimation of tumor volume by TRUS has been shown to be inaccurate. Likewise, as previously mentioned, the detection and staging accuracy of TRUS for prostate cancer have been shown to be too inaccurate to advocate its use as a screening modality. Further advances in equipment and transducer technology with increased resolution and operator experience may alter these previously reported disappointing results

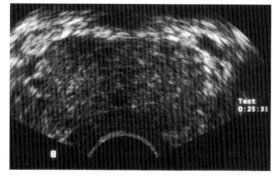

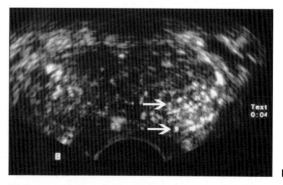

Figure 10–13 (A) 61-year-old male with prostate cancer (Gleason score 6) along the left side of the prostate from base to apex and elevated prostate specific antigen (9.1 ng/mL). Transverse baseline sonographic image reveals homogeneous echotexture. (Reprinted with permission from Halpern EJ, Verkh L, Forsberg F, Gomella LG, Mattrey RF, Goldberg BB. AJR Am J Roentgenol 2000;174:1575–1580)

(B) Same patient as in **Fig. 10–12.** Contrast-enhanced intermittent image with 2-second interscan delay shows focal enhancement at the site of cancer in the left base (*arrows*). (Reprinted with permission from Halpern EJ, Verkh L, Forsberg F, Gomella LG, Mattrey RF, Goldberg BB. AJR Am J Roentgenol 2000;174:1575–1580)

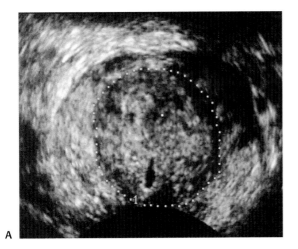

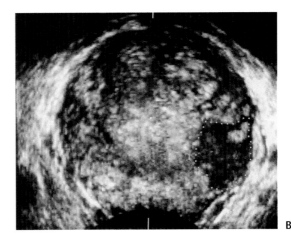

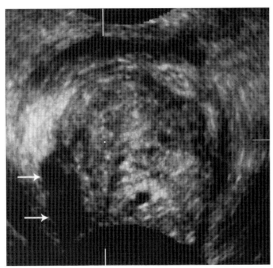

Figure 10–14 **(A)** Coronal reconstruction of a three-dimensional volume acquisition ultrasound (US) in a patient with elevated prostate-specific antigen and benign prostate hyperplasia (BPH). The coronal image allows excellent delineation of the area of BPH (dotted circle). Summation of multiple coronal slices was used to measure the volume of BPH. (Reprinted with permission from Hamper UM, Trapanotto V, DeJong MR, et al. Three-Dimensional Ultrasound of the Prostate: Early Experience. Radiology 1999;212:719–723) **(B)** Coronal three-dimensional (3-D) image in a patient with a left-sided, biopsy-proven peripheral zone nodule adenocarcinoma (dotted circle). Three-dimensional ultrasound (US) predicted confinement of tumor to the gland, which was confirmed at surgery. (Reprinted with permission from Hamper UM, Trapanotto V, DeJong MR, et al. Three-dimensional ultrasound of the prostate: early experience. Radiology 1999;212:719–723) **(C)** Coronal 3-D image in a patient with a right-sided, biopsy-proven peripheral zone nodule adenocarcinoma (*arrows*). Three-dimensional US predicted extension of tumor outside of the gland, which was confirmed at surgery. (Reprinted with permission from Hamper UM, Trapanotto V, DeJong MR, et al. Three-dimensional ultrasound of the prostate: early experience. Radiology 1999;212:719–723)

regarding the detection and staging of prostate carcinoma; however, because of the currently tight economic climate in the health care industry and declining funding by government or other agencies, prospective multicenter studies will be difficult to perform in the future.

Summary

Screening and detection of prostate cancer with PSA, DRE, and/or TRUS remains a controversial and complex issue with many open and still unanswered questions. The data suggest that the use of PSA testing in the past detected more and earlier cancers; however, no data are available to demonstrate improved survival for men with prostate cancer. The combination of DRE and PSA markedly improves sensitivity and has represented the least costly detection approach to potentially decrease the mortality from prostate cancer. Serum PSA was related to prostate cancer 20 years ago. However, in the last 5 to 6 years serum PSA has only been related to BPH. Therefore, there is urgent

need for serum markers that reflect the size and grade of this common tumor. For the future, the availability of a more cancer-specific PSA assay, other cancer-related proteins, or molecular staging will become the most potent factor in lowering prostate cancer detection costs.

Currently, a combination of tests is probably still the best way to detect prostate cancer. TRUS with or without biopsy should be reserved for those patients with abnormal test results. Local staging with magnetic resonance endorectal coils seems most accurate. In experienced hands, its staging accuracy should approach 80% or more. Further staging with nuclear medicine, particularly PET imaging as well as bone scans and tests such as CT or MRI, can be performed to detect lymph node and distant metastases prior to implementation of definitive therapy.[83] Today's screening and diagnostic tools, even with biopsy, however, still have limits. Most importantly, it is essential that we have yet to prove through prospective studies that early diagnosis of prostate cancer actually leads to an improvement in morbidity and reduction in mortality in patients with the disease.[9]

References

1. Cancer Facts and Figures 2006. *American Cancer Society*, Atlanta, GA 2004; 17–19.
2. Catalona WJ, Smith DS, Ratliff TL, Basler JW. Detection of organ-confined prostate cancer is increased through prostate-specific antigen-based screening. JAMA 1993;270:948–954
3. Catalona WJ, Richie JP, Ahmann FR, et al. Comparison of digital rectal examination and serum prostate specific antigen in the early detection of prostate cancer: results of a multicenter clinical trial of 6,630 men. J Urol 1994;151:1283–1290
4. Stamey TA, Yang N, Hay AR, et al. Prostate-specific antigen as a serum marker for adenocarcinoma of the prostate. N Engl J Med 1987;317:909–916
5. Han M, Gann PH, Catalona WJ. Prostate-specific antigen and screening for prostate cancer. Med Clin North Am 2004;88:245–265
6. Clark TWI, Goldenberg SL, Cooperberg PL, Wong AD, Singer J. Stratification of prostate-specific antigen level and results of transrectal ultrasonography and digital rectal examination as predictors of positive prostate biopsy. Can Ass Radiol J 1997;48:252–258
7. So A, Goldenberg L, Gleave ME. Prostate specific antigen: an updated review. Can J Urol 2003;10:2040–2050
8. Stamey TA, Caldwell M, McNeal JE, Nolley R, Hemenez M, Downs J. The prostate specific antigen era in the United States is over for prostate cancer: what happened in the last 20 years? J Urol 2004;172:1297–1301
9. Carter HB. Prostate cancers in men with low PSA levels: must we find them? N Engl J Med 2004;350:2292–2294
10. Catalona WJ, Smith DS, Ratliff TL, et al. Measurement of prostate-specific antigen in serum as a screening test for prostate cancer. [published erratum appears in N Engl J Med 1991;325:1324] N Engl J Med 1991;324:1156–1161
11. Rietbergen JBW, Kranse R, Kirkels WJ, De Koning HJ, Schroder FH. Evaluation of prostate-specific antigen, digital rectal examination and transrectal ultrasonography in population-based screening for prostate cancer: improving the efficiency of early detection. Br J Urol 1997;79:57–63
12. Wang MC, Valenzuela LA, Murphy GP, Chu TM. Purification of a human prostate specific antigen. Invest Urol 1979;17:159–163
13. Ellis WJ, Chetner MP, Preston SD, Brawer MK. Diagnosis of prostatic carcinoma: the yield of serum prostate specific antigen, digital rectal examination and transrectal ultrasonography. J Urol 1994;152:1520–1525
14. Mochtar CA, Kiemeney LA, van Riemsdijk MM, et al. Prostate-specific antigen as an estimator of prostate volume in the management of patients with symptomatic benign prostatic hyperplasia. Eur Urol 2003;44:695–700
15. Lange PH, Ercole CJ, Lightner DJ, Fraley EE, Vessella R. The value of serum prostate specific antigen determinations before and after radical prostatectomy. J Urol 1989;141:873–879
16. Mettlin C, Murphy GP, Ray P, et al. American Cancer Society–National Prostate Cancer Detection Project: results from multiple examinations using transrectal ultrasound, digital rectal examination, and prostate specific antigen. Cancer 1993;71:891–898
17. Thompson IM, Pauler DK, Goodman PJ, et al. Prevalence of prostate cancer among men with a prostate-specific antigen level < or = 4.0 ng per milliliter. N Engl J Med 2004;350:2239–2246
18. Van Iersel MP, Witjes WP, de la Rosette JJ, Oosterhof GO. Prostate-specific antigen density: correlation with histological diagnosis of prostate cancer, benign prostatic hyperplasia and prostatitis. Br J Urol 1995;76:47–53
19. Gretzer MB, Partin AW. PSA markers in prostate cancer detection. Urol Clin North Am 2003;30:677–686
20. Canto E, Shariat SF, Slawin KM. Molecular diagnosis of prostate cancer. Curr Urol Rep 2004;5:203–211
21. Moul JW, Merseburger AS, Srivastava S. Molecular markers in prostate cancer: the role in preoperative staging. Clin Prostate Cancer 2002;1:42–50
22. Mikolajczyk S, Song Y, Wong JR, Matson RS, Rittenhouse HG. Are multiple markers the future of prostate cancer diagnostics? Clin Biochem 2004;37:519–528
23. Rommel FM, Augusta VE, Breslin JA, et al. The use of prostate specific antigen density to enhance the predictive value of intermediate levels of serum prostate specific-antigen. J Urol 1994;151:88–93
24. Lee F, Littrup PJ, Loft-Christensen L, et al. Predicted prostate specific antigen results using transrectal ultrasound gland volume: differentiation of benign prostatic hyperplasia and prostate cancer. Cancer 1992;70:211–220
25. Brawer MK, Aramburu EA, Chen GL, Preston SD, Ellis WJ. The inability of prostate specific antigen index to enhance the predictive the value of prostate specific antigen in the diagnosis of prostatic carcinoma. J Urol 1993;150:369–373
26. Benson MC, Whang IS, Pantuck A, et al. Prostate specific antigen density: a means of distinguishing benign prostatic hypertrophy and prostate cancer. J Urol 1992;147:815–816
27. Littrup PJ, Sparschu R. Transrectal ultrasound and prostate cancer risks: the "tailored" prostate biopsy. Cancer 1995;75:1805–1813
28. Littrup PJ, Goodman AC. Economic considerations of prostate cancer: the role of detection specificity and biopsy reduction. CA Cancer J Clin 1995;75:1987–1993
29. Carter HB, Pearson JD, Metter EJ, et al. Longitudinal evaluation of prostate-specific antigen levels in men with and without prostate disease. JAMA 1992;267:2215–2220
30. Oesterling JE, Jacobsen SJ, Chute CG, et al. Serum prostate-specific antigen in a community-based population of healthy men: establishment of age-specific reference ranges. JAMA 1993;270:860–864
31. Canto EI, Singh H, Shariat SF, Lamb DJ, Mikolajczak SD, Linton JH. Serum BPSA outperforms both total PSA and free PSA as a predictor of prostatic enlargement in men without prostate cancer. Urology 2004;63:905–910
32. Partin AW, Carter HB. The use of prostate specific antigen and free/total PS in the diagnosis of localized prostate cancer. Urol Clin North Am 1996;23:531–540
33. Bangma CH, Riebergen JB, Ranse R, et al. The free-to-total prostate specific antigen ratio improves the specificity of prostate specific antigen in screening for prostate cancer in the general population. J Urol 1997;157:2191–2196
34. Van Cangh PJ, De Nayer P, De Vischer L, et al. Free to total prostate-specific antigen (PSA) ratio improves the discrimination between prostate cancer and benign prostatic hyperplasia (BPH) in the diagnostic gray zone of 1.8 to 10 ng/mL total PSA. Urology 1996;48:67–70
35. Partin AW, Brawer MK, Subong ENP, et al. Prospective evaluation of percent free-PSA and complexed PSA for early detection of prostate cancer. Prostate Cancer Prostatic Dis 1998;1:197–203
36. Filella X, Truan D, Alcover J, et al. Comparison of several combinations of free, complexed, and total PSA in the diagnosis of prostate cancer in patients with urologic symptoms. J Urology 2004;63:1100–1103
37. Aus G, Becker C, Lilja H, Khatami A, Phil CG, Hugosson J. Free-to-total prostate-specific antigen ratio as a predictor of non-organ-confined prostate cancer. Scand J Urol Nephrol 2003;37:466–470
38. Seiden MV, Kantoff PW, Krithivas K, et al. Detection of circulating tumor cells in men with localized prostate cancer. J Clin Oncol 1994;12:2634–2639

39. Katz AE, Olsson CA, Raffo AJ, et al. Molecular staging of prostate cancer with the use of an enhanced reverse transcriptase-PCR assay. Urology 1994;43:765–775

40. Mitsiades CS, Lembessis P, Sourla A, Milathianakis C, Tsintavis A, Koutsilieris M. Molecular staging by RT-PCR analysis for PSA and PSMA in peripheral blood and bone marrow samples is an independent predictor of time to biochemical failure following radical prostatectomy for clinically localized prostate cancer. Clin Exp Metastasis 2004;21:495–505

41. Li J, White N, Zhang Z, et al. Detection of prostate cancer using serum proteomics patter in a histologically confirmed population. J Urol 2004;171:1782–1787

42. Burnett AL, Chan DW, Brendler CB, Walsh PC. The value of serum enzymatic acid phosphatase in the staging of localized prostate cancer. J Urol 1992;148:1832–1834

43. Cooner WH. Rectal examination and ultrasonography in the diagnosis of prostate cancer. Prostate Suppl 1992;4:3–10

44. Lee F, Littrup PJ, Torp-Pedersen ST, et al. Prostate cancer: comparison of transrectal US and digital rectal examination for screening. Radiology 1988;168:389–394

45. Rifkin MD, Zerhouni EA, Gatsonis CA, et al. Comparison of magnetic resonance imaging and ultrasonography in staging early prostate cancer: results of a multiinstitutional cooperative trial. N Engl J Med 1990;323:621–626

46. Wang L, Mullerad M, Hui-Ni C, et al. Prostate cancer: incremental value of endorectal MR imaging findings for prediction of extracapsular extension. Radiology 2004;232:133–139

47. Comet-Batlle J, Vilanova-Busquets JC, Saladie-Roig JM, Gelabert-Mas A, Barcelo-Vidal C. The value of endorectal MRI in the early diagnosis of prostate cancer. European Urology 2003;201–204

48. Huncharek M, Muscat J. Serum prostate-specific antigen as a predictor of radiographic staging studies in newly diagnosed prostate cancer. Cancer Invest 1995;13:31–35

49. Hersh MR, Knapp EL, Choi J. Newer imaging modalities to assess tumor in the prostate. Cancer Control 2004;11:353

50. Schoder H, Larson SM. Positron emission tomography for prostate, bladder, and renal cancer. Semin Nucl Med 2004;34:274–292

51. DeWeese TL, van der Poel H, Li S, et al. A phase I trial of CV706, a replication-competent, PSA selective oncolytic adenovirus, for the treatment of locally recurrent prostate cancer following radiation therapy. Cancer Res 2001;61:7464–7472

52. Freedland SJ, Mangold LA, Epstein JI, Partin A. Biopsy indication: a predicator of pathologic stage among men with preoperative serum PSA levels of 4.0 ng/mL or less and Tic disease. Urology 2004;63:887–891

53. Fink KG, Hutarew G, Pytel A, et al. One 10-core prostate biopsy is superior to two sets of sextant prostate biopsies. BJU Int 2003;92:385–388

54. Newman JS, Bree RL, Rubin JM. Prostate cancer: diagnosis with color Doppler sonography with histologic correlation of each biopsy site. Radiology 1995;195:86–90

55. Wilson NM, Masoud AM, Barsoum HB, Refaat MM, Moustafa MI, Kamal TA. Correlation of power Doppler with microvessel density in assessing prostate needle biopsy. Clin Radiol 2004;59:946–950

56. Passavanti G, Pizzuti V. Power Doppler ultrasonography as an additional tool to increase reliability of systematic biopsy of the prostate; a brief evaluation. Arch Ital Urol Androl 2004;76:110–112

57. Epstein JI, Walsh PC, Carmichael M, Brendler CB. Pathological and clinical findings to predict tumor extent of nonpalpable (stage T1 c) prostate cancer. JAMA 1994;271:368–374

58. deVries SH, Raaijmakers R, Kranse R, Blijenberg BG, Schroder FH. Prostate cancer characteristics and prostate specific antigen changes in screening detected patients initially treated with a watchful waiting policy. J Urol 2004;172:2193–2196

59. Keetch DW, Catalona WJ, Smith DS. Serial prostatic biopsies in men with persistently elevated serum prostate specific antigen values. J Urol 1994;151:1571–1574

60. Johansson JE, Adami HO, Andersson SO, et al. High 10-year survival rate in patients with early, untreated prostatic cancer. JAMA 1992;267:2191–2196

61. Dahnert WF, Hamper UM, Walsh PC, Eggleston JC, Sanders RC. Prostatic evaluation by transrectal sonography with histopathologic correlation: The echogenic appearance of early carcinoma. Radiology 1986;158:97–102

62. Lee F, Gray JM, McLeary RD, et al. Prostatic evaluation by transrectal sonography: criteria for diagnosis of early carcinoma. Radiology 1986;158:91–95

63. Salo JO, Rannikko S, Makinen J, Lehtonen T. Echogenic structure of prostatic cancer imaged on radical prostatectomy specimens. Prostate 1987;10:1–9

64. Hamper UM, Sheth S, Walsh PC, Epstein JI. Bright echogenic foci in early prostatic carcinoma: sonographic and pathologic correlation. Radiology 1990;176:339–343

65. Rifkin MD, Choi H. Implications of small, peripheral hypoechoic lesions in endorectal US of the Prostate. Radiology 1988;166:619–622

66. Sheth S, Hamper UM, Walsh PC, Holtz PM, Epstein JI. Transrectal ultrasonography in stage A adenocarcinoma of the prostate: a sonographic–pathologic correlation. Radiology 1991;179:35–39

67. Hamper UM, Sheth S, Walsh PC, Holtz PM, Epstein JI. Stage B adenocarcinoma of the prostate: transrectal US and pathologic correlation of nonmalignant hypoechoic peripheral zone lesions. Radiology 1991;180:101–104

68. Hamper UM, Sheth S, Walsh PC, Holtz PM, Epstein JI. Carcinoma of the prostate: value of transrectal sonography to detect extension into the neurovascular bundle. AJR Am J Roentgenol 1990;155:1015–1019

69. Alexander AA. To color Doppler image the prostate or not: that is the question. Radiology 1995;195:11–13

70. Kelly IM, Lees WR, Rickards D. Prostate cancer and the role of color Doppler US. Radiology 1993;189:153–156

71. Rifkin MD, Sudakoff GS, Alexander AA. Prostate: techniques, results, and potential applications of color Doppler US scanning. Radiology 1993;186:509–513

72. Folkman J, Cotran R. Relation of vascular proliferation to tumor growth. Int Rev Exp Pathol 1976;16:207–248

73. Newman JS, Bree RL, Rubin JM. Prostate cancer: diagnosis with color Doppler sonography with histologic correlation of each biopsy site. Radiology 1995;195:86–90

74. Weidner N, Semple JP, Welch WR, Folkman J. Tumor angiogenesis and metastasis-correlation in invasive breast carcinoma. N Engl J Med 1991;324:1–8

75. Karaman CZ, Unsal A, Akdilli A, Taskin F, Erol H. The value of contrast enhanced power Doppler ultrasonography in differentiating hypoechoic lesions in the peripheral zone of prostate. Eur J Radiol 2005;54:148–155

76. Yuen JS. Re: contrast enhanced color Doppler endorectal sonography of the prostate: efficiency for detecting peripheral zone tumors and role for biopsy procedure. J Urol 2004;171:2384

77. Frauscher F, Klauser A, Halpern EJ. Advances in ultrasound for the detection of prostate cancer. Ultrasound Q 2002;18:135–142

78. Roy C, Buy X, Lang H, Saussine C, Jacqmin D. Contrast enhanced color Doppler endorectal sonography of prostate: efficiency for de-

tecting peripheral zone tumors and role for biopsy procedure. J Urol 2003;170:69–72

79. Frauscher F, Klauser A, Volgger H, et al. Comparison of contrast enhanced color Doppler targeted biopsy with conventional systematic biopsy: impact on prostate cancer detection. J Urol 2002;167: 1648–1652

80. Halpern EJ, Frauscher F, Rosenberg M, Gomella LG. Directed biopsy during contrast-enhanced sonography of the prostate. AJR Am J Roentgenol 2002;178:915–919

81. Mehta SS, Azzouzi AR, Hamdy FC. Three-dimensional ultrasound and prostate cancer. World J Urol 2004;22:339–345

82. Hamper UM, Trapanotto V, DeJong MR, Sheth S, Caskey Cl. Three-dimensional US of the prostate: early experience. Radiology 1999;212:719–723

83. Frauscher F, Halpern EJ, Klauser A. Use of MRI to detect lymph-node metastases in prostate cancer. N Engl J Med 2003;349:1185–1186

11 Intraoperative Ultrasound

Robert A. Kane

Intraoperative ultrasound is a dynamic and highly interactive imaging study and is one of the most rapidly developing areas within ultrasonography. Unfortunately, many radiologists have been reluctant to spend a significant portion of time out of the department during the workday to perform and interpret intraoperative ultrasound studies, fearing that they will lose 1 or 2 hours of work time while waiting in the operating suite until the surgeon is ready for the scans to be performed. However, the information obtained during intraoperative ultrasound is often crucial for accurate diagnostic assessment and planning of surgical approaches to resection of the disease processes. Studies have shown that the impact of intraoperative ultrasound imaging on surgical decision making justifies the time and effort involved in terms of both efficacy and cost-benefit.[1] Our opinion, as well as that of many others with experience in the field, is that the benefits gained by intraoperative ultrasound imaging justify the time spent by the radiologists performing the procedure.

Technique for Efficient Performance of Intraoperative Ultrasound

We have evolved several means to improve the radiologists' efficiency when performing intraoperative ultrasound scans. These strategies typically allow a radiologist to perform the intraoperative ultrasound and return to the radiology department in ~30 minutes. The most effective strategies are as follows:

1. Intraoperative ultrasound studies are booked in advance with the ultrasound section whenever possible, which allows more planning and manipulation of the work schedule within the ultrasound section, and anticipation of the approximate time for performing the study.
2. Prepositioning of the intraoperative ultrasound scanner in the operating suite in advance of the examination may save a few minutes' waiting time for elevators.
3. The radiologist who will perform the examination may choose to work in surgical scrubs, thereby eliminating the need to change into scrubs when the call from the operating room arrives.
4. Mutual cooperation and respect between the surgeons and radiologists has resulted in an agreement that the surgeons will call for the intraoperative ultrasound

scan 10 to 15 minutes before they are actually ready for scanning, and the radiologists and technologists guarantee their readiness to perform the scan within 10 to 15 minutes of the telephone call. This arrangement is usually successful in avoiding any unnecessary waiting by either the surgical team or the radiological team and thus maximizes efficiency.

In our institution, the radiologist scrubs in on the case and is gowned and gloved and performs the actual scanning. A typical intraoperative study can be completed within 5 to 10 minutes, assuming that the sonologist is experienced. Scanning performed by the surgeon with the radiologist observing at the bedside or by remote teleradiography is less optimal compared with the radiologist actually performing the scan. Scanning provides important hand-to-eye information, and the scanning technique of most surgeons cannot compare with that of a skilled and experienced sonologist. Even though intraoperative ultrasound scanning has removed many of the noise-generated barriers to excellent image quality, proper scanning technique, understanding of image artifacts, and recognition of subtle findings such as isoechoic tumor nodules are best achieved by someone with extensive experience in ultrasonography. In a busy hospital setting, with frequent utilization of intraoperative ultrasonography, a remote teleradiography linkage to the intraoperative ultrasound images may be an acceptable alternative, providing that the surgeon performing the intraoperative scans has sufficient experience at intraoperative scanning.

If possible, it is optimal to sterilize the intraoperative ultrasound probes before the operation. We have had excellent success using gas sterilization with ethylene oxide for many of our intraoperative probes. However, many manufacturers are reluctant to allow gas sterilization, fearing that the transducers will be damaged by the high temperatures of aeration that are required by ethylene oxide gas sterilization, although we have not experienced any problems. Some operating suites will allow prolonged immersion in Cidex (glutaraldehyde; Johnson & Johnson, Arlington, Texas) as an adequate method of probe sterilization, but other institutions do not consider this sufficiently sterile for open intraoperative use, and there have been some adverse patient contrast reactions to the glutaraldehyde if it has not been sufficiently rinsed prior to patient exposure. In our institution, direct patient contact with glutaraldehyde-soaked equipment is not allowed, and therefore sterile probe covers are utilized. The application of probe covers may add 1 or 2 minutes to the time of the procedure as the cover is being applied, and there is some risk of compromise of sterile technique should the probe cover rip, which can occur occasionally. Therefore, when using equipment with sterile probe covers, we soak the probes in glutaraldehyde for 30 minutes before the procedure in case there is a break in sterile technique. The probes are thoroughly rinsed and, as an additional precaution, sterile gel is used inside the probe cover. It is preferable to use specifically designed transducer sheaths that fit snugly over the transducer head because loose-fitting covers may cause imaging artifacts due to trapped gas or folds in the sheath. Standard endoscopic sheathes can be used to cover the entire transducer cord.

Our preferred method of sterilization currently utilizes the Sterrad system (Advanced Sterilization Products, Irvine, California), which is gas-plasma technology using low-temperature sterilization, thereby avoiding some of the problems with the high-temperature ethylene oxide systems. Sterilization is adequate to allow direct patient contact with the probes, thereby avoiding the necessity for probe covers. There are no hazardous emissions and, hence, sterilization time is shorter because prolonged aeration and ventilation are not required.

Application of Intraoperative Ultrasound

Intraoperative ultrasound has many uses, and the applications are extensive and growing. In neurosurgery, intraoperative ultrasound is used effectively in surgery on the brain and spinal cord, and, in intraabdominal surgery, the uses are principally in the liver, biliary tract, and pancreas. Intraoperative assessment of vascular surgical disease and intraoperative ultrasound imaging post endarterectomy or reconstructive procedures is now on the increase. Other newly developing areas of use include intraoperative localization of breast tumors; applications in the genitourinary systems, such as evaluation of small renal cell carcinomas; as well as in gynecologic surgery; and, finally, to provide guidance for interventional procedures, such as prostate cryosurgery and tumor ablations in the liver. One of the most exciting and rapidly developing new areas is that of laparoscopic ultrasound (LUS) imaging, which is being applied to assessment of diseases of the liver, pancreas, and biliary tract within the abdomen and has also been used to help detect lung tumors during thoracoscopic resections. Another new and exciting application is the use of catheter-mounted, high-frequency ultrasound transducers for endoluminal intraoperative use in the bile ducts and ureters, for gynecologic procedures, and for vascular intraluminal assessment. Given the limitations of space, this discussion focuses on selected neurosurgical and intraabdominal applications.

Neurosurgical Applications

Brain

Intraoperative ultrasound scans of the brain can be obtained through a burr hole, using specially designed small burr hole probes or endoluminal probes, such as are used for prostate or transvaginal scanning. More commonly, intraoperative ultrasound scans are obtained through an open craniotomy flap. Excellent images can be obtained transdurally as well as directly on the brain surface after incision of the dura. The optimal frequency for brain imaging ranges from 5 to 7.5 MHz in frequency, and the best probe configuration is found in the endfire sector type probes, either mechanical or electronic convex array or phased array probes. The dura or brain surface is moistened with a small amount of sterile saline solution, which provides acoustic coupling for the transducer. Meticulous scanning technique is essential, with particular care to avoid applying significant pressure on the brain. A very light contact with the moistened dura or brain surface is sufficient for adequate acoustic coupling.

The principal use of intraoperative ultrasound is to accurately locate and localize masses within the brain substance that cannot be visualized directly by the neurosurgeon, and of course the brain cannot be palpated. Even masses a few millimeters deep to the cortical surface are difficult or impossible to detect visually. The vast majority of primary and metastatic brain tumors are markedly hyperechoic in comparison with the surrounding normal brain structures.[2] The sulcal convolutions on the brain surface are somewhat echogenic, but most of the brain substance is of relatively low and homogeneous echogenicity. Consequently, most tumors

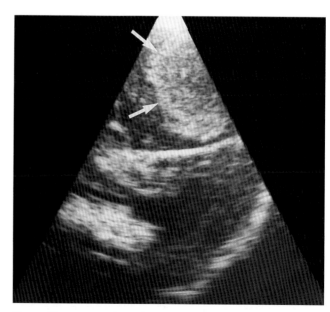

Figure 11–1 Hyperechoic glioma. Ultrasound scan shows a glioma (arrows) in the occipital lobe.

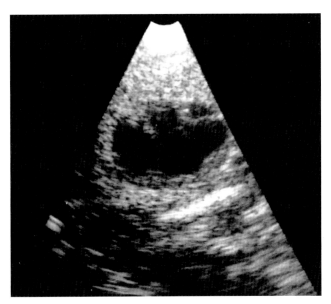

Figure 11–2 Predominantly cystic astrocytoma. Ultrasound scan clearly shows mural nodularity and septation.

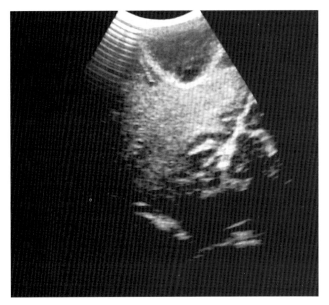

Figure 11–3 Poorly differentiated brain metastasis from primary lung carcinoma. Ultrasound scan shows an echogenic rim, but the central portion is hypoechoic due to liquefaction necrosis. Note the gyral and sulcal detail, which is obliterated by brain edema surrounding the tumor nodule.

stand out dramatically as hyperechoic lesions against a relatively hypoechoic background (**Fig. 11–1**). The reactive edema associated with brain tumors can decrease even further the echogenicity of brain substance and increase the conspicuity of focal masses.[3] Meningiomas are the most highly echogenic primary brain tumors, and usually have a relatively smooth contour and sharp margination. Calcifications within meningiomas occur frequently and result in a further increase in echogenicity. Glioblastomas are also markedly hyperechoic and are often well marginated, but may have less well-defined margins when they are aggressive and invasive.[4] Cystic degeneration may occur in glioblastomas as well as in cystic astrocytomas (**Fig. 11–2**), and the septations, cyst cavities, and areas of solid tumor and mural nodularity are well depicted by intraoperative ultrasound.[5,6] The complex nature of these cystic neoplasms is more completely portrayed with intraoperative ultrasound than with other imaging modalities, including computed tomography (CT) and even magnetic resonance imaging (MRI). Complete definition of the various spaces and cystic compartments may be important to guide surgical decompression of cystic tumors by aspiration. Most brain metastases are also hyperechoic and well circumscribed (**Fig. 11–3**), with an appearance similar to meningiomas and gliomas.[7] Liquefaction necrosis, which may occur spontaneously or as the result of therapy, may diminish the echogenicity of tumors centrally (**Fig. 11–3**). Low-grade astrocytomas can present a much more difficult imaging problem because they tend to be less echogenic and also to have very poorly defined infiltrative margins, insinuating into the adjacent brain substance in a very ill-defined manner.[8,9] In addition, chronic edema associated with low-grade astrocytomas

may actually increase brain echogenicity adjacent to the tumor, thus making tumor margins even more poorly defined.[10]

In addition to defining the tumor site and assessing margins, intraoperative ultrasound is helpful to the neurosurgeon in selecting an approach to resection of the tumor that will hopefully minimize damage to surrounding functional brain tissue. Following resection, intraoperative ultrasound can be utilized to evaluate completeness of surgical resection by rescanning after filling the surgical cavity with sterile saline and seeking any residual tumor nodules.

Intraoperative ultrasound imaging is also very helpful in guiding biopsy procedures, again with the goal of minimizing trauma to adjacent brain tissues.[11] Specially designed probes can be used through a modified burr hole to allow precise needle placement with minimal patient trauma.[12] Biopsies can be performed with electronic real-time biopsy guides, or freehand under direct real-time visualization.[13] High-resolution endfire endoluminal probes have been quite useful to perform accurate real-time biopsies through small craniotomy sites utilizing electronic biopsy guidance (**Fig. 11–4**). Utilization of color flow imaging may help to choose a path for the biopsy needle that will minimize disruption of major blood vessels between the cortical surface and the tumor site.

Real-time guidance can also be successfully used for tumor ablative techniques, placement of ventricular shunt catheters, and drainage of intracranial fluid collections and

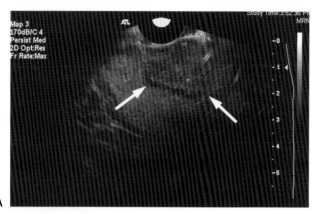

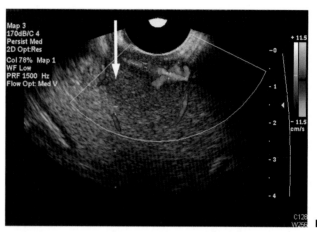

Figure 11–4 (A) Left temporal glioblastoma (arrows). **(B)** Color flow imaging helps target a safe, less vascular path for biopsy. The linear cursor (arrow) demarks the planned position of the biopsy needle.

abscesses (**Fig. 11–5**).[14] Following ultrasound-guided needle biopsies, we routinely rescan the patient for several minutes after the biopsy to assess for any bleeding within the lesion. Acute bleeding may appear as a small, highly echogenic focus within the mass or in the surrounding brain parenchyma. Occasionally, fluid/fluid levels may be seen, particularly when there is bleeding into a mass with cystic degeneration (**Fig. 11–6**). Scanning for several minutes is usually sufficient to ensure that any bleeding has stabilized.

Gray-scale, Doppler, and color flow imaging have been used in neurosurgical approaches to aneurysms and arteriovenous malformations (AVMs).[15] Assessment of blood flow is important during clipping or resection of aneurysms. Many AVMs are poorly visualized on gray-scale intraoperative ultrasound imaging, but the use of color flow imaging has been very helpful in defining their location and boundaries.

Many neurosurgical procedures now utilize frame-based or nonframe-based image guidance systems utilizing preoperative image information derived from MRI or CT scans, as a guide to surgical exploration and resection. However, brain tissue movement during surgery can be a significant source of error during image-guided surgical interventions. To compensate for this tissue motion, intraoperative ultrasound has been utilized to detect brain deformation during neurosurgery. Interactive image overlay systems allow projection of the region of interest on

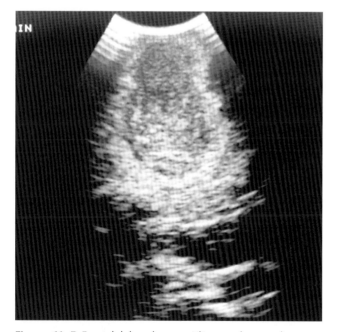

Figure 11–5 Frontal lobe abscess. Ultrasound scan shows an echogenic rim and centrally located, moderately echogenic purulent material. Ultrasound-guided aspiration and evacuation of the abscess was performed.

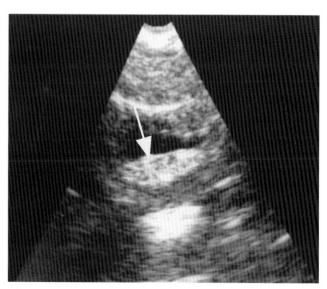

Figure 11–6 Astrocytoma. Ultrasound scan shows fluid-blood level (arrow) within the cystic cavity of an astrocytoma after needle biopsy.

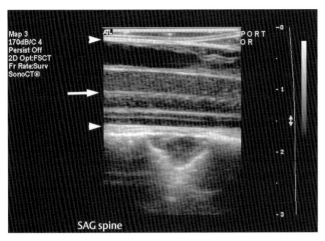

Figure 11–7 Thoracic cord. Sagittal ultrasound scans show the central spinal canal (arrow) as a paired linear echogenic structure. The dura (arrowheads) is well seen posteriorly and anteriorly.

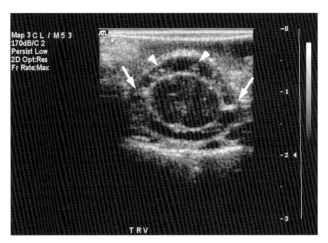

Figure 11–8 Transverse ultrasound scan of the cervical cord demonstrates dentate ligaments (arrows) and several nerve roots cut in cross section (arrowheads) within the posterior dural sac.

intraoperative ultrasound to overlay an associated MR image, helping the surgeon correlate the ultrasound anatomy to the more familiar MR images. The small discrepancies between the ultrasound and preoperative MR images can thus be utilized to assess tissue motion during neurosurgery.[16] Indeed, even today, there are advocates for intraoperative ultrasound as a much simpler, less expensive, and equally efficacious technique for guiding intraoperative procedures in comparison with the elegant, but highly complex and exceedingly expensive intraoperative MRI systems.[17]

Spine

The uses of intraoperative ultrasound imaging in the evaluation of spinal cord abnormalities are similar to those for brain imaging. Endfire probes are essential and the optimal frequency would be in the 7 to 10 MHz range, although 5 MHz probes can be successfully utilized. Electronic curved array or linear array probes are preferable because they allow concomitant utilization of color flow imaging, but mechanical endfire probes can also be utilized. The surgical laminectomy site is filled with sterile degassed saline to provide an acoustic coupling medium. The probe is then placed onto the pool of degassed saline solution. Images are usually obtained through the dura without direct contact with the spinal cord.

Both axial and sagittal planes are utilized. The spinal cord itself has a relatively low to moderate echogenicity and is quite homogeneous in texture.[18] The central spinal canal or indentation of the cord at the site of the central canal can be visualized as an echogenic single or paired set of lines relatively central within the spinal cord, which is otherwise featureless (**Fig. 11–7**). The central spinal canal is an important normal landmark that is frequently disrupted by pathological conditions within the cord. The arachnoid membrane is difficult to visualize, but the dura is well seen both dorsally and ventrally, and a small amount of fluid is usually present between the dura and the arachnoid. The dentate ligaments are well visualized in axial views (**Fig. 11–8**). They arise from the dorsal and lateral margins of the sac and extend laterally to the adjacent spinal canal. Nerve roots are inconsistently imaged in the cervical and thoracic spine, but are well seen at the conus medullaris and distally in the region of the cauda equina. Nerve roots appear to be hypoechoic or anechoic, but are readily visualized within the spinal fluid by highly reflective dorsal and ventral margins, appearing as two parallel echogenic lines. Pulsations can be imaged in real time from the anterior spinal artery, which is deep to the cord. Color flow imaging and power Doppler imaging will show the vascularity in a more complete fashion.

Assessment of the location and extent of masses is one of the principal uses of spinal intraoperative ultrasound. Lesion location can be assessed as intramedullary or extramedullary, and intradural and extradural components can be evaluated.[19] This capability can be particularly useful in depicting tumors such as neurofibromas, which may have both intradural and extradural components. The spinal cord cannot be retracted extensively, and intraoperative ultrasound imaging can provide important information as to the full extent of such tumors.[20] Many intramedullary tumors of the cord, including ependymomas, dermoids, and many metastases, are hyperechoic. Astrocytomas, however, are frequently isoechoic with extremely ill-defined margins, and consequently are very poorly visualized. These lesions may be recognized by effacement of the landmark echoes from the central spinal canal, as well as by fusiform swelling of the cord. Other nonneoplastic inflammatory and posttraumatic conditions can also cause swelling of the cord and may not be readily distinguishable from astrocytomas.[21] Astrocytomas may show cystic degeneration, which can also be seen in ependymomas and hemangioblastomas

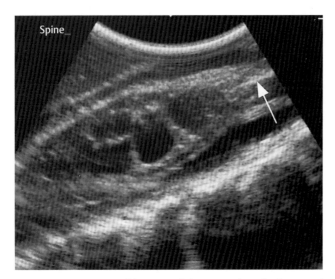

Figure 11–9 Hemangioblastoma of the cervical cord. Ultrasound scan shows multiple cystic components and interruption of the central spinal canal (arrow), which indicates the presence of an intramedullary mass.

(**Fig. 11–9**). These tumors can form fairly large cystic cavities and simulate syringomyelia. However, the presence of solid masses, mural nodules, or irregularly thickened septations will help to distinguish cystic tumors from a benign syrinx.[22,23]

Extramedullary tumors include meningiomas (**Fig. 11–10**), neurofibromas, lipomas, and dermoids, as well as malignant tumors, which are most often metastatic. Other conditions can also produce an extramedullary mass effect, including protruding discs, bony lesions (spurs and fracture fragments), hematomas, abscesses, and arachnoid cyst. Most of the neoplastic lesions appear as moderately echogenic masses with displacement or compression of the adjacent spinal cord and displacement of other struc-

tures, including nerve roots. Bony spurs and fragments are highly echogenic and may be associated with acoustic shadow. Herniated disc fragments are moderately echogenic, but substantially less so than bony spurs.[24] Hematomas appear hyperechoic acutely,[25] but may have a variable appearance, depending on their age and degree of liquefaction, whereas most abscesses and cysts have predominantly fluid components and increased transmission of sound through the fluid.

Intraoperative ultrasound is very useful in evaluating the extent of surgical resections,[26,27] as well as in guiding biopsies, particularly biopsies of tumors with extensive cystic or necrotic components. Intraoperative ultrasound and color flow imaging can be useful in identifying the more viable solid components of the tumor, thereby avoiding the necrotic components and diminishing the number of biopsies required to establish a diagnosis. Drainage of epidural abscesses and hematomas can also be aided by ultrasound guidance, as well as the drainage of cystic tumor cavities and the cavities of syringomyelia, both by real-time guidance of needle placement into the various component cavities and assessment of completeness of evacuation of cyst fluid. Finally, placement of intracystic shunt catheters within a syrinx can also be facilitated by intraoperative ultrasound guidance, and intraoperative ultrasound can demonstrate the adequacy of neural tissue decompression when spinal fractures are treated with Harrington rod fixation.[28]

Abdominal Applications

Gallbladder and Bile Ducts

Intraoperative imaging of the gallbladder and extrahepatic bile ducts is best performed using an endfire probe with a center frequency of 7 or 7.5 MHz. Either linear array or

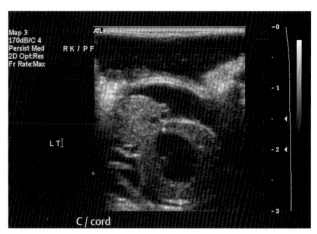

Figure 11–10 Cervical hemangioblastoma. **(A)** Transverse scan demonstrating the intramedullary portion of this tumor (arrow), including a small cystic component (arrowhead). A secondary syrinx (S) is noted centrally in the cord. **(B)** A scan at a slightly different level reveals the large extramedullary intradural component of this mass.

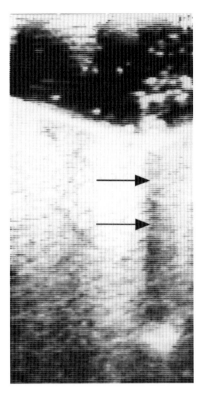

Figure 11–11 Gallbladder stones. Intraoperative ultrasound scan of the gallbladder shows numerous tiny, submillimeter stones not seen on preoperative studies. Arrows indicate acoustic shadowing from the conglomeration of these tiny stones.

sector formats are acceptable. Imaging at 5 MHz is probably also acceptable, but may require a standoff mechanism, such as filling the abdominal cavity with sterile saline or using a water-filled glove, to avoid near-field artifacts which may detract from imaging these structures. Scanning is performed directly in contact with the common bile duct or gallbladder, and scanning can be performed in any anatomical plane desired. If a complete study requires

imaging of the intrahepatic bile ducts, then the endfire probe may be satisfactory for the central ducts, but a complete evaluation of the peripheral ducts may require a sidefire liver-type probe. Intraoperative ultrasound of the gallbladder is not frequently required because preoperative ultrasound studies are usually more than adequate. Routine screening for gallstones is performed on patients with morbid obesity who are undergoing gastric bypass or stapling procedures because these patients frequently develop acute cholecystitis after substantial weight loss. Therefore, if stones are present, then the gallbladder is usually removed at the time of gastric surgery. These patients may be difficult, if not impossible, to image adequately because of their body habitus and, therefore, if the preoperative study is unsatisfactory, intraoperative ultrasound imaging of the gallbladder can be rapidly performed and may be capable of demonstrating stones that were not visualized preoperatively (**Fig. 11–11**).[29]

Intraoperative ultrasound may be useful in assessing gallbladder masses discovered incidentally at surgery or to assess the extent of a known gallbladder carcinoma (**Fig. 11–12**), particularly regarding potential invasion into the adjacent liver bed, which would require a more aggressive surgical resection.[30] Intraoperative ultrasound is nearly as accurate as frozen section to determine the depth of invasion.[31] If the tumor is resectable but also invading the liver, most surgeons would advocate a wedge resection of liver parenchyma to obtain a tumor-free margin at the time of intraoperative ultrasound. A careful search for more distant hepatic metastases or lymph node metastases should be performed to avoid unnecessary radical surgery in patients with advanced metastatic disease.

Intraoperative ultrasound of the bile ducts has been regarded by several surgical groups as a competitive or possibly superior modality to radiographic intraoperative cholangiography.[32,33] There is also a substantial amount of interest in the use of laparoscopic ultrasound

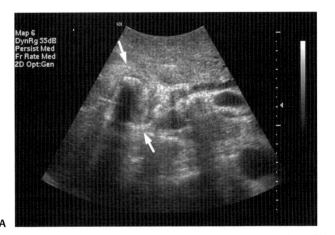

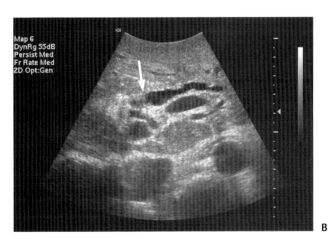

Figure 11–12 Gallbladder carcinoma. **(A)** Large solid mass in the gallbladder fossa (arrows), engulfing a gallstone that exhibits posterior acoustic shadowing. **(B)** Small isoechoic metastasis (arrow) causing obstruction and dilatation of the left hepatic bile duct.

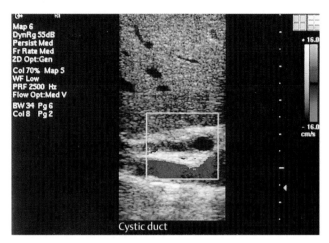

Figure 11–13 Transverse view of the common duct. Color flow Doppler image allows distinction of the biliary ducts from the adjacent portal vein (red) and hepatic artery (blue). This image shows the entry of the cystic duct into the common duct.

imaging for bile duct assessment in patients with potential choledocholithiasis undergoing laparoscopic cholecystectomy. The common bile duct, common hepatic duct, and intrahepatic bile ducts can be well visualized with both open and laparoscopic intraoperative ultrasound (**Fig. 11–13**).[34,35] Therefore, intraoperative ultrasound or LUS can be quite effective in demonstrating bile duct stones, and because laparoscopic cholangiography is somewhat arduous and difficult to perform, LUS may provide a superior alternative,[36] although no directly comparative studies have been performed. Routine use of LUS for every laparoscopic cholecystectomy is unwarranted due to the low yield of unsuspected pathology.[37] In our own institution, however, when choledocholithia-

sis is suspected clinically, endoscopic retrograde cholangiopancreatography is performed preoperatively both for diagnosis and, when positive, for therapeutic intervention via endoscopic sphincterotomy and stone extraction. If this approach is undertaken, the need for any form of intraoperative bile duct evaluation is substantially diminished.

Benign strictures and malignant obstructions in the biliary tract can be well evaluated by intraoperative ultrasound or LUS imaging to define the precise site and extent of the obstruction and help plan the type of biliary bypass procedure to be performed.[38] The sclerosing form of cholangiocarcinoma can be difficult to fully assess even with intraoperative ultrasound imaging because the tumor is an infiltrative and intensely sclerosing type lesion with poorly identified margins. Other forms of cholangiocarcinoma, particularly the papillary types, can be well defined by intraoperative ultrasound imaging (**Fig. 11–14**). In patients with central Klatskin type cholangiocarcinomas, we have occasionally been asked to scan the liver to identify large dilated intrahepatic ducts that might prove suitable for a peripheral hepaticojejunostomy, when a central decompression is mechanically impossible. This has been successfully accomplished in particular in the left lobe along the ligamentum teres, where large ducts draining segments 2 and 3 can, at times, be identified. More frequently now, however, patients with this large central type tumor are drained externally by percutaneous or endoscopic techniques.

Liver

Intraoperative ultrasound of the liver is most frequently performed on patients who are undergoing possible surgical resection of liver cancer, either primary or metastatic.

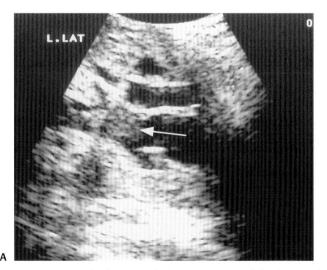

A

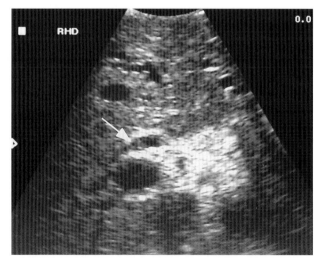

B

Figure 11–14 Klatzkin-type cholangiocarcinoma. **(A)** Ultrasound scan shows dilatation of the left hepatic duct, with tumor invasion (arrow). **(B)** Ultrasound scan shows dilatation of the peripheral ducts in the left medial segment, but the right hepatic duct (arrow) has a normal caliber and is free of tumor. This finding allowed a left hepatectomy and right hepaticojejunostomy to be performed.

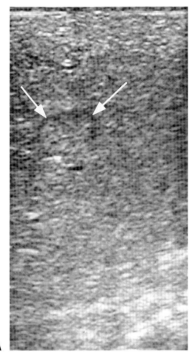

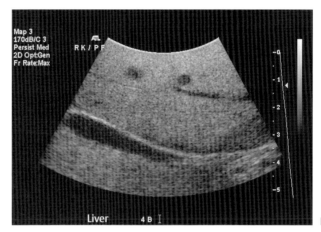

Figure 11–15 Occult liver metastases seen only with intraoperative ultrasound imaging. **(A)** A 1.2 cm isoechoic colon metastasis visible only because of the hypoechoic rim (arrows). **(B)** Two out of seven additional occult breast metastases identified at intraoperative ultrasound, each measuring 4 mm in diameter.

This examination is best performed using a side-fire probe with center frequency of 5 MHz, which allows full penetration of the liver from front to back, even in the right lobe where 12 cm of tissue can be adequately imaged. Although higher center frequencies of 7 or 7.5 MHz are excellent for biliary pancreatic imaging, only ~6 cm of liver can be effectively imaged at this higher frequency, and therefore a complete examination of the liver would be significantly lengthened in time and made more difficult because scans along the undersurface of the liver are less satisfactory due to the irregular contours and possible adhesions. A sidefire linear array or convex array configuration is also important to fit the probe between the liver and the diaphragm or the liver and the lateral rib cage, where there is very little space. By cradling the sidefire probe in the fingers, all portions of the liver can be adequately reached and scanned even without full mobilization of the liver. Scanning is optimal in the transverse plane beginning at the dome of the left edge of the liver and proceeding from cephalad to caudad. The next field should slightly overlap the original field while moving from left to right across the liver. With this overlapping field of view, the entire liver can be adequately assessed in 5 to 10 minutes.[39] The principal advantages of intraoperative ultrasound imaging of the liver are as follows:

1. The most complete detection of primary and metastatic tumors in the liver

2. Real-time definition of lobar and segmental liver anatomy as well as normal and aberrant vascular supply and drainage
3. Assessment of the feasibility of resection, planning of the most appropriate type of resection, and identification of deep tumor margins in patients undergoing nonsegmental wedge-type resections
4. Real-time guidance for tumor biopsy procedures and aspiration of fluid collections
5. Real-time guidance for ablative techniques such as cryosurgery, radiofrequency ablation, or alcohol ablation

The spatial resolution of intraoperative ultrasound imaging in the liver is unsurpassed, allowing for imaging of cysts as small as 1 to 3 mm and solid lesions as small as 3 to 5 mm (**Fig. 11–15**). Until the advent of multidetector CT and faster MRI allowing multiple-phase contrast imaging, intraoperative ultrasound would routinely detect 25 to 30% more lesions.[40] The vast majority of lesions detected by intraoperative ultrasound, but not by preoperative imaging studies or palpation are 1 cm or less in diameter, which in part, reflects the spatial resolution limits of preoperative studies.[41] CT arterial portography can definitely increase the sensitivity for detection of liver lesions to the range of 85 to 90%,[42] but this results in somewhat less specificity, particularly in attempts to detect lesions well under 1 cm in size. False-positive results for CT arterial portography

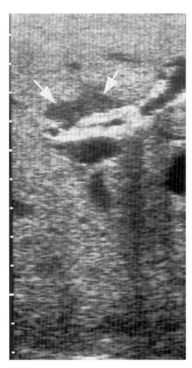

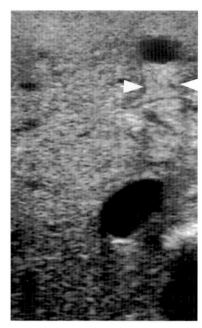

Figure 11–16 Diffuse fatty infiltration of the liver. Ultrasound scan shows diffuse fatty infiltration with sparing (arrows) at the porta hepatis. This sparing caused false-positive results on computed tomographic arterial portography.

Figure 11–17 Hepatic cyst. Ultrasound scan shows an enhanced 5 mm cyst (arrowheads), which caused a false-positive computed tomographic reading.

are encountered with some frequency due to perfusion abnormalities (**Fig. 11–16**) and small hepatic cysts (**Fig. 11–17**).[43,44] Recent advances in MRI, multidetector CT, and positron emission tomographic (PET) scanning have reduced the additional intraoperative ultrasound lesion detection rate to 5 to 10%.[45–47]

In our institution and others, patients who may be candidates for resection of liver tumors initially undergo laparoscopy to attempt to identify patients with diffusely

metastatic disease outside the liver, which would render the patient inoperable. Laparoscopic ultrasound of the liver can be combined with this approach to identify the maximum number of detectable liver lesions because additional tumors detected by LUS, but not on preoperative imaging, may also render a patient inoperable due to multiplicity of lesions or involvement of multiple lobes of the liver. LUS has the same capacity for detecting small liver lesions as open intraoperative ultrasound and is even more important in this situation because the surgeon is unable to palpate the liver, and only a minority of small liver tumors can be directly visualized with the laparoscope.[48,49] LUS is technically more challenging and much more time consuming than open intraoperative ultrasound imaging of the liver and may have slightly less sensitivity for lesion detection, as has been suggested in preliminary studies.

However, with further evolution of the technique and improvement in the equipment for laparoscopic ultrasound imaging, the small differences in sensitivity may diminish. State-of-the-art intraoperative ultrasound equipment allows the use of color flow or power Doppler imaging to assess the vascularity of liver tumors (**Fig. 11–18**). In addition, careful assessment of the vascular supply of the liver can have a major impact on surgical approach (**Fig. 11–19**). The presence of an accessory inferior right hepatic vein, which drains into the inferior vena cava distal to the hepatic confluence, may allow performance of a more extensive left trisegmentectomy. Similarly, an accessory or replaced left hepatic artery arising from the left gastric artery (**Fig. 11–20**), or a right hepatic artery arising from the superior mesenteric artery may influence the type of resection

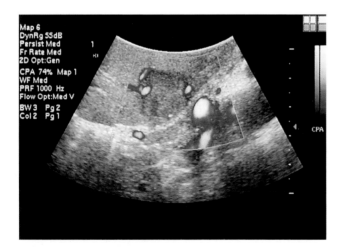

Figure 11–18 Colorectal metastasis. Power Doppler image demonstrates a hypovascular tumor with vessels being displaced around the periphery of the tumor nodule.

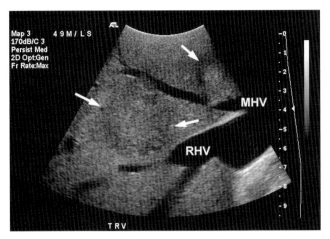

Figure 11–19 Two large isoechoic colorectal metastases (arrows) with deformity of the middle hepatic vein (MHV) and immediate contiguity to the right hepatic vein (RHV). The involvement or immediate proximity to the hepatic veins made resection technically impossible.

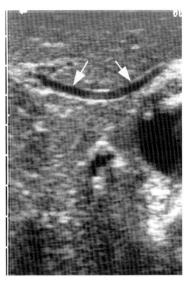

Figure 11–20 Replaced left hepatic artery. Ultrasound scan shows the point at which the left hepatic artery (arrows) enters the liver, along the ligamentum venosum.

performed.[50] The demonstration of major vessels surrounding masses or cystic lesions may influence the direct surgical approach to excision, drainage, or unroofing of a cyst (**Fig. 11–21**).

Lymphadenopathy can be readily assessed both in the porta hepatis as well as in the peripancreatic and celiac nodal groups. Demonstration of enlarged nodes in these areas may be important (**Fig. 11–22**) in determining resectability of a liver lesion because metastatic lymphadenopathy would generally render the patient inoperable for cure. Confirmation of lymph node metastases can be obtained directly by ultrasound-guided lymph node biopsies. Intraoperative ultrasound is not effective in demonstrating serosal implants or seeding of the mesentery by tumor, but this type of metastatic disease is often well detected by palpation or direct visual inspection or inspection via the laparoscope.

In patients with primary hepatocellular carcinoma, venous invasion is a frequent occurrence and is well detected both in the portal venous system as well as in the hepatic venous system.[51] Hepatic venous invasion can be life threatening at the time of surgery if the clot extends into the inferior vena cava or into the right atrium. Careful assessment of the full extent of venous invasion is therefore essential. Occasionally, during assessment of a patient with liver tumor of unknown origin, the site of the primary tumor may be visualized. In particular, the pancreas

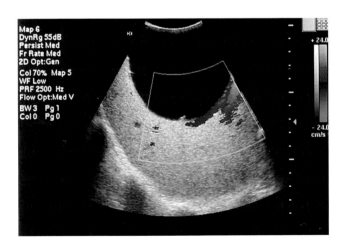

Figure 11–21 Hepatic cyst. Color flow imaging demonstrates displacement of the hepatic vasculature deep to the large hepatic cyst, distant from the area of planned surgical unroofing.

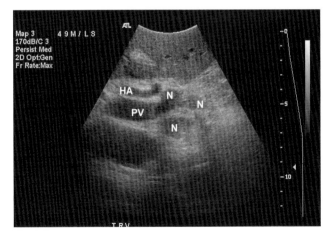

Figure 11–22 Metastatic lymphadenopathy. Multiple enlarged lymph nodes (N) were identified at intraoperative ultrasound and confirmed by biopsy to represent metastatic colorectal cancer. Planned hepatic metastasectomy was thereby canceled. HA, hepatic artery; PV, portal vein.

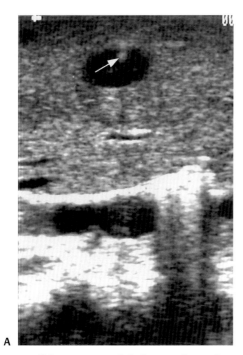
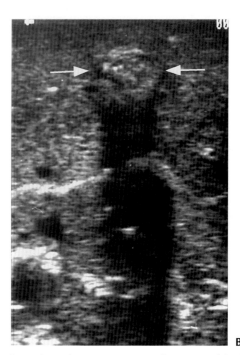

A   B

Figure 11–23 Hepatocellular carcinoma. **(A)** Ultrasound scan shows needle tip (arrow) penetrating a small tumor nodule. **(B)** On ultrasound scan, the nodule (arrows) is echogenic, with acoustic shadowing, after ethanol injection for tumor ablation.

should be closely assessed as a possible source of an unknown primary adenocarcinoma.

Most interventional intraoperative ultrasound-guided procedures, including biopsies, aspirations, and drainages, can be successfully performed with freehand real-time ultrasound guidance. Tumor ablation techniques, such as cryosurgery, radiofrequency, and ethanol injection (**Fig.**

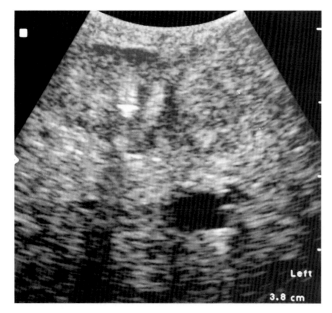

Figure 11–24 Hepatocellular carcinoma. During freehand laparoscopic ultrasound-guided biopsy, ultrasound scan shows the needle tip as an echogenic line within the tumor nodule.

11–23) are successfully performed and monitored under real-time intraoperative ultrasound guidance. At present however, guidance for procedures under laparoscopic ultrasound control is much more difficult. There are no commercially available systems equipped with electronic biopsy guidance systems similar to those used extensively and successfully in the diagnostic ultrasound laboratory. Consequently, LUS-guided interventional procedures are much more difficult, whether they involve biopsies, drainages, or tumor ablations. Freehand biopsies can be performed with LUS guidance (**Fig. 11–24**) by using specially designed long needles that puncture through the abdominal wall and enter the liver adjacent to the LUS probe, with the angle and depth of penetration controlled with real-time guidance. The degree of difficulty in performing these procedures is substantially greater than with open intraoperative ultrasound imaging, however, particularly for small, deep-seated lesions. It is hoped that eventually electronic biopsy guidance systems or interactive, stereotactic fusion imaging with preoperative CT or MRI will be developed by the manufacturers for use with LUS probes.

Pancreas

Intraoperative ultrasound imaging of the pancreas requires an endfire probe, either linear or sector format, with a center frequency ranging from 5 to 7.5 MHz. The sidefire configuration, which serves well for liver imaging, is unsuited for imaging the pancreas because this configuration will not allow satisfactory contact with the pancreas, particularly in large, deep abdominal cavities. The sector format is favored because it shows a wider area of anatomy in each image section. When intraoperative ultrasound is used to evaluate neoplastic lesions in the pancreas, the liver should also be scanned for evidence of metastatic disease, which is commonly seen in ductal adenocarcinoma as well as in islet cell tumors of the pancreas.

Virtually all islet cell tumors of the pancreas produce hormones that can be detected by pathological studies using special stains or electron microscopy, but only a subset of these tumors produce clinical symptomatology. Patients with symptomatic islet cell tumors often have extremely small-sized tumors that are difficult to image by preoperative techniques. Many competitive and complementary strategies have evolved, including the use of multidetector CT, MRI with gadolinium, octreotide nuclear scans, superselective angiographic techniques, and portal venous sampling as well as endoscopic ultrasound imaging. Although each technique has its advocates, none is wholly satisfactory, with sensitivities ranging from 70 to 85%. Intraoperative ultrasound imaging is the single most effective technique for detection of functioning islet cell tumors[52,53] and, at times, can detect even nonpalpable lesions as small as 3 to 5 mm. Most islet cell tumors are homogeneous and therefore hypoechoic; they are thus well detected against the background of hyperechoic pancreatic parenchyma. Most islet cell tumors have smooth well-marginated borders, whether benign or malignant, because these tumors are seldom locally aggressive, even when malignant.

The pancreas can be scanned from the head and uncinate process to the tail in a matter of minutes, either before or after mobilization techniques have been performed. It may be useful to fill the abdominal cavity with degassed saline solution to serve as an acoustic window, although excellent images can often be obtained with direct contact imaging or even by scanning through compressed bowel and mesentery. Occasionally, the lateral segment of the liver may provide an acoustic window to the pancreatic body and tail. As with the liver and biliary tract, a systematic imaging study with overlapping fields is essential to evaluate the entire pancreas.

Insulinomas are usually solitary (**Fig. 11–25**) and benign,[54] but all islet cell tumors have malignant potential. Gastrinomas are also frequently extrapancreatic in location,[55] lying in the so-called gastrinoma triangle between the common duct, head of the pancreas, and second and third portions of the duodenum. In patients with the multiple endocrine neoplasia syndrome (MEN-1), the insulinomas may also be multiple.[56] In fact, these tumors often arise in the wall of the duodenum or in extrapancreatic tissues and adjacent lymph nodes (**Fig. 11–26**). Malignant islet cell tumors frequently involve local lymph nodes in the pancreatic, portal, and celiac beds. Liver metastases are also frequent and may be widespread and very small, exhibiting either a decreased or increased echogenicity. Glucagonomas and somatostatinomas are often somewhat larger than the other functional islet cell tumors and are

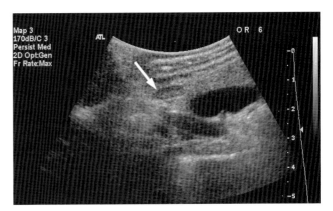

Figure 11–25 Insulinoma. This nonpalpable 3 × 7 mm insulinoma (arrow) in the head of the pancreas is well demonstrated at intraoperative ultrasound.

frequently located more distally in the pancreas, are usually solitary, and are also most often malignant. The so-called nonfunctional islet cell tumors (those that do not produce clinical symptomatology) often present as very large pancreatic masses, which usually exhibit locally benign behavior even when malignant and metastatic. Therefore, these tumors are usually well marginated, with passive displacement of surrounding vessels and infrequent vascular or neural invasion (**Fig. 11–27**).

Laparoscopic ultrasound of the pancreas has also been described as a sensitive and successful method in localizing insulinomas.[57] This method may be particularly important for small lesions localized to the body or tail of the pancreas because laparoscopic partial pancreatic resections

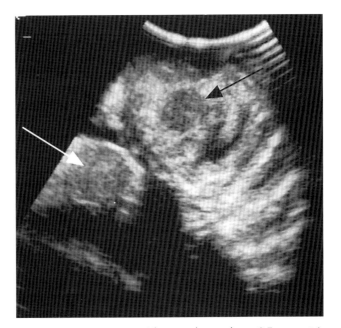

Figure 11–26 Gastrinoma. Ultrasound scan shows 0.7 cm gastrinoma arising in the wall of the duodenum (black arrow), with adjacent 1.2 cm metastasis (white arrow) in the lymph node.

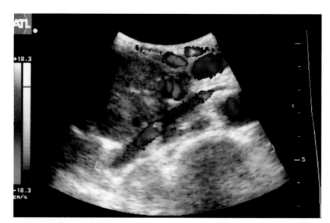

Figure 11–27 Nonfunctioning pancreatic islet cell tumor. Color flow Doppler imaging demonstrates passive displacement of the pancreatic vasculature around the large 5 cm hypoechoic mass, without evidence of vascular invasion. These tumors tend to be locally nonaggressive, even when malignant.

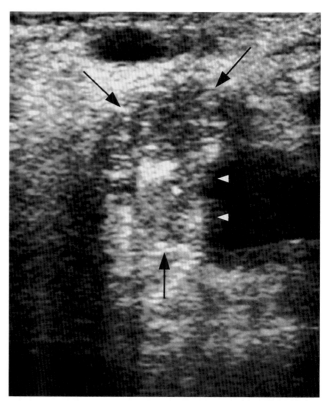

Figure 11–28 Pancreatic ductal adenocarcinoma. Ultrasound scan shows a mass (black arrows), which has invaded the lateral wall of the superior mesenteric vein (arrowheads). This invasion makes the tumor unresectable.

can be performed, thus avoiding a more prolonged hospitalization and recovery time from an open surgical resection. The LUS approach to the pancreas is best performed by utilizing a right upper or left upper quadrant port, allowing the probe to be oriented along the long axis of the pancreas in a relatively transverse plane. This allows for better orientation than attempting to image in the sagittal oblique plane across the short axis of the pancreas. At times, however, the head/neck and uncinate processes of the pancreas are better imaged in a more sagittal approach from a periumbilical port, which may also be more useful in allowing concurrent imaging of the liver for potential metastatic disease.

Intraoperative ultrasound imaging is seldom required for detection of ductal adenocarcinoma of the pancreas because this lesion is usually readily palpable, although identification of tumor by palpation can be difficult when there is extensive surrounding pancreatitis and, in this setting, intraoperative ultrasound imaging may be of help. Intraoperative and especially laparoscopic ultrasound imaging can be useful to assess for signs of unresectability in small pancreatic adenocarcinomas.[58] Preoperative imaging studies, especially high-quality multidetector CT arteriography, can be very accurate in predicting unresectability, but these techniques are still evolving and are not yet widely available. In many settings, laparoscopy is performed before open laparotomy and resection[59] to visually assess for metastatic disease in the mesentery and peritoneal surfaces, as well as on the surface of the liver. LUS can be utilized in conjunction with this approach to assess local resectability of pancreatic tumors (**Fig. 11–28**) by assessing the integrity of the pancreatic vasculature, particularly the superior mesenteric vein (SMV), splenic vein, as well as the superior mesenteric artery (SMA) and celiac artery. Direct vascular invasion of the SMV/portal vein confluence or the celiac artery or SMA would render the patient inopera-

ble. As with other types of tumors, assessment of metastatic disease to local lymph nodes and to the liver can also be performed. A combination of the visual laparoscopic and LUS techniques can help to minimize the number of patients subjected to open laparotomy, only to prove ultimately unresectable.[60,61]

Intraoperative ultrasound can also be used in assessing cystic neoplasms of the pancreas.[62] Serous microcystic adenomas of the pancreas, which are almost always benign, can be well assessed by intraoperative ultrasound imaging (**Fig. 11–29**). The cyst cavities should be thin walled, as well as the septations, and most of the cysts are under 1 to 2 cm in size, many as small as a few millimeters in diameter. Conversely, the presence of thick, irregular septa, mural nodules, or solid components is most consistent with a mucinous cystadenoma or cystadenocarcinoma (**Fig. 11–30**), both of which require surgical resection because malignancy cannot be excluded by imaging criteria, and even the benign cystadenoma is considered premalignant. Intraductal papillary mucinous neoplasms (IPNM) of the pancreas often present difficulties in surgical judgment as to the exact extent of the neoplasm and, therefore, the extent of required pancreatic resection. Intraoperative ultrasound provides an excellent means of assessing patients with IPNM, particularly in defining small hyperechoic masses within the main pancreatic duct or branch

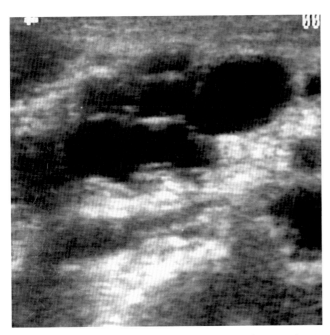

Figure 11–29 Microcystic pancreatic adenoma. Ultrasound scan shows multiple thin-walled cysts, all well under 2 cm in size, with no septal thickening or nodularity.

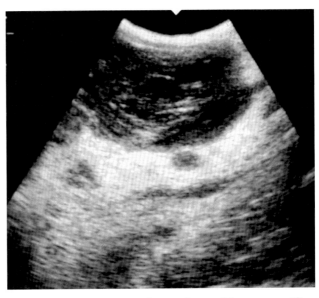

Figure 11–30 Mucinous cystadenocarcinoma of the pancreas. Ultrasound scan shows a large 3 cm cystic mass with thickened irregular septations and an adjacent small solid nodule.

ducts, as well as more accurately defining the extent of multifocal lesions, proving more sensitive than endoscopic retrograde cholangiopancreatography (ERCP) and endoscopic ultrasonography and thereby proving valuable for planning surgical strategy.[63]

Intraoperative ultrasound imaging can be useful in patients with pancreatitis who are undergoing surgery for biliary bypass or pancreatic drainage procedures (**Fig. 11–31**). The extent of pseudocysts and pancreatic

ductal abnormalities can be well demonstrated as well as the potential communications between the pancreatic duct and the pseudocyst cavities.[64,65] If the pancreatic duct is obstructed, drainage of the pseudocysts may prove inadequate and drainage of the pancreatic duct itself may be required for adequate therapy. The pancreatic duct may be difficult to localize by palpation in an enlarged, fibrotic, and rock-hard pancreas, whereas identification of the dilated pancreatic duct is simple and highly accurate with

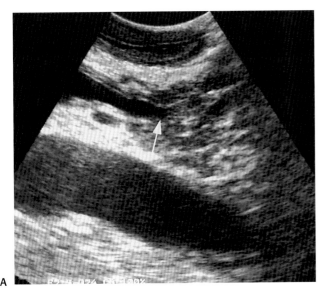

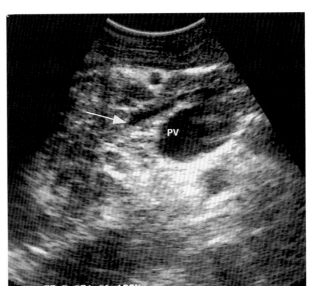

Figure 11–31 Calcific pancreatitis. **(A)** Sagittal ultrasound scan demonstrates a stricture of the common bile duct (arrow) at the entrance of an enlarged head of the pancreas. **(B)** Transverse ultrasound scan shows an obstruction of the pancreatic duct (arrow).

Pancreatitis rather than neoplasm was suggested by the lack of a hypoechoic mass and by diffuse enlargement with calcification. This diagnosis was confirmed by multiple biopsies. A biliary bypass was performed, and pancreatic resection was avoided. PV, portal vein.

intraoperative ultrasound, thereby identifying the optimal site for incision and drainage via a Puestow procedure. The use of color flow imaging and power Doppler can be important in evaluating focal peripancreatic fluid collections to assess for possible pseudoaneurysms. Intraoperative ultrasound guidance can also be employed for biopsy of pancreatic masses, drainage of fluid collections, and diagnostic punctures of the pancreatic duct.

Conclusion

Intraoperative ultrasound is an important and rapidly expanding field. The demand from surgeons for access to this highly effective modality is growing continuously. The rapidly developing capacity of laparoscopic surgery is adding further to increased demand for ultrasound imaging via laparoscopic approaches.

The techniques and applications presented in this chapter will hopefully increase the interest of radiologists in performing and interpreting intraoperative ultrasound and LUS studies, as well as to assist them in a more efficient use of their time when performing these studies. Intraoperative ultrasound studies have a profound impact on patient care and strongly influence surgical decision making. The necessity for high-quality intraoperative ultrasound scans is unquestionable and, in this author's opinion, the best-quality scans will be obtained when the radiologist scrubs in and both performs and interprets the study using the scanning skills and observational ability that can only be acquired by years of experience with ultrasound imaging studies.

References

1. Kane RA, Hughes LA, Cua EJ, et al. The impact of intraoperative ultrasonography on surgery for liver neoplasms. J Ultrasound Med 1994;13:1–6
2. Knake JE, Chandler WF, McGillicuddy JE, et al. Intraoperative sonography for brain tumor localization and ventricular shunt placement. AJR Am J Roentgenol 1982;139:733–738
3. Enzmann DR, Wheat R, Marshall WH, et al. Tumors of the central nervous system studied by computed tomography and ultrasound. Radiology 1985;154:393–399
4. Rubin JM, Dohrmann GJ. Intraoperative neurosurgical ultrasound in the localization and characterization of intracranial masses. Radiology 1983;148:519–524
5. Latchaw RE, Gold LHA, Moore JS Jr, et al. The nonspecificity of absorption coefficients in the differentiation of solid tumors and cystic lesions. Radiology 1977;125:141–144
6. Kjos BO, Brant-Zawadzki M, Kucharczyk W, et al. Cystic intracranial lesions: magnetic resonance imaging. Radiology 1985;155:363–369
7. Lange SC, Howe JF, Shuman WP, et al. Intraoperative ultrasound detection of metastatic tumors in the central cortex. Neurosurgery 1982;11:219–222
8. Knake JE, Chandler WJ, Gabrielson TO, et al. Intraoperative sonographic delineation of low-grade brain neoplasms defined poorly by computed tomography. Radiology 1984;151:735–739
9. Hatfield MK, Rubin JM, Gebarski SS, et al. Intraoperative sonography in low-grade gliomas. J Ultrasound Med 1989;8:131–134
10. Smith SJ, Vogelzang RL, Marzano MI, et al. Brain edema: ultrasound examination. Radiology 1985;155:379–382
11. Tsutsumi Y, Andoh Y, Inoue N. Ultrasound-guided biopsy for deep-seated brain tumors. J Neurosurg 1982;57:164–167
12. Berger MS. Ultrasound-guided stereotactic biopsy using a new apparatus. J Neurosurg 1986;65:550–554
13. Sutcliffe JC, Battersby RD. Intraoperative ultrasound-guided biopsy of intracranial lesions: comparison with freehand biopsy. Br J Neurosurg 1991;5:163–168
14. Shanley DJ, Eline MJ. Intracerebral hematoma localization and removal using intraoperative ultrasound. Milit Med 1992;157:622–624
15. Black KL, Rubin JM, Chandler WF, et al. Intraoperative color flow Doppler imaging of AVMs and aneurysm. J Neurosurg 1988;68:635–639
16. Comeau RM, Fenster A, Peters TM. Intraoperative US in interactive image-guided neurosurgery. Radiographics 1998;18:1019–1027
17. Rubin JM, Quint DJ. Intraoperative US versus intraoperative MR imaging for guidance during intracranial neurosurgery. Radiology 2000;215:917–918
18. Rubin JM, Dohrmann GJ. Intraoperative ultrasonography of the spine. Radiology 1983;146:173–175
19. Platt JF, Rubin JM, Chandler WF, et al. Intraoperative spinal sonography in the evaluation of intramedullary tumors. J Ultrasound Med 1988;7:317–325
20. Quencer RM, Montalvo BM, Green BA, et al. Intraoperative spinal sonography of soft-tissue masses of the spinal cord and spinal canal. AJR 1984;143:1307–1315
21. Post MJD, Quencer RM, Montalvo MB, et al. Spinal infection: evaluation with magnetic resonance imaging and intraoperative ultrasound. Radiology 1988;169:765–771
22. Hutchins WW, Vogelzang RL, Neiman HL, et al. Differentiation of tumor from syringohydromyelia: intraoperative neurosonography of the spinal cord. Radiology 1984;151:171–174
23. Quencer RM, Montalvo BM, Naidich TP, et al. Intraoperative sonography and spinal dysraphism and syringohydromyelia. AJR Am J Roentgenol 1987;148:1005–1013
24. Montalvo BM, Quencer RM, Brown MD, et al. Lumbar disk herniation and canal stenosis: value of intraoperative sonography in diagnosis and surgical management. AJR Am J Roentgenol 1990;154:821–830
25. Mirvis SE, Geisler FH. Intraoperative sonography of cervical spinal cord injury: results in 30 patients. AJR Am J Roentgenol 1990;155:603–609
26. Lunardi P, Acqui M, Ferrante L, Fortuna A. The role of intraoperative ultrasound imaging in the surgical removal of intramedullary cavernous angiomas. Neurosurgery 1994;34:520–523
27. Dempsey RJ, Moftakhar R, Pozniak M. Intraoperative Doppler to measure cerebrovascular resistance as a guide to complete resection of arteriovenous malformations. Neurosurgery 2004;55:155–161
28. Quencer RM, Montalvo BM, Eismont FJ, Green BA. Intraoperative spinal sonography in thoracic and lumbar fractures: evaluation of Harrington rod instrumentation. AJR Am J Roentgenol 1985;145:343–349
29. Herbst CA, Mittlestaedt CA, Staab EV, et al. Intraoperative ultrasonography evaluation of the gallbladder in morbidly obese patients. Ann Surg 1984;200:691–692
30. Machi J, Sigel B, Zaren HA, Kurohiji T, Yamashita Y. Operative ultrasonography during hepatobiliary and pancreatic surgery. World J Surg 1993;17:640–645

31. Azuma T, Yoshikawa T, Araida T, et al. Intraoperative evaluation of the depth of invasion of gallbladder cancer. Am J Surg 1999;178: 381–384

32. Sigel B, Coelho JCU, Nyhus LM, et al. Comparison of cholangiography and ultrasonography in the operative screening of the common bile duct. World J Surg 1982;6:440–444

33. Sigel B, Machi J, Beitler JG, et al. Comparative accuracy of operative ultrasonography and cholangiography in detecting common duct calculi. Surgery 1983;94:715–720

34. Yamashita Y, Kurohiji T, Hayashi J, et al. Intraoperative ultrasonography during laparoscopic cholecystectomy. Surg Laparosc Endosc 1993;3:167–171

35. Stiegmann GV, McIntyre R, Yamamoto M, et al. Laparoscopy-guided intracorporeal ultrasound accurately delineates hepatobiliary anatomy. Surg Endosc 1993;7:325–330

36. Jakimowicz J. Laparoscopic intraoperative ultrasonography, equipment, and technique. Semin Laparosc Surg 1994;(1):52–61

37. Rothlin MA, Schlumpf R, Largiader F. Laparoscopic sonography. Arch Surg 1994;129:694–700

38. vanDelden OM, deWit LT, vanDijkum EJMN, et al. Value of laparoscopic ultrasonography in staging of proximal bile duct tumors. J Ultrasound Med 1997;16:7–12

39. Kane RA. Intraoperative ultrasound. In: Wilson SR, Charboneau JW, Leopold GR, eds. Ultrasound: A Categorical Course Syllabus. San Francisco, CA: American Roentgen Ray Society; 1993:341–350

40. Clarke MP, Kane RA, Steele DG, et al. Prospective comparison of preoperative imaging and intraoperative ultrasonography in the detection of liver tumors. Surgery 1989;106:849–855

41. Kane RA, Longmaid HE, Costello P, Finn JP, Roizental M. Noninvasive imaging in patients with hepatic masses: a prospective comparison of ultrasound, CT and MR imaging [abstract]. Am J Roentgenol 1993;160(Suppl):133

42. Soyer P, Levesque M, Elias D, Zeitoun G, Roche A. Detection of liver metastases from colorectal cancer: comparison of intraoperative US and CT during arterial portography. Radiology 1992;183: 541–544

43. Matsui O, Takahashi S, Kadoya M, et al. Pseudolesion in segment IV of the liver at CT during arterial portography: correlation with aberrant gastric venous drainage. Radiology 1994;193:31–35

44. Nelson RC, Thompson GH, Chezmar JL, Harned RK, Fernandez MP. CT during arterial portography: diagnostic pitfalls. Radiographics 1992;12:705–718

45. Sahani DV, Kalva SP, Tanabe KK, et al. Intraoperative US in patients undergoing surgery for liver neoplasms: comparison with MR imaging. Radiology 2004;232:810–814

46. Milson JW, Jerby BL, Kessler H, et al. Prospective, blinded comparison of laparoscopic ultrasonography vs. contrast-enhanced computerized tomography for liver assessment in patients undergoing colorectal carcinoma surgery. Dis Colon Rectum 2000;43:41–49

47. Rydzewski B, Dehdashti F, Gordon BA, et al. Usefulness of intraoperative sonography for revealing hepatic metastases from colorectal cancer in patients selected for surgery after undergoing FDG PET. AJR Am J Roentgenol 2002;178:353–358

48. Kane RA, Roizental M, Kruskal JB, et al. Preliminary investigation of liver and biliary imaging with a dedicated laparoscopic US system [abstract]. Radiology 1994;193(P):287

49. John TG, Greig JD, Crosbie JL, Miles WF, Garden OJ. Superior staging of liver tumors with laparoscopy and laparoscopic ultrasound [comments]. Ann Surg 1994;220:711–719

50. Kruskal JB, Kane RA. Intraoperative ultrasonography of the liver. Crit Rev Diagn Imaging 1995;36:175–226

51. Kruskal JB, Kane RA. Correlative imaging of malignant liver tumors. Semin Ultrasound CT MR 1992;13:336–354

52. Gorman B, Charboneau JW, James EM, et al. Benign pancreatic insulinoma: preoperative sonographic localization. AJR Am J Roentgenol 1986;147:929–934

53. Zeiger MA, Shawker TH, Norton JA. Use of intraoperative ultrasonography to localize islet cell tumors. World J Surg 1993;17:448–454

54. Charboneau JW, Gorman B, Reading CC, et al. Intraoperative ultrasonography of pancreatic endocrine tumors. In: Rifkin MD, ed. Intraoperative and Endoscopic Ultrasonography. New York, NY: Churchill Livingstone; 1987:123–134

55. Sugg SL, Norton JA, Fraker DL, et al. A prospective study of intraoperative methods to diagnose and resect duodenal gastrinomas. Ann Surg 1993;218:138–144

56. Akerstrom G, Johansson H, Grama D. Surgical treatment of endocrine pancreatic lesions in MEN-1 (review). Acta Oncol 1991;30: 541–545

57. Lo CY, Lo CM, Fan ST. Role of laparoscopic ultrasonography in intraoperative localization of pancreatic insulinoma. Surg Endosc 2000;14:1131–1135

58. Alberti A, Dattola P, Littori F, et al. [Intraoperative ultrasonography in the staging of pancreatic head neoplasms] L'ecografia intraoperatoria nella stadiazione delle neoplasie cefalopancreatiche. Chir Ital 2002;54:59–64

59. John TG, Greig JD, Carter DC, Garden OJ. Carcinoma of the pancreatic head and periampullary region: tumor staging with laparoscopy and laparoscopic ultrasonography. Ann Surg 1995;221:156–164

60. Hann LE, Conlon KC, Bach AM, Dougherty EC, et al. Laparoscopic sonography of peripancreatic tumors: preliminary experience. Am Roentgenol 1997;169:1257–1262

61. vanDelden OM, Smits NJ, Bemelman WA, et al. Comparison of laparoscopic and transabdominal ultrasonography in staging of cancer of the pancreatic head region. J Ultrasound Med 1996;15:207–212

62. Kubota K, Noie T, Sano K, et al. Impact of intraoperative ultrasonography on surgery for cystic lesions of the pancreas. World J Surg 1997;21:72–76

63. Kaneko T, Nakao A, Inoue S, et al. Intraoperative ultrasonography by high-resolution annular array transducer for intraductal papillary mucinous tumors of the pancreas. Surgery 2001;129: 55–65

64. Sigel B, Machi J, Ramos JR, et al. The role of ultrasound imaging during pancreatic surgery. Ann Surg 1984;200:486–493

65. Printz H, Klotter HJ, Nies C, et al. Intraoperative ultrasonography in surgery for chronic pancreatitis. Int J Pancreatol 1992;12:233–237

12 Leg Swelling with Pain or Edema

Edward I. Bluth

Patients who present with leg swelling with pain or edema are of great clinical concern because they are at risk for having acute deep venous thrombosis (DVT). Acute DVT is an important public health problem because it affects over 20 million individuals yearly in the United States. Estimates of the incidence of DVT range from between 100 and 180 per 100,000 persons per year.[1] DVT occurs in both sedimentary outpatients as well as hospital inpatients, although rarely in children. Among the predisposing factors are prolonged congestive heart failure, pelvic and lower extremity surgery, pregnancy, obesity, inactivity, airplane travel, coagulopathy, and paraplegia.[2]

The diagnosis of DVT has other significant implications as well. It has been known for more than a century that DVT may be a presenting feature of an occult neoplasm. Recently, a definite association between DVT and a subsequent clinically occult cancer has been shown, particularly in the first 6 to 12 months of follow-up.[3] However, in the study by Sorensen et al 40% of the patients diagnosed with cancer within 1 year of the diagnosis of DVT had distant metastases. As a result, it is uncertain whether an extensive search for an occult neoplasm would be cost-effective or warranted because early diagnosis may not change outcomes. The types of cancers most strongly associated with DVT in this Swedish study of more than 15,000 patients were cancer of the pancreas, ovary, liver (primary hepatic cancer), and brain.[3]

Presently, it is important to diagnose acute DVT because of its relationship with acute pulmonary embolism. The presence of DVT does not equate with pulmonary embolism, but detecting DVT may prevent pulmonary embolism from developing. It is reported that when significant acute venous thrombosis is diagnosed but not treated, pulmonary embolism is likely to occur in up to 50% of the cases.[4] More importantly, it is believed that in up to 30% of the episodes of pulmonary embolism the outcome is death.[4] Pulmonary embolism is reported to be the cause of death in more than 10,000 hospitalized patients each year in the United States.[5] Mortality can be significantly reduced when acute DVT is treated with anticoagulation. Because an estimated 90% of pulmonary emboli arise from the lower extremities, there is a great clinical need to accurately assess the venous system of the lower extremities when there is clinical suspicion of acute DVT.

Accuracy of Presentation in Diagnosing Deep Venous Thrombosis

Patients who present with the clinical symptomatology of leg swelling with pain or edema certainly are at risk for acute DVT. However, the clinical accuracy of diagnosing this entity is known to be very poor. Every clinical sign

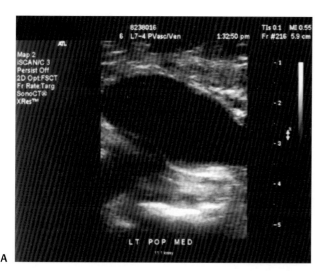

A

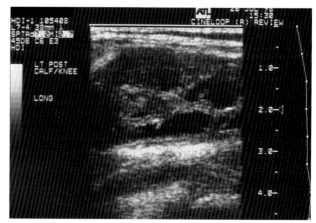

B

Figure 12–1 (A) Oblique view of a large sonolucent mass located in the popliteal fossa separate and apart from the artery and vein on sagittal color flow Doppler imaging. This is consistent with a Baker's cyst. **(B)** Oblique image of a complex mass in the popliteal space of another patient. This mass is separate and medial to the artery and vein and is characteristic of a ruptured Baker's cyst.

attributed to DVT has been statistically analyzed and found to be of no value in reliably determining the presence or absence of DVT.[6] The location of signs and symptoms of pain or swelling is usually unrelated to the extent or location of clot within the veins. Symptoms localized to the calf may have an etiology in the femoral veins, and thigh pain may be related to occlusion of calf veins.[7] The specificity for clinical diagnosis is low because the symptomatology associated with acute DVT can have, among other causes, a musculoskeletal or lymphatic basis. Furthermore, asymptomatic DVT can commonly occur, and the sequelae can even be severe enough to cause death by pulmonary embolism.

In patients who present with bilateral leg symptoms, in the absence of significant risk factors (such as malignancy, paralysis, bed rest of more than 3 days, major surgery, strong family history of DVT, or leg, thigh, or calf swelling)[8] the first assumption should be that the etiology is cardiac disease or chronic peripheral vascular disease.[9] However, in patients with risk factors, the possibility of bilateral clot must be seriously considered, and a bilateral ultrasound examination is warranted.

Accuracy of D-Dimer Test in Diagnosing Deep Venous Thrombosis

D-dimer has emerged as a clinically useful serological test. D-dimer represents a breakdown of the cross-linked fibrin clot. It is elevated in almost all patients with acute DVT, having a sensitivity of 97%, but it is nonspecific (less than 50%). D-dimer is also elevated in patients who have had recent surgery, trauma, sepsis, and malignancy.[1] However, it is very useful in excluding DVT having a negative predictive value of 97%.[10] In certain patient groups, D-dimer combined with clinical assessment has been shown to safely reduce or eliminate the need for noninvasive testing.[10]

Differential Diagnosis

The differential diagnosis for the symptoms of leg swelling with pain or edema includes acute DVT, Baker's (popliteal) cyst, cellulitis, lymphedema, chronic venous insufficiency, superficial thrombophlebitis, popliteal venous aneurysm, popliteal artery aneurysm, iliac artery aneurysm, femoral artery pseudoaneurysm, enlarged lymph nodes extrinsically compressing the veins, heterotopic ossification, hematoma, muscular tears, and diabetic muscle infarction.[7,11–19] The appropriate use of imaging studies, and, in particular, the appropriate use of ultrasound, enables us to distinguish which of these clinical entities is present.

Baker's cysts appear as sonolucent or complex masses more commonly medial than lateral. When they rupture,

the surface margins become irregular (**Fig. 12–1A,B**). They appear separate and distinct from the popliteal artery or vein. The normal popliteal artery measures less than 1 cm. Veins and arteries should taper normally, and an outpouching would suggest aneurysmal dilatation (**Fig. 12–2**). Frequently, thrombus may surround the residual lumen of an arterial aneurysm. Aneurysms or pseudoaneurysms, owing to their expanded size, can compress the venous structures that surround them, resulting in swelling or edema of the distal extremity. The visualization of a concomitant vascular abnormality should, therefore, not preclude further evaluation of the more distal venous structures because the resultant stasis may be a predisposing factor to the development of DVT (**Fig. 12–3**). Patients with superficial thrombophlebitis have an increased risk of progressing to DVT. In one report, 11% of patients who initially had isolated superficial venous thrombus progressed to DVT.[20] In another study, 23% of patients with superficial thrombophlebitis had occult DVT of the lower extremities.[21] As a result, if superficial venous thrombosis is noted, then the deep venous system should be carefully studied. Similarly, enlarged lymph nodes can also extrinsically compress adjacent venous structures, resulting in lower extremity symptoms (**Fig. 12–4**). This has been noted in patients with acquired immunodeficiency syndrome (AIDS). On rare occasions, pain or swelling of the lower extremity may be the presenting symptom of lymphoma. Lymph nodes appear separate from the vascular structures and are easily distinguished using color flow Doppler imaging (CFDI). Hematomas are also separate and distinct from the arteries and veins and, depending on their age, appear as either complex or sonolucent masses.

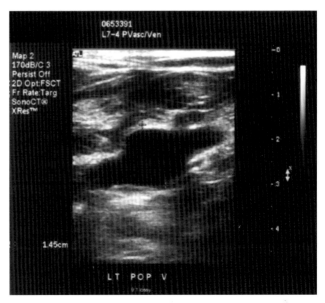

Figure 12–2 Sagittal color flow Doppler imaging of a 1.5 cm popliteal venous aneurysm.

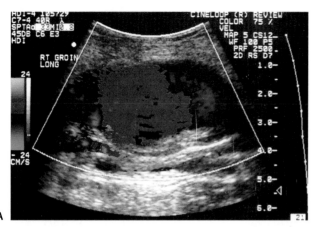

A

B

Figure 12–3 (A) Large pseudoaneurysm of the right common femoral artery (CFA) postcardiac catheterization compressing the common femoral vein (CFV). **(B)** Transverse image showing the more expanded hypoechoic noncompressible proximal superficial femoral vein (SFV) consistent with acute thrombus. PFV, profunda femoral vein.

Diagnostic Imaging Evaluation

Tests to evaluate the lower extremities include contrast venography, venous ultrasound including CFDI and Doppler spectral analysis, impedance plethysmography (IPG), various radionuclide approaches, magnetic resonance (MR) venography, computed tomography (CT), nonimaging continuous wave Doppler, and thermography. All evaluation methods were studied by the Cardiovascular Appropriateness Panel of the American College of Radiology (ACR), and each of these methods was rated for appropriateness in 1995 and reassessed in 1999 (**Table 12–1**).[22]

Contrast venography has been the gold standard by which other examination methods have been rated; however, in 5 to 10% of patients it may not give a reliable result, and because it also requires the use of intravenous contrast with the associated risks of renal failure, extravasation, chemical-induced thrombophlebitis, and idiopathic contrast reactions, its appropriateness rating was only intermediate. In contrast, duplex Doppler compression ultrasound received the highest possible rating and, therefore, now should be used as the study of choice to evaluate symptomatic patients.

The panel reported also that thermography and nonimaging continuous wave Doppler analysis were inappropriate and should not be performed. IPG was given an intermediate appropriateness rating as was MR venography. The accuracy of IPG is reported to be close to 90% for DVT above the knees, but it requires meticulous technique. Heijboer et al reported that serial ultrasonography is a more accurate means of detecting DVT than is IPG. An abnormal IPG had a positive predictive value of 83% for DVT compared with a 94% rate for an ultrasound abnormality in patients with DVT.[23]

Radionuclide venography was given a lower intermediate rating. The accuracy of detecting large obstructive thrombi is reported to be close to 90%. Another approach that can be used and appears best to diagnose DVT below the knee or in the lower thigh is the active uptake of radionuclide-labeled fibrinogen, platelets, peptides, fibrin, and plasmin by thrombi. New imaging agents may also be helpful in differentiating acute recurrent from chronic DVT. CT is most useful for imaging thrombosis related to the iliac veins and is not particularly suitable for studying the femoropopliteal veins. It is also valuable in identifying sources of extrinsic compression of the iliac veins. Recently, CT venography has been recommended as a quick and safe means to evaluate the deep venous system after multidetector row CT (MDCT) angiography of the pulmonary arteries (within the same examination), particularly if the patient is clinically unstable and requires immediate diagnosis.[24,25] This methodology has a reported sensitivity ranging between 71 and 100%, specificity between 93 and 97%, positive predictive value between 53 and 92%, and negative predictive value between 92 and 97%.[24,26,27] However, the estimated median cumulative effective radiation dose is 8.26 mSv

Figure 12–4 Solid mass density in the right inguinal area separate and apart from the common femoral artery and common femoral vein. On biopsy this mass of nodes was diagnosed as non-Hodgkin's lymphoma.

Table 12–1   American College of Radiology ACR Appropriateness Criteria for Clinical Condition: Suspected Lower Extremity Deep Vein Thrombosis

	Clinical Condition	
Radiologic Procedure	**Appropriateness Rating**	**Comments**
US, lower extremity, duplex Doppler compression	9	
MRI, venography, lower extremity	6	Demonstrated to be useful, but insufficient supporting data so far.
INV, venography, pelvis	6	When other studies equivocal or an intervention is planned.
CT, pelvis, with contrast	6	As an adjunct to CTPA done for suspected PE.
INV, venography, lower extremity	5	When other studies equivocal or an intervention is planned.
CT, venography, lower extremity (following arm injection)	5	As an adjunct to CTPA done for suspected PE.
NM, venography (MAA), lower extremity	3	
IPG, lower extremity	2	
X-ray, lower extremity	2	
Continuous wave Doppler (nonimaging), lower extremity	1	

Appropriateness Criteria Scale:
1 = Least appropriate, 9 = Most appropriate
INV = interventional venography

[compared with 2.5 mSv for CT angiography (CTA) of pulmonary arteries] for all patients with an effective gonadal dose of 3.87 mSv. This dose is more than 300% of the median effective dose for CTA of the pulmonary arteries (2.5 mSv). This dose must be significantly reduced before it could become a routine clinical method to evaluate for DVT in clinically stable patients, particularly for those who are young.

MR venography has also been suggested as a useful technique to detect DVT in the lower extremities.[28,29] It appears to be particularly useful in detecting femoral and iliac vein thrombi and may be particularly valuable in determining the proximal extent of disease in these vessels. Newer techniques such as venous enhanced subtracted peak arterial (VESPA) MR venography,[30] flow-independent MR venography,[5] and direct thrombus MR imaging,[31,32] may allow MR to play a more significant role in DVT imaging in the future.

One major limitation of both MR and CT is the significant increase in cost relative to ultrasound. Presently, both may be most useful for evaluating the more proximal venous structures when a satisfactory study is not achieved with ultrasound. But when considering the overall sensitivities, specificities, and costs of the various testing options, ultrasound remains the screening test of choice for lower extremity DVT.

Ultrasound Imaging

Evaluating patients with symptoms of leg swelling with pain or edema should involve using all the capabilities of ultrasound when available, including Doppler spectral analysis, CFDI, transducer compression, and high-resolution B-mode imaging. The examination should integrate all these methodologies into the complete study of the venous structures of the lower extremity. Extended field of view sonography, a new option of some machines, may be useful in demonstrating more easily the full extent of disease. The use of contrast agents and harmonic imaging may be helpful, in the future, in cases in which the complete occlusion of vessels is uncertain.

Normal Findings

With Doppler spectral analysis and CFDI, three parameters of normal lower extremity veins can be identified: respiratory phasicity, spontaneous flow, and augmentation (**Fig. 12–5A–E**). During the respiratory cycle, the change in venous flow is termed respiratory phasicity (**Fig. 12–5A**). During inspiration, an increase in intraabdominal pressure causes compression of the inferior vena cava and a decrease in the Doppler signal. In expiration, there is an increase in visualized flow and in the Doppler spectral analysis signal (**Fig. 12–5B**). The Valsalva maneuver leads to stasis and venous dilatation. The normal physiological response of the femoral vein is a 50 to 200% increase in diameter. At the end of the Valsalva maneuver, augmented venous flow normally occurs (**Fig. 12–5C**). In a normal venous system, augmentation also occurs with distal mechanical compression (**Fig. 12–5B,D,E**). Spontaneous venous flow is easily detected in the large leg vessels, but is frequently not seen in some of the smaller calf vessels. Augmentation will frequently be required to prove patency.

A normal vein also demonstrates compressibility, has unidirectional flow, and is free of internal echoes. Compressibility is best demonstrated when the transducer is

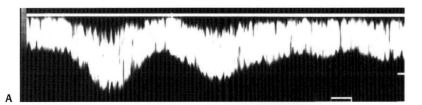

A

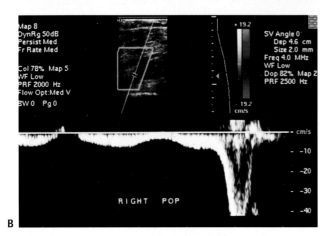

B

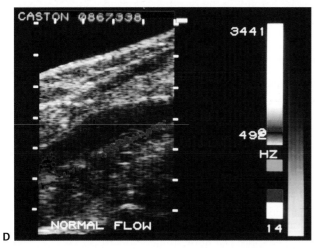

C

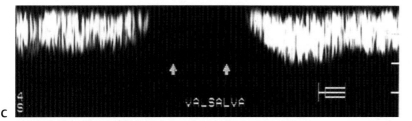

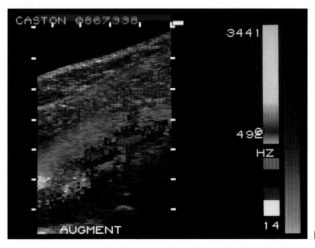

D

E

Figure 12–5 (A) Normal parameters of lower extremity veins include respiratory phasicity, **(B)** augmentation following distal compression, and **(C)** absence of flow during the Valsalva maneuver and then slight augmentation following the maneuver. These are demonstrated with Doppler spectral analysis. **(D)** Augmentation can also be demonstrated with color flow Doppler imaging following **(E)** distal compression.

held in the transverse position relative to the vein because the transducer will not roll off the vessel (**Fig. 12–6A,B**). An adequate amount of pressure sufficient to dimple the overlying skin should be applied with the transducer to visualize the normal sonographic finding of a collapsed venous lumen. Unidirectional flow is best identified with CFDI.

Technique

The choice of transducers for studying the lower extremities depends on the patient's body habitus and the depth of the vessel being studied. For the average patient, a 5 to 10 MHz linear transducer is most appropriate. Vessels ranging in size

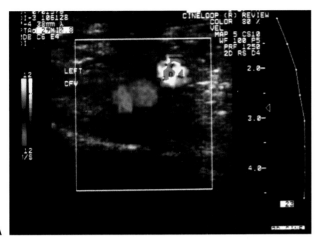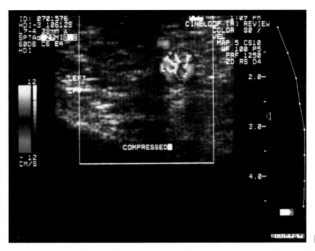

A   B

Figure 12–6 (A) Transverse color flow Doppler imaging demonstrating the normal common femoral vein (CFV–blue) and the common femoral artery (CFA–red) without and **(B)** with compression. Note the collapse of the normal vein.

from 1 mm to slightly over 1 cm can be clearly visualized over a depth of 6 cm. For large-body-habitus patients, transducers of lower MHz can be used. Linear array transducers permit long segments of vessels to be imaged more rapidly and are therefore preferred. Transducers will frequently

need to be switched when the examiner moves from the inguinal region to the thicker thigh or the calf veins.

Vessels that can be studied include the common femoral veins; saphenous veins; superficial femoral veins (SFVs); popliteal veins; calf veins, including the anterior tibial, posterior tibial, and peroneal veins; and if possible, the iliac veins (**Fig. 12–7**). The external iliac, common femoral, saphenous, and superficial femoral veins are best evaluated with the patient supine. The popliteal veins can be studied in any of three different positions: with the patient prone and the leg flexed 20 to 30 degrees, with the patient decubitus and the study side up, and by elevating the foot and leg and scanning from below. At times, a combination of these techniques is necessary. Flow augmentation of the calf veins can be achieved by having the patients plantar flex the foot. This self-augmentation technique helps in better visualization of these vessels. Some have advocated studying the calf veins by having the patient sitting up and dangling the legs over the side of the examining table.

The calf veins can be studied by using either an anterolateral or a posteromedial approach (**Fig. 12–8**). To evaluate the posterior tibial veins, it is recommended to turn the foot outward and place the probe posterior medial to the medial malleolus (**Fig. 12–9**). The color box can also be directed to the left to optimize flow. For the study of the peroneal and anterior tibial veins, the foot should be turned inward and the probe should be placed parallel with the fibula and tilted outward (**Fig. 12–9**). Additionally, the color box can be directed straight to better visualize the veins. Also, if a linear probe is not technically adequate, a curved array transducer can be substituted. Additionally, it has been noted that if the posterior tibial and peroneal veins are patent, it is exceedingly rare to have an isolated thrombus in the anterior fibial vein. Therefore, if the other two venous pairs are patent, examination for the anterior tibial vein is unnecessary.

Figure 12–7 Vessels commonly visualized when evaluating the veins of the lower extremities.

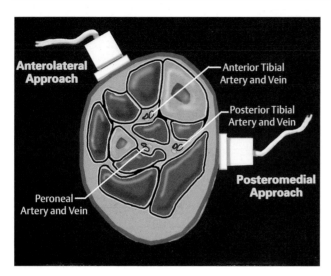

Figure 12–8 Diagram demonstrating practical anatomical approaches used to study the calf veins.

Sonographers and sonologists should carefully scan the femoral veins to look for duplicated vessels. In a recent report, Screaton et al demonstrated that multiple femoral veins were present in 177 (46%) of 381 venograms.[33] This is much more than the generally accepted frequency of duplication of 20 to 25%.[34] However, even with this high frequency of duplication, Screaton et al demonstrated only a 6% false-negative rate for DVT, which was not statistically significant compared with the 1% (4/402 patients) false-negative rate found in patients with single femoral veins. Quinlan et al also demonstrated that variations in lower limb venous anatomy were common, showing that in 31% of 404 bilateral venograms, the SFV was duplicated.[35] For the inexperienced, it is important to realize that the incidence of duplication for femoral veins is significant and,

therefore, special attention must be directed to insure that a duplicated thrombosed vessel is not ignored.

Examination Protocol

Recently, there has been considerable debate about what constitutes an adequate and appropriate examination. The traditional protocol described in the American College of Radiology Standard for Performance of the Peripheral Venous Ultrasound Examination adopted in 1993 and reassessed in 1999 and 2005 calls for the careful examination of the full length of the common femoral vein, superficial femoral vein, and popliteal vein.[22] Images with and without compression should be recorded at the common femoral, midsuperficial femoral, and midpopliteal veins. We use CFDI as an adjunct in nearly all our examinations because it helps speed identification of vessels. Power Doppler imaging can sometimes be useful in identifying early recanalization, but because there is no directionality of flow, it is not as useful as CFDI alone. Doppler spectral analysis is useful in assessing phasicity and augmentation responses and is particularly helpful as a secondary means of evaluating the patency of the iliac veins. Some centers also include the study of the greater saphenous vein where it enters the common femoral vein as part of the routine examination because of the risk of superficial thrombophlebitis extending into the deep system. In the future, ultrasound contrast may be included as a means to improve indeterminate or uncertain studies.

Limited Compression Examinations

Pezzullo, Perkins, and Cronan reported in a prospective study of 53 symptomatic patients and a retrospective study of 155 symptomatic patients that a limited compression

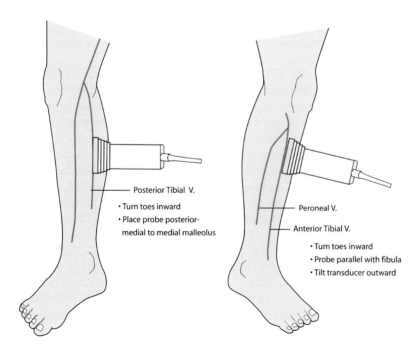

Figure 12–9 How to evaluate calf veins.

examination of the common femoral (from the inguinal ligament to the takeoff of the profunda femoral vein) and of the popliteal vein (above and below the knee) depicted each case of DVT that was detected with the traditional more complete examination.[36] Additionally, they found a 54% reduction in examination time (9.7 min) with the limited study. As a result, they recommended studying just the common femoral and popliteal veins and repeating the study in 2 to 5 days if the patient was still symptomatic. In reaction, Frederick et al prospectively studied 721 symptomatic patients and determined after 755 examinations that DVT limited to a single vein occurs with sufficient frequency that the study could not be abbreviated without loss of diagnostic accuracy.[37] They found that DVT was limited to the common femoral vein in eight studies (6.1%), to the superficial femoral vein in six studies (4.6%), and to the popliteal vein in 14 studies (10.7%). They found no statistically significant difference between the frequency of isolated thrombus in any of these three veins. Maki et al, in a study of 2704 lower extremities, found that acute DVT was isolated to the superficial femoral vein in 22.3% of those patients who had DVT.[38] Considering these two major studies, a limited examination is not recommended.

Scanning Calf Veins

The issue of what to do about studying the calf veins is also controversial. The ACR standard does not require the study of calf veins. Gotlieb et al found no significant adverse outcomes between patients who participated in a study in which the calf veins were only evaluated if physical signs or symptoms were present.[39] However, although most calf vein thromboses resolve spontaneously, ~20% extend to the proximal venous system.[10,36] This suggests that if symptoms persist or worsen, a repeat study should be performed even if an initial study was negative. In 2% of patients who had an initial normal examination, abnormalities were evident on serial testing due to extension of calf vein thrombosis.[8] Even in the most careful and detailed examination of the calf veins, it is difficult to be certain that all of the possibly duplicated vessels are free of thrombus. Reported rates on nondiagnostic studies vary in the literature from 19.3% to 82.7%.[10] Additionally, as a result, some have suggested repeating a negative ultrasound in 7 days to look for propagation of thrombus.[40] It has been suggested, however, that a negative ultrasound combined with a normal plasma D-dimer value or low pretest risk factor probability can exclude DVT without further tests.[8] With the more recent aggressive interventional approaches to thrombolytic therapy for treating DVT, the accurate identification of calf vein thrombosis that might propagate proximally is becoming increasingly important. Additionally, with the advent of low molecular weight heparin/warfarin and the introduction of the safer fixed dose ximelgratan, which does not require coagulation monitoring, some clinicians are now beginning to advocate treating isolated calf vein thrombo-

sis and rescanning in 1 week to determine if there is a need to continue therapy or if the calf thrombosis has resolved.[41,42] Including the calf veins in the assessment of the lower extremity therefore is advisable when possible.

Although not yet included in most protocols, the identification of occluded distended communicating and perforating veins, most particularly the gastrocnemius and soleal veins, is important to note. Perforating veins greater than 3 mm in size are considered abnormal. Some clinicians are beginning to treat acutely thrombosed gastrocnemius and soleal veins in the same manner as acute thrombosis of the three paired calf veins.

Microbubble ultrasound contrast agents are reported to be particularly useful in improving the evaluation of calf veins. Bucek et al reported that the use of Levovist (Schering, Berlin, Germany) reduced the rate of indeterminate examinations from 55 to 20% and improved the specificity for detection of calf vein DVT from 25 to 67% without compromising sensitivity (10 to 86%).[43] Contrast was thought to be particularly helpful in improving the quality of difficult examinations caused by significant leg swelling and patient obesity.

How to Scan Carefully

How carefully the vessels are studied depends on the history and symptomatology. Usually, it is adequate to scan every 1 to 2 cm of the veins. In most symptomatic patients, the clot usually involves multiple or whole venous segments. However, orthopedic patients, particularly those who had hip fractures and joint replacements, have short and focal segments of thrombus above the knee and extensive thrombus in the calf veins. As a result, if the calf veins are not studied, the examiner should study the veins above the knee in shorter intervals than they might otherwise plan to do. Additionally, absent flow augmentation tells the examiner that there should be an obstruction between the site of Doppler sampling and the site of augmentation, and, therefore, a detailed study of this area should be performed.

Several studies have recently reported that in orthopedic patients with joint replacements (hips and knees) and in postoperative foot and ankle surgical patients, although calf DVT may be present, the thrombus disappears spontaneously without developing more significant proximal propagation or embolization when the patient is appropriately anticoagulated.[44–46] Therefore, careful assessment of the calf veins is important in these patients when possible so appropriate therapy can be instituted.

Unilateral or Bilateral Scanning

Another controversial issue regarding technique is whether to study both lower extremities, which has traditionally been done. However, in a recent article, Naidich et al[47] showed that in only 1% of patients was the thrombus found in the asymptomatic leg when evaluation of the

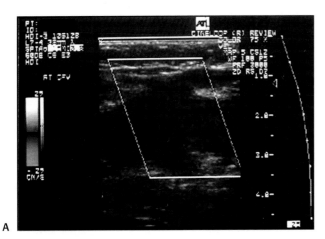
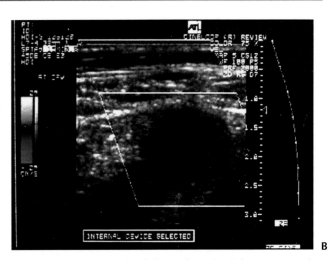

Figure 12–10 (A) Sagittal and **(B)** transverse images of the right common femoral vein (CFV) and profunda femoral vein (PFV) demonstrating hyperexpanded vessels filled with hypoechoic thrombus consistent with acute deep venous thrombosis.

symptomatic leg was negative. Cronan[9] described that the likelihood of finding clots solely in the asymptomatic leg was between 0 and 1% and therefore questioned the routine evaluation of the asymptomatic leg. However, the status of the venous structures is important, particularly in differentiating acute recurrent thrombus from chronic venous thrombus. Therefore, routine bilateral studies are probably worthwhile, if for no other reason than as a baseline for future comparison.

Benefits of Ultrasound

Classic Findings of Acute Deep Venous Thrombosis

When classic findings are present, acute venous thrombosis appears to be hypoechoic. On CFDI it can be demonstrated as an intraluminal defect or color void. Acute DVT expands the venous lumen; it is noncompressible, does not

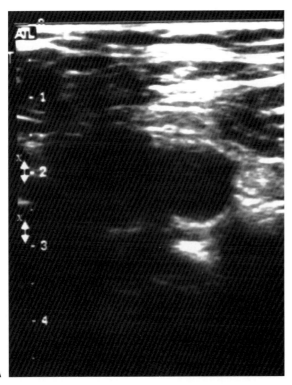
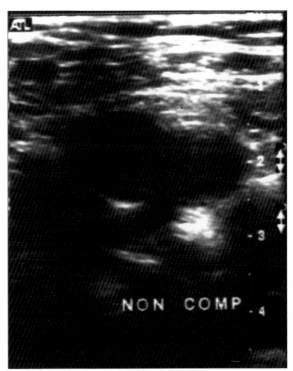

Figure 12–11 (A) Transverse images without and **(B)** with compression of a popliteal vein. The vein **(B)** remains hyperexpanded and is filled with hypoechoic plaque. It does not collapse, consistent with acute deep venous thrombosis.

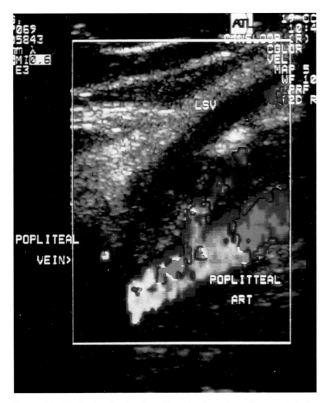

Figure 12–12 Sagittal color flow Doppler imaging of an acutely occluded popliteal vein (PV) and lesser saphenous vein (LSV). Note that the thrombosed veins appear expanded and hypoechoic.

demonstrate augmentation, and, as an indirect sign, the distal vein demonstrates nonvariable venous signals or loss of phasicity (**Fig. 12–10A,B, Fig. 12–11, Fig. 12–12, Fig. 12–13, Fig. 12–14**). The latter finding is particularly important when the iliac veins are not well visualized and they can only be secondarily evaluated by interrogating the common femoral veins (**Fig. 12–15A–D**). As an early manifestation of acute DVT, irregularities corresponding to acute thrombus can be noted on the venous valves (**Fig. 12–13**).

Accuracy

Loss of compressibility of the veins is the most important of the criteria and is the most universally accepted as being highly accurate (**Fig. 12–11A,B**). Cronan pooled the results of several series that totaled 1619 lower extremities and compared compression ultrasonography with ascending venography. This pooling resulted in a 95% sensitivity and a 98% specificity for compression ultrasound.[6] Many studies have similarly shown the high accuracy of compression sonography in diagnosing acute DVT. The sensitivities range from 88 to 100% and the specificities from 92 to 100%.[23,48–60] Additionally, in several outcome studies, patients who had negative compression ultrasounds and therefore were followed but not treated with anticoagulation did not have any evidence of developing pulmonary emboli.[61,62] This adds further credence to the accuracy of

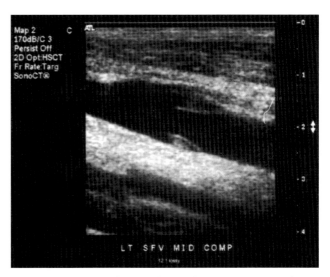

Figure 12–13 Gray-scale sagittal image demonstrating acute thrombus developing along a posterior leaflet of a venous valve. Resolution of thrombus involving valves can result in valve destruction leading to venous incompetence and the venous insufficiency syndrome.

this technique. With CFDI, the normal vessels are usually completely filled in with color, indicating patency. Additionally, compression, phasicity, and augmentation responses can be studied. Several studies have reported that CFDI was comparable to compression sonography.[63,64] Lewis et al reported a sensitivity of 95%, a specificity of 99%, an accuracy of 98%, a positive predictive value of 95%, and a negative predictive value of 99%.[65] For isolated calf vein thrombosis, the sensitivity is significantly lower, ranging between 60 and 80%. Lewis et al also reported that the rate for indeterminate results in their patients was 6% with CFDI, which was comparable to the rate of indeterminate examinations reported for compression sonography.

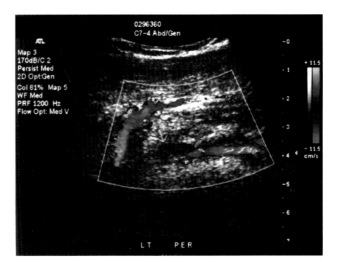

Figure 12–14 Nonoccluding acute thrombus located in the anterior tibial and peroneal veins. Note the calf vessels are hyperexpanded and the acute thrombus is hypoechoic. Color flow does not extend to the outer margin of the vessels.

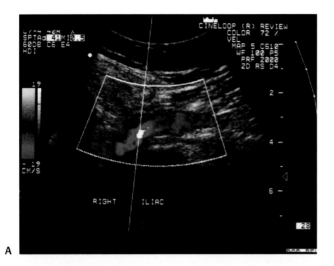

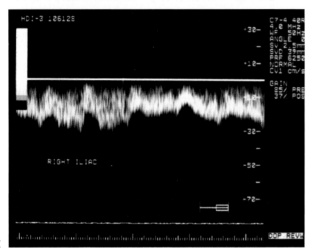

Figure 12–15 (A) Sagittal color flow Doppler imaging of the right and **(B)** left iliac veins demonstrating flow. **(C)** There is loss of respiratory phasicity in the right common femoral vein Doppler spectral analysis pattern compared with **(D)** the normal left, indicating a more proximal obstruction on the right.

It is hoped that in the future, accuracy can be improved with the use of ultrasound contrast agents.[43]

Although with the use of careful techniques and state of the art equipment and with the potential use of ultrasound contrast the accuracy of lower extremity venous ultrasound will remain excellent, it is unlikely for it to be 100%. As in all tests, false-negatives can occur. Theodorou et al reported that the pulmonary embolism rate was 1.6% even after a negative ultrasound was performed in a laboratory that had a sensitivity of 93%, specificity of 98%, and accuracy of 97%.[66] Sonography, similar to all tests, is not foolproof.

Complications

There are very few complications attributed to ultrasound. Although no complications are generally assumed to be the result of compression ultrasound, a few case reports have described documented cases of a pulmonary embolism developing as a result of a compression study of a

superficial femoral vein.[67] Gentle compression is therefore advised, particularly when acute thrombus is present.

Limitations

The limitations of this technique include proximal obstruction by an extrinsic mass such as adenopathy, hematoma, or tumor, which may, therefore, limit compressibility of the venous structures and suggest a false-positive diagnosis. Additionally, congestive heart failure with secondary venous distension may also lead to an inaccurate assessment and false-positive diagnosis.

Other significant problems relate to differentiating chronic thrombus from an acute exacerbation. This is particularly difficult in patients with chronic DVT who have residual changes of a thickened venous wall and who have decreased compliance. When recurrent thrombus occurs in these patients, the venous wall cannot acutely expand, and diagnostic certainty decreases.

False-negative examinations can occur in obese patients and patients with edematous extremities, which are therefore difficult to examine. Small nonocclusive thrombi less than 3 cm in length in the profunda femoral vein and the distal popliteal vein in particular are prone to being missed.[63,64] The presence of nonocclusive thrombus can be identified by noting subtle changes in respiratory phasicity while maintaining the augmentation response (**Fig. 12–16**). Additionally, careful attention to detail relative to technical optimization can help in visualization, particularly in the calf (**Fig. 12–14**). Nevertheless, nonobstructing thrombus may lead to false-negative examinations if collateral vessels are present, and as a result there are no changes in blood flow patterns. The adductor canal is a particularly difficult site to produce a technically adequate examination, but, luckily, isolated

thrombus in this location is rare.[50] Another pitfall is to mistake a patent lesser saphenous vein at the saphenopopliteal junction for a distal popliteal vein that is thrombosed (**Fig. 12–12**). Usually, the saphenous vein is more superficial and is smaller than the 3 to 4 mm popliteal vein.

Frequently, iliac veins are difficult to visualize, but if careful attention is paid to the spectral analysis patterns of the visualized portions of the distal iliac and femoral veins and loss of phasicity is noted, a secondary sign of proximal thrombosis will not be missed and the correct diagnosis will be suggested (**Fig. 12–15**). Collateral vessels can also be mistaken for occluded vessels. Collaterals can be differentiated by appreciating the fact that the true venous structure is adjacent to the artery, whereas collateral veins have a more random relationship (**Fig. 12–17**). Lastly, the

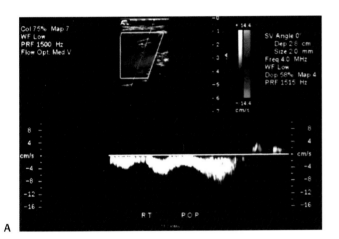

A

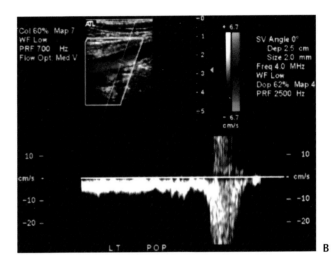

B

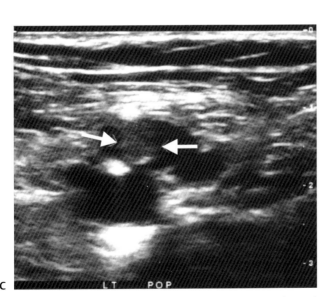

C

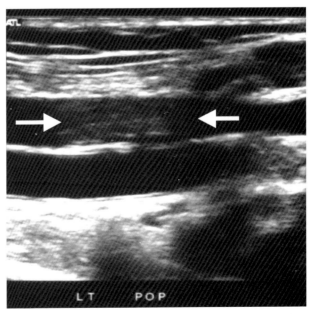

D

Figure 12–16 (A) Sagittal color flow Doppler imaging and Doppler spectral analysis of the right and **(B)** left popliteal veins. Note normal respiratory phasicity on the right and subtle decrease in phasicity on the left. This suggests proximal thrombus. However, there is good augmentation response on the left **(B),** indicating that the thrombus is nonoccluding. **(C)** Corresponding transverse and **(D)** sagittal grayscale images demonstrate nonoccluding thrombus in the more proximal left popliteal vein.

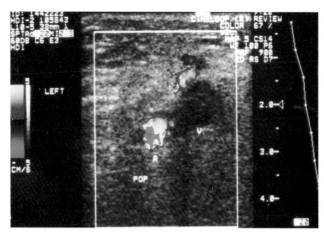

Figure 12–17 Large collateral vessel adjacent to an occluded popliteal vein. Note that the collateral vein is not immediately adjacent to the artery.

venous structures are frequently duplicated, and this duplication cannot always be visualized, even with CFDI. Thrombosis in one of these duplicated vessels may go undetected. In the future, it is hoped that the use of ultrasound contrast agents may reduce these limitations.

Diagnosing Chronic Venous Thrombosis

Cronan has reported that after 6 months of acute DVT, 48% of veins will still have demonstrable abnormalities on ultrasound examination. In this study, 14% of the abnormal veins remained completely occluded.[6] A larger number of

veins recanalized to some extent, but remained with residual clot as organized thrombus material along the vein wall. This organized fibrous intimal venous thickening results from an ingrowth of inflammatory cells, which begins to occur soon after acute thrombus adheres to the venous endothelium. This thickened vein will now resist compression, causing confusion with nonocclusive thrombosis, and can lead to the incorrect diagnosis of acute recurrent thrombosis.

Some findings that can help distinguish chronic from acute thrombosis include the fact that chronic thrombus does not expand the venous lumen, that chronic thrombus is generally more echogenic than acute thrombus, that collateral vessels when seen particularly with CFDI suggest a chronic etiology, and that flow is seen within the central venous lumen with CFDI and the wall changes may be better appreciated (**Fig. 12–18, Fig. 12–19**). Linkins et al reported success in diagnosing DVT by comparing the change in thrombus length over two ultrasound examinations.[68] A change in length of 9 cm or greater is supportive of a diagnosis of recurrent DVT. Less than 9 cm was reported to be measurement error. However, in many cases, distinguishing recurrent acute venous thrombosis from chronic thrombosis is a very difficult diagnostic dilemma. Perhaps there may be a role for radionuclide imaging or MR in some of these indeterminate cases. In a small study, Fraser et al showed that VESPA MR venography demonstrated contrast enhancement of the vessel wall in cases of acute thrombosis, but not in cases of chronic thrombosis. If confirmed, this may mean that this technique could be used to resolve nondiagnostic ultrasound cases.[30]

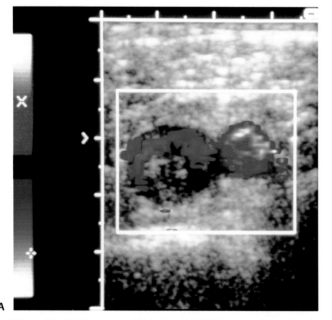

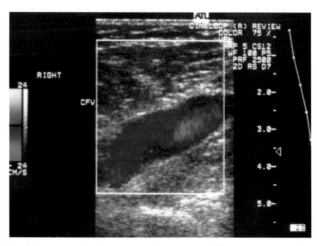

A   B

Figure 12–18 Transverse **(A)** and sagittal **(B)** images demonstrating recanalized flow around chronic thrombus in two different patients. The vein is not expanded and the thrombus is echogenic.

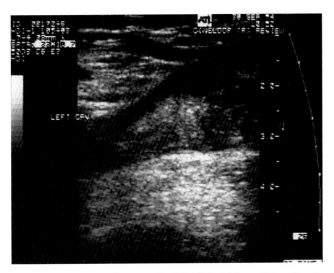

Figure 12–19 Sagittal image of a left CFV which contains chronic residual thrombus from a previous episode of DVT but now has superimposed acute recurrent thrombosis as evidenced by the expanded noncompressible CFV.

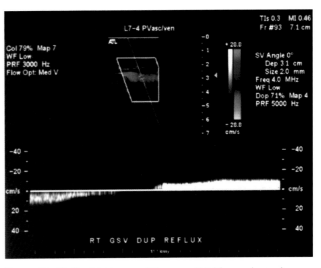

Figure 12–20 Sagittal image of the superficial femoral vein demonstrating reversal of flow after a Valsalva maneuver lasting several seconds. This is characteristic of venous reflux.

Diagnosing Chronic Venous Insufficiency Syndrome and Ultrasound-Guided Treatment

The chronic venous insufficiency syndrome occurs as a result of destruction of venous valves secondary to acute DVT, allowing blood to flow from the deep to the superficial venous system (**Fig. 12–13**). The resulting volume overload and distension or obstruction of these veins produces a clinical picture of pain, swelling, skin changes, necrosis, and superficial ulcerations. This syndrome can be identified by seeing reverse flow with CFDI for more than 1 second when the patient performs the Valsalva maneuver (**Fig. 12–20**). Other methods to test for reflux include applying compression to the limb above the area being evaluated and producing augmentation by squeezing the calf with the patient standing and then observing the venous response.[69] Johnson et al reported that after an episode of DVT, 41% of patients developed features of the chronic venous insufficiency syndrome, although only 13% of patients developed skin complications.[70] The magnitude of the reflux detected by ultrasound appears to be related to the likelihood of developing ulcerations.[69]

Radiofrequency ablation and laser ablation of the refluxing greater saphenous vein (GSV) have been introduced as a new option for treatment of complications of venous reflux, particularly varicosities. Ultrasound is used for mapping the GSV, for guidance in cannulating the GSV, and for positioning the tip of the interventional catheter within 1 cm of the origin of the inferior epigastric vein (the first GSV tributary) to perform the procedure. Hingorani et al have reported that DVT was noted in 16% of 66 patients

treated (12 of 73 limbs). Eleven had extension of the occlusive clot into the proximal GSV and one had one calf DVT. None of these patients developed pulmonary embolism, however.[71] Early postoperative venous ultrasound of the lower extremities is therefore essential and should be performed in all patients undergoing noninvasive closure of the GSV.

Summary

Ultrasound continues to be recognized as the first and most appropriate study to perform when a patient presents with symptomatic lower extremities suggesting acute venous thrombosis. There are numerous advantages to performing a sonographic study of the lower extremities. These evaluations can be performed portably, generally cause no complications, and generally do not involve the use of contrast media or radiation. In ~10% of patients, other abnormalities such as Baker's cysts, arterial aneurysms, or hematomas can be detected and can explain the symptoms (**Fig. 12–2, Fig. 12–4**). The limitations of ultrasound are that it requires experienced operators, it is frequently hard to define the iliac and calf veins, it is difficult to distinguish chronic from acute recurrent thrombosis, and the presence of duplicated vessels can be a significant challenge to achieving an accurate study. In the future, with the introduction of contrast agents, some of these limitations should be resolved or eliminated. Nonetheless, at the present time, because it is the study of choice, it is important for all those involved in diagnostic ultrasound to be comfortable in performing and interpreting these examinations.

References

1. Jacobson AF. Diagnosis of deep venous thrombosis: a review of radiologic, radionuclide, and non-imaging methods. Q J Nucl Med 2001;45:324–333

2. Foley WD. Extremity venous disease. In: Foley WD, ed. Color Doppler Flow Imaging. Reading, MA: Andover Press; 1991:129–151

3. Sorensen HT, Mellemkjaer L, Steffensen FH, Olsen JH, Nielsen GL. The risk of a diagnosis of cancer after primary deep venous thrombosis or pulmonary embolism. N Engl J Med 1998;338:1169–1173

4. Needleman L, Polak J. Suspected lower extremity deep vein thrombosis. In: American College of Radiology Appropriateness Criteria for Imaging and Treatment Decisions. Reston VA: ACR; 1995: CV-8.1–8.6

5. Gallix B, Achard-Lichere C, Dauzat M, Bruel JM, Lopez FM. Flow-independent magnetic resonance venography of the calf. J Magn Reson Imaging 2003;17:421–426

6. Cronan JJ. Venous thromboembolic disease: the role of US. Radiology 1993;186:619–630

7. Hirsh J, Hull RD. Venous thromboembolism: natural history, diagnosis and management. In: Hirshi J, Hull RD, eds. Diagnosis of Venous Thrombosis. Boca Raton, FL: CRC Press; 1987:23–28

8. Ginsberg JS. Management of venous thromboembolism. N Engl J Med 1996;335:1816–1828

9. Cronan JJ. Controversies in venous ultrasound. Semin Ultrasound CT MR 1997;18:33–38

10. Fraser JD, Anderson DR. Venous protocols, techniques, and interpretations of the upper and lower extremities. Radiol Clin North Am 2004;42:279–296

11. Melikian N, Bingham J, Goldsmith DJ. Diabetic infarction: an unusual cause of acute limb swelling in patients on hemodialysis. Am J Kidney Dis 2003;42:1102–1103

12. Bluth EI, Merritt CR, Sullivan MA. Gray-scale evaluation of the lower extremities. JAMA 1982;247:3127–3129

13. Borgstede JP, Clagett GE. Types, frequency, and significance of alternative diagnoses found during duplex Doppler venous examinations of the lower extremities. J Ultrasound Med 1992;11:85–89

14. Sandler DA, Mitchell JR. How do we know who has had deep venous thrombosis? Postgrad Med J 1989;65:16–19

15. Grice GD III, Smith RB III, Robinson PH, Rheudasil JM. Primary popliteal venous aneurysm with recurrent pulmonary emboli. J Vasc Surg 1990;12:316–318

16. Ross GJ, Violi L, Barber LW, Vujic I. Popliteal venous aneurysm. Radiology 1988;168:721–722

17. Lutter KS, Kerr TM, Roedersheimer LR, Lohr JM, Sampson MG, Cranley JJ. Superficial thrombophlebitis diagnosed by duplex scanning. Surgery 1991;110:42–46

18. Ikeda M, Fujimori Y, Tankawa H, Iwata H. Compression syndrome of the popliteal vein and artery caused by popliteal cyst. Angiology 1984;35:245–251

19. Swett HA, Jaffe RB, McIff EB. Popliteal cysts: presentation as thrombophlebitis. Radiology 1975;115:613–615

20. Chengelis DL, Bendick PJ, Glover JL, Brown OW, Ranval TJ. Progression of superficial venous thrombosis to deep vein thrombosis. J Vasc Surg 1996;24:745–749

21. Jorgensen JO, Hanel KC, Morgan AM, Hunt JM. The incidence of deep venous thrombosis in patients with superficial thrombophlebitis of the lower limbs. J Vasc Surg 1993;18:70–73

22. American College of Radiology. ACR Standards for Performance of the Peripheral Venous Ultrasound Examination. Reston, VA: ACR; 1993

23. Heijboer H, Buller HR, Lensing AW, Turpie AG, Colly LP, ten Cate JW. A comparison of real-time compression ultrasonography with impedance plethysmography for the diagnosis of deep venous thrombosis in symptomatic outpatients. N Engl J Med 1993;329: 1365–1369

24. Begemann PG, Bonacker M, Kemper J, et al. Evaluation of the deep venous system in patients with suspected pulmonary embolism with multi-detector CT: a prospective study in comparison to Doppler sonography. J Comput Assist Tomogr 2003;27: 399–409

25. Loud P, Katz D, Bruce D, Klippenstein D, Grossman Z. Deep venous thrombosis with suspected pulmonary embolism: detection with combined CT venography and pulmonary angiography. Radiology 2001;219:498–502

26. Duwe KM, Shiau M, Budorick NE, Austin JH, Berkmen YM. Evaluation of the lower extremity veins in patients with suspected pulmonary embolism: a retrospective comparison of helical CT venography and sonography. 2000 ARRS Executive Council Award I. American Roentgen Ray Society. AJR Am J Roentgenol 2000;175: 1525–1531

27. Peterson DA, Kazerooni EA, Wakefield TW, et al. Computed tomographic venography is specific but not sensitive for diagnosis of acute lower-extremity deep venous thrombosis in patients with suspected pulmonary embolus. J Vasc Surg 2001;34: 798–804

28. Evans AJ, Sostman HD, Knelson MH, et al. Detection of deep venous thrombosis: prospective comparison of MR imaging with contrast venography. AJR Am J Roentgenol 1993;161:131–139

29. Spritzer CE, Norconk JJ Jr, Sostman HD, Coleman RE. Detection of deep venous thrombosis by magnetic resonance imaging. Chest 1993;104:54–60

30. Fraser DG, Moody AR, Davidson IR, Martel AL, Morgan PS. Deep venous thrombosis: diagnosis by using venous enhanced subtracted peak arterial MR venography versus conventional venography. Radiology 2003;226:812–820

31. Fraser DGW. Using magnetic resonance direct thrombus imaging to diagnose deep-vein thrombosis in the lower legs. Ann Intern Med 2002;136:I26

32. Fraser DGW, Moody AR, Morgan PS, Martel AL, Davidson I. Diagnosis of lower-limb deep venous thrombosis: a prospective blinded study of magnetic resonance direct thrombus imaging. Ann Intern Med 2002;136:89–98

33. Screaton NJ, Gillard JH, Berman LH, Kemp PM. Duplicated superficial femoral veins: a source of error in the sonographic investigation of deep vein thrombosis. Radiology 1998;206:397–401

34. Cronan JJ. Venous duplex US of the lower extremities: effect of duplicated femoral veins [editorial]. Radiology 1998;206:308–309

35. Quinlan DJ, Alikhan R, Gishen P, Sidhu PS. Variations in lower limb venous anatomy: implications for US diagnosis of deep vein thrombosis. Radiology 2003;228:443–448

36. Pezzullo JA, Perkins AB, Cronan JJ. Symptomatic deep venous thrombosis: diagnosis with limited compression US. Radiology 1996;198:67–70

37. Frederick MG, Hertzberg BS, Kliewer MA, et al. Can the US examination for lower extremity deep venous thrombosis be abbreviated? A prospective study of 755 examinations. Radiology 1996; 199:45–47

38. Maki DD, Kumar N, Nguyen B, Langer JE, Miller WT Jr, Gefter WB. Distribution of thrombi in acute lower extremity deep venous thrombosis: implications for sonography and CT and MR venography. AJR Am J Roentgenol 2000;175:1299–1301

39. Gottlieb RH, Voci SL, Syed L, et al. Randomized prospective study comparing routine versus selective use of sonography of the complete calf in patients with suspected deep venous thrombosis. AJR Am J Roentgenol 2003;180:241–245

40. Kraaijenhagen RA, Piovella F, Bernardi E, et al. Simplification of the diagnostic management of suspected deep vein thrombosis. Arch Intern Med 2002;162:907–911

41. Fiessinger JN, Huisman MV, Davidson BL, et al. Ximelagatran vs low-molecular-weight heparin and warfarin for the treatment of deep vein thrombosis. JAMA 2005;293:681–689

42. Gurewich V. Ximelagatran: promises and concerns. JAMA 2005; 293:736–739

43. Bucek RA, Kos T, Schober E, et al. Ultrasound with Levovist in the diagnosis of suspected calf vein thrombosis. Ultrasound Med Biol 2001;27:455–460

44. Elias A, Cadene A, Elias M, et al. Extended lower limb venous ultrasound for the diagnosis of proximal and distal vein thrombosis in asymptomatic patients after total hip replacement. Eur J Vasc Endovasc Surg 2004;27:438–444

45. Wang CJ, Wang JW, Weng LH, Hsu CC, Lo CF. Outcome of calf deepvein thrombosis after total knee arthroplasty. J Bone Joint Surg Br 2003;85:841–844

46. Solis G, Saxby T. Incidence of DVT following surgery of the foot and ankle. Foot Ankle Int 2002;23:411–447

47. Naidich JB, Torre JR, Pellerito JS, Smalberg IS, Kase DJ, Crystal KS. Suspected deep venous thrombosis: is US of both legs necessary? Radiology 1996;200:429–431

48. Rosner NH, Doris PE. Diagnosis of femoropopliteal venous thrombosis: comparison of duplex sonography and plethysmography. AJR Am J Roentgenol 1988;150:623–627

49. White RH, McGahan JP, Daschbach MM, Hartling RP. Diagnosis of deep-vein thrombosis using duplex ultrasound. Ann Intern Med 1989;111:297–304

50. Vogel P, Laing FC, Jeffrey RB Jr, Wing VW. Deep venous thrombosis of the lower extremity: US evaluation. Radiology 1987;163:747–751

51. Cronan JJ, Dorfman GS, Scola FH, Schepps B, Alexander J. Deep venous thrombosis: US assessment using vein compression. Radiology 1987;162(1 Pt 1):191–194

52. Cronan JJ, Dorfman GS, Grusmark J. Lower-extremity deep venous thrombosis: further experience with and refinements of US assessment. Radiology 1988;168:101–107

53. George JE, Smith MO, Berry RE. Duplex scanning for the detection of deep venous thrombosis of lower extremities in a community hospital. Curr Surg 1987;44:202–204

54. Appelman PT, De Jong TE, Lampmann LE. Deep venous thrombosis of the leg: US findings. Radiology 1987;163:743–746

55. Lensing AWA, Prandoni P, Brandjes D, et al. Detection of deep venous thrombosis by real-time B-mode ultrasonography. N Engl J Med 1989;320:342–345

56. Froehlich JA, Dorfman GS, Cronan JJ, Urbanek PJ, Herndon JH, Aaron RK. Compression ultrasonography for the detection of deep venous thrombosis in patients who have a fracture of the hip: a prospective study. J Bone Joint Surg Am 1989;71:249–256

57. O'Leary DH, Kane RA, Chase BM. A prospective study of the efficacy of B-scan sonography in the detection of deep venous thrombosis in the lower extremities. J Clin Ultrasound 1988;16:1–8

58. Aitken AGF, Godden DJ. Real-time ultrasound diagnosis of deep vein thrombosis: a comparison with venography. Clin Radiol 1987;38:309–313

59. Killewich LA, Bedford GR, Beach KW, Strandness DE Jr. Diagnosis of deep venous thrombosis: a prospective study comparing duplex scanning to contrast venography. Circulation 1989;79:810–814

60. Becker DM, Philbrick JT, Abbitt PL. Real-time ultrasonography for the diagnosis of lower extremity deep venous thrombosis: the wave of the future? Arch Intern Med 1989;149:1731–1734

61. Vaccaro JP, Cronan JJ, Dorfman GS. Outcome analysis of patients with normal compression US examinations. Radiology 1990;175: 645–649

62. Sarpa MS, Messina LM, Smith M, et al. Significance of a negative duplex scan in patients suspected of having acute deep venous thrombosis of the lower extremity. J Vasc Tech 1989;13:222–226

63. Rose SC, Zweibel WJ, Nelson BD, et al. Symptomatic lower extremity deep venous thrombosis: accuracy, limitations, and role of color duplex flow imaging in diagnosis. Radiology 1990;175:639–644

64. Foley WD, Middleton WD, Lawson TL, Erickson S, Quiroz FA, Macrander S. Color Doppler ultrasound imaging of lower extremity venous disease. AJR Am J Roentgenol 1989;152:371–376

65. Lewis BD, James EM, Welch TJ, Joyce JW, Hallet JW, Weaver AL. Diagnosis of acute deep venous thrombosis of the lower extremities: prospective evaluation of color flow Doppler imaging versus venography. Radiology 1994;192:651–655

66. Theodorou SJ, Theodorou DJ, Kakitsubata Y. Sonography and venography of the lower extremities for diagnosing deep vein thrombosis in symptomatic patients. Clin Imaging 2003;27:180–183

67. Perlin SJ. Pulmonary embolism during compression US of the lower extremity. Radiology 1992;184:165–166

68. Linkins LA, Pasquale P, Paterson S, Kearon C. Change in thrombus length on venous ultrasound and recurrent deep vein thrombosis. Arch Intern Med 2004;164:1793–1796

69. Polak JA. Peripheral artery and veins: contributions of CFDI. In: Bluth EI, Divon MY, Laurel MD, eds. Update in Duplex, Power and Color Flow Imaging. American Institute of Ultrasound in Medicine; 1996:51–62

70. Johnson BF, Manzo RA, Bergelin RO, Strandness DE Jr. Relationship between changes in the deep venous system and the development of the postthrombotic syndrome after an acute episode of lower limb deep venous thrombosis: a one- to six-year follow-up. J Vasc Surg 1995;21:307–313

71. Hingorani AP, Ascher E, Markevich N, et al. Deep venous thrombosis after radiofrequency ablation of greater saphenous vein: a word of caution. J Vasc Surg 2004;40:500–504

13 Biopsy, Drainage, and Percutaneous Treatment of a Mass

Gerald D. Dodd III and Hayden Head

The process to biopsy or drain a mass or to perform percutaneous treatment such as radiofrequency ablation (RFA) of a tumor begins with a consultation request. This clinical request is part of a consultation between the requesting physician and the radiologist who will perform the procedure. This consultation should include a review of the patient's pertinent clinical history, the objectives of the requested procedure, a review of pertinent imaging studies, an assessment of whether the procedure is indicated and technically feasible, the determination of the disposition of any tissue or fluid obtained, and an assessment of the patient's willingness and ability to tolerate the procedure. After the decision to perform the procedure has been made, the radiologist must choose a method of guidance.

Mode of Image Guidance for Percutaneous Treatment

Three primary modalities can be used to guide percutaneous interventional procedures: fluoroscopy, computed tomography (CT), and sonography. In a few situations, the pathological condition or the patient's anatomy may dictate a particular method of guidance. In most instances, however, sonographic guidance has proved to be quicker and easier than the other methods. In Asia and in many parts of Europe, sonography is the dominant method used to guide the performance of most nonvascular and interventional procedures. At several academic and private hospitals in the United States, sonography is used to guide 95% of all biopsies and drainages of abdominal, pelvic, pleural, and mediastinal masses. The advantages of sonography include real-time guidance, multidirectional imaging, identification and avoidance of major vessels, portability, excellent anatomical resolution, and reduced cost. The cost savings of sonography result from the lower capital expenses and operating costs of sonographic equipment and the potential use of CT scanners for diagnostic purposes, rather than for intervention.

Ultrasound-Guided Percutaneous Treatment

Methods

The two primary methods of performing sonographically guided intervention are the free-hand technique and the attached-guide technique. Advocates of the free-hand technique claim it allows for greater freedom in choosing needle placement and better needle visibility. Advocates of guides claim that they provide greater accuracy for deep biopsies, quicker needle localization, diminished teaching time, and improved coordination in procedures performed with nonradiologists. Because few companies manufacture needle guides for high-frequency probes, most near-field biopsies are performed with the free-hand technique. However, we believe that use of an attachable guide makes a biopsy or drainage of a mass more than 5 cm deep easier and quicker.

The success of sonographic guidance depends highly on optimization of the sonographic equipment. Important parameters that should be controlled are the type of probe, the gray scale, the field of view, and the focus. All of these variables have a direct effect on the visualization of the pathological condition and the needle. For near-field biopsies, the best results are usually obtained with 7 to 10 MHz linear probes. Most abdominal biopsies are best performed with 3.5 or 2.5 MHz sector probes. The field of view should be chosen to maximize visualization of the pathological condition and the needle. As a general rule, the field of view should be adjusted so that the needle traverses at least one third of the image. Under no circumstances should a large field of view be used when performing a biopsy of a small near-field lesion. The probes should be focused at the level at which the needle is expected to enter the lesion. Visualization of the needle can be improved by needle motion (use of an in-and-out motion with approximately a 1 cm excursion) and a slight rocking motion of the probe. This rocking motion can bring a needle that has deviated slightly out of the ultrasound plane back into the field of view.

With the attached-guide technique, the speed and success of the procedure can be improved by using two sets of hands: one person holds the probe and corrects it, and the second person places the needle catheter. Although the use of two people requires precise communication, it can produce less traumatic and more accurate results. In academic centers, the second person is usually a resident or fellow. In private practice, the most logical choice for the second person would be a sonographer. The most crucial task in the two-person technique is holding the probe, which is usually performed by the attending radiologist. The delivery of the anesthetic and placement of the needle are easier tasks and are usually done by the second person.

Technique

Percutaneously guided intervention may seem difficult and dangerous; however, in most instances, it is relatively simple and safe. Its success requires adherence to a few basic principles:

1. Check for and correct coagulopathy in all patients with a prothrombin time greater than 15 seconds, a partial thromboplastin time greater than 45 seconds, or fewer than 50,000/mm³ platelets.
2. Defer the procedure if the patient has taken aspirin during the prior week.
3. Use abundant amounts of local anesthetic for procedures performed with needles larger than 22 gauge.
4. Do not use a local anesthetic for simple 22 gauge aspirations.
5. Confirm the location of all needle or catheter tips before obtaining a biopsy specimen or deploying drainage catheters.
6. Avoid crossing major vessels.
7. Do not aspirate potentially sterile fluid collections through the bowel.
8. Use a subcostal approach when possible.

The following discussion provides examples of the standard approaches used to perform a biopsy or to drain masses.

Percutaneous Biopsy

When performing percutaneous biopsies, we use only a 20 gauge end-cutting needle and an 18 gauge core biopsy gun. After the patient has been prepared for the procedure, the probe is covered with a sterile sheath, and a biopsy guide is attached. The pathological condition is located, and the path of the biopsy chosen. When possible, a subcostal approach is used to prevent the potential complications (pneumothorax, contaminated pleural space, and lacerated intercostal artery) of an intercostal approach. If the procedure is a biopsy of a liver tumor, then every attempt is made to perform the biopsy through a mantle of normal liver parenchyma. This precaution reduces the risk of bleeding because normal liver tissue is less likely to bleed than a tumor. Additionally, by choosing a biopsy path through the least vascular portion of the tumor, the risk of bleeding can be further reduced. Anesthetic is administered through the biopsy guide with a 10 cm long, 22 gauge spinal needle. Conceptually, an attempt is made to create a cylinder of anesthesia from the skin to the mass or organ from which the biopsy specimen is to be obtained. A traditional skin wheal is not raised. No skin nick is made. When the 20 gauge biopsy needle is used, the needle is placed into the lesion, and the stylet removed. The specimen is obtained by moving the needle back and forth across the lesion without aspiration. When using the 18 gauge gun, the tip of the needle is advanced to a location ~5 mm from the margin of the lesion and then fired across the transition zone. Care is taken to ensure that there is adequate room for needle excursion.

Percutaneous Catheter Drainage

Catheters are placed using either the trocar or Seldinger technique. With either technique, copious amounts of anesthetic are administered both through the guide and as a skin wheal. A skin nick is made and blunt dissection is performed. Because it is difficult to pass a catheter through the thoracic or abdominal fascia, adequate dissection is often the key to successful catheter placement. The trocar technique is best reserved for large "cannot-miss" fluid collections. This conviction is based on the poor sonovisibility of most catheters, which makes confirmation of location difficult, and on the marked risk associated with making multiple passes with a large-diameter trocar catheter. The Seldinger technique is used to place catheters in fluid collections that are small or hard to reach. The advantage of this technique is that it uses small-diameter, echogenic access needles. Small access needles can be placed and repositioned with a greater margin of safety than trocar drainage catheters. After satisfactory access has been obtained, a drainage catheter is exchanged over a wire. The use of locking loop catheters markedly decreases the frequency of accidental catheter removal. We do not use any of the commercially available fasteners to secure a catheter to a patient; we prefer to suture the catheter in place. Physician's orders for the care of indwelling catheters should include an in-and-out flushing of the catheter with 10 mL of sterile saline solution every 8 hours and monitoring the input and output of the catheter.

Paracentesis and Thoracentesis

Diagnostic aspirations of localized fluid collections, pleural effusions, and ascites are performed without anesthetic. A single 22 gauge needle is placed in one pass into the fluid collection. If no fluid is obtained with this puncture, however, lidocaine is administered along the needle tract as the initial needle is withdrawn. When a 22 gauge aspiration fails (that is, when the needle is in the area of interest, but no fluid has been obtained), an 18 gauge needle is used for aspiration. If the 18 gauge needle fails to obtain fluid, the procedure may be canceled or continued with a drainage catheter.

General Applications

The general techniques just described can be used to evaluate a wide spectrum of pathological conditions. Obvious applications include random biopsies of the liver or

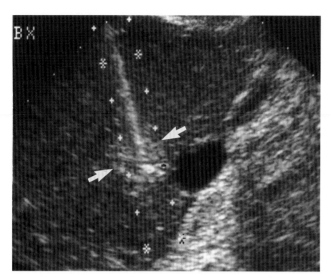

Figure 13–1 Liver mass biopsy. Transverse ultrasound scan of the liver shows a 1 cm hyperechoic nodule (arrows) with an echogenic needle traversing most of its diameter.

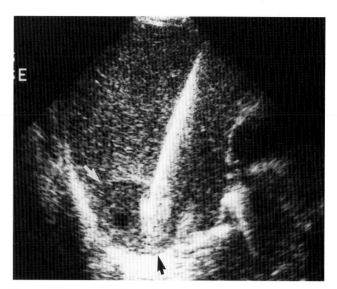

Figure 13–2 Hepatic abscess drainage. Transverse ultrasound scan shows 4 cm abscess (arrows) in the posterior right lobe of the liver. Note the presence of the needle and wire.

kidneys, biopsies of hepatic or renal masses (**Fig. 13–1**), and aspiration or drainage of fluid collections of the solid organs or peritoneal cavity of the abdomen (**Fig. 13–2, Fig. 13–3**).[1,2] Less obvious applications, such as the guidance of percutaneous transhepatic cholangiography, nephrostomy (**Fig. 13–4**), and cholecystotomy (**Fig. 13–5**), are more easily performed with sonography than with fluoroscopy.[3] Why puncture a patient five to 20 times under fluoroscopic guidance, hoping for a chance encounter of the needle with a bile duct or the urinary collecting system? Why ir-

radiate both the patient and the medical personnel needlessly? With sonography, the desired anatomy can be directly visualized and often punctured only once.

Sonography is underused for the biopsies or the aspiration of pulmonary or mediastinal masses. Most pulmonary masses that abut the pleura can be visualized and biopsy performed with sonography (**Fig. 13–6**). Likewise, mediastinal masses that can be visualized by sonography are easily and safely sampled using sonographic guidance (**Fig. 13–7**).[4] In these instances, the two-dimensional

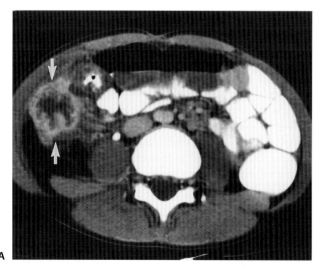

A

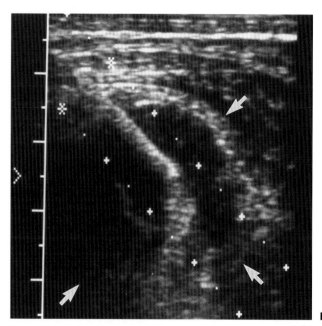

B

Figure 13–3 Periappendiceal abscess drainage. **(A)** Computed tomographic image of the lower abdomen shows a 3 cm heterogeneous periappendiceal abscess (arrows). **(B)** Transverse ultrasound scan of the right lower quadrant obtained from the same patient shows a spherical abscess (arrows), with the needle in the cavity.

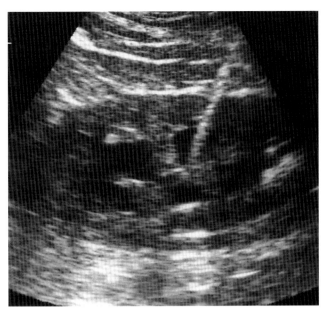

Figure 13–4 Nephrostomy. Posterior oblique ultrasound scan through the right kidney shows marked hydronephrosis. The needle is puncturing one of the middle calyces.

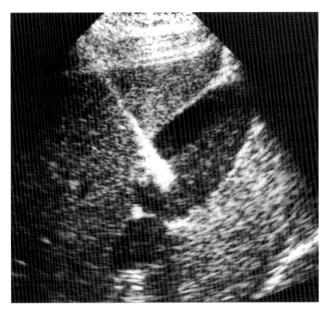

Figure 13–5 Percutaneous cholecystostomy. Sagittal ultrasound scan of the right upper quadrant shows the needle traversing the anterior aspect of the liver to enter the gallbladder lumen.

resolution and real-time imaging capability of sonography provide a much greater safety margin than CT or fluoroscopy.

After general confidence in the use of sonographic guidance has been achieved, the technique can be applied more aggressively to perform procedures traditionally believed to be outside the realm of sonography. The biopsy of

small retroperitoneal lymph nodes is a good example. We have found that biopsies of most retroperitoneal lymph nodes can be successfully performed using sonographic guidance. This success is independent of the patient's size. We have successfully performed biopsies of numerous 1 cm paraaortic lymph nodes in markedly obese patients and rarely needed to switch to CT guidance because we

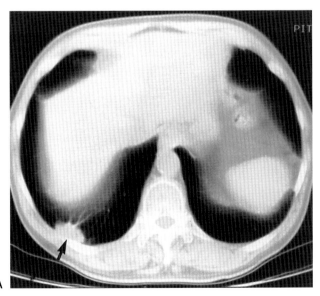

A

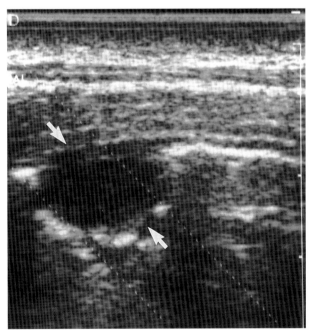

B

Figure 13–6 Biopsy of the lung. **(A)** Computed tomographic image of the lower thorax shows a 2 × 3 cm lung mass (arrow) abutting the pleura in the right lower lobe. **(B)** Corresponding oblique intercostal ultrasound scan clearly shows the lung mass (arrows). A biopsy was performed under sonographic guidance. Its results showed the mass to be a metastatic tumor.

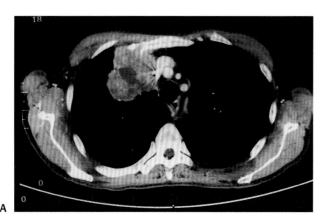

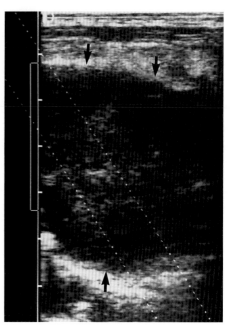

A   B

Figure 13–7 Lung mass invading mediastinum. **(A)** Axial computed tomographic image of the upper thorax shows a large heterogeneous anterior mass that abuts the pleura and projects laterally beyond the lateral sternal margin. **(B)** Corresponding intercostal parasternal ultrasound scan clearly shows the mass (arrows). A biopsy was performed under sonographic guidance.

were unable to see the node (**Fig. 13–8**).[5] Another aggressive, but ultimately simple procedure is the biopsy or drainage of a pelvic mass with the transvaginal or transrectal approach (**Fig. 13–9**).[6] Both procedures are easy to perform and are well tolerated by patients.

Tumor Ablation

With the advent of percutaneous ablation for solid tumors, a new role has opened up for ultrasound-guided intervention. In the past several years, an increasing number of physicians worldwide have adopted novel image-guided local ablative techniques for treatment of solid tumors of the abdomen and thorax, and ablation has gained considerable attention as an alternative to surgery with some tumors, especially those of the liver.[7-9]

Similar to percutaneous interventional procedures in general, several modalities of image guidance can be utilized for ablation; namely CT, magnetic resonance imaging (MRI), and sonography. The choice of the image guidance modality to use depends on the training and preference of the individual physician and the resources available at a

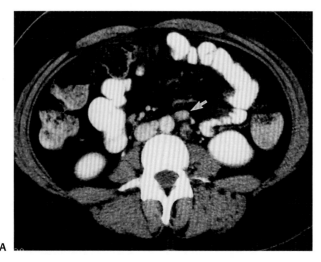

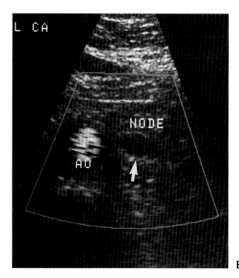

A   B

Figure 13–8 Biopsy of the retroperitoneal lymph nodes. **(A)** Axial computed tomographic image of the lower abdomen shows a 1 cm para-aortic lymph node (arrow). **(B)** Corresponding transverse ultrasound scan through the lower abdomen shows a hyperechoic node (arrow) adjacent to the aorta (AO).

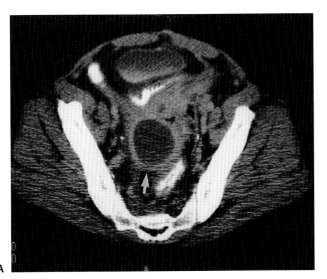

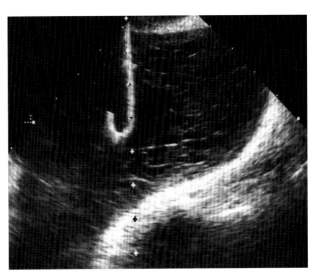

Figure 13–9 Transvaginal drainage of a pelvic abscess. **(A)** Axial computed tomographic image of the pelvis demonstrates a 4 cm pelvic abscess (arrow), just anterior to the rectum. **(B)** Corresponding transvaginal ultrasound scan shows a J wire in a complex cavity of the abscess.

given medical center. Each modality offers potential advantages over the others. At some centers, CT and MRI guidance are preferred over sonography. Both techniques yield better depiction of the final extent of the ablation zone, and MRI is the only modality that allows real-time monitoring of tissue temperatures. However, to date, there is no proof that the potential advantages translate into altered patient survival. Also, both CT and MRI guidance add considerable expense to the procedure that is unwarranted when treating most small tumors. Given this, we use the least invasive approach that allows an adequate and safe ablation. In most cases, sonography has proven optimal.

It is important to note, however, that the percutaneous approach is not appropriate for ablation of all tumors. Percutaneous ablation may be used when patients have fewer than five tumors, each measuring < 5 cm, all visible by sonography (or CT or MRI) with a safe route of access. Otherwise, an intraoperative approach by laparoscopy or laparotomy may be needed in patients with tumors measuring > 5 cm, tumors not adequately visualized by imaging, tumors that are inaccessible percutaneously, and tumors directly adjacent to bowel.

Many practitioners worldwide use sonography to guide needle placement and monitor the ablation procedure. We have used sonography almost exclusively to guide percutaneous ablation since our program began in 1996. For tumor ablation, in contrast to routine biopsies and drainages, we employ the free-hand technique discussed earlier because of the inherently better control of needle placement. Furthermore, depending on the complexity of the ablation case, numerous needle adjustments may be required, and the flexibility of the free-hand technique in needle repositioning is crucial in these situations.

At our facility, and in the medical community at large, radiofrequency ablation (RFA) is by far the most commonly used ablation technique, and the greatest ablation experience is with tumors of the liver.[10] RFA produces thermal injury in living tissue via an alternating electric current in the radiofrequency range (460 to 500 kHz). The tip of a shielded needle electrode conducts the current and concentrates energy in tissue, causing local ionic agitation and subsequent frictional heat. Temperatures in excess of 50°C produce tissue coagulation. Currently, three RFA devices are widely used in the United States. The first two are designed as multitined expandable electrodes (**Fig. 13–10A,B**). Each consists of a central straight-needle cannula that is used to deploy an array of curved electrode tines from the tip into the adjacent tissues. The configurations of the electrode arrays are designed to produce large spherical ablation zones. The third device consists of a straight, internally cooled needle electrode (**Fig. 13–10C**). The internal cooling is designed to prevent charring of the adjacent tissues and thus create a larger ablation zone. This applicator may be used alone or as a triangular three-needle cluster electrode. All RFA devices require the use of two or more dispersive electrodes in the form of adhesive pads that attach to either or both the patient's back and legs.

Successful RFA of liver tumors depends on inducing coagulation of the entire tumor as well as a 1 cm thick margin of normal liver around the 360 degree perimeter of the tumor. Sonography has an important advantage in this regard—the ability to monitor the ablation in real time. Under ultrasound, RFA produces a roughly spherical transient hyperechoic zone that extends perpendicular to the exposed electrode tip or tines (**Fig. 13–11**). This hyperechoic reaction is caused by the production of microbubbles as water in the heated tissue vaporizes. The hyperechoic zone has been shown to correspond roughly to the actual zone of gross tissue necrosis.[11] Because current equipment reliably produces ablations of ~3 cm surrounding the needle tip,

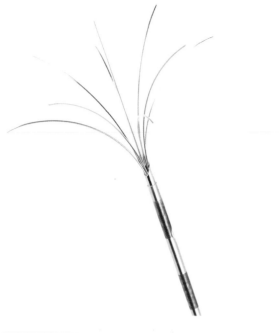

A

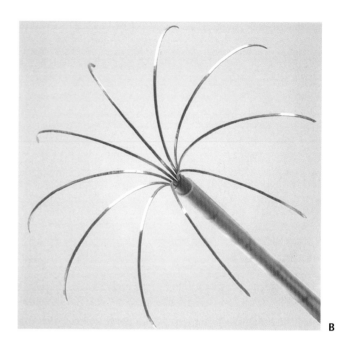

B

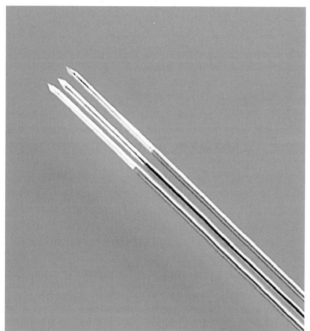

C

Figure 13–10 Current radiofrequency ablation needle electrodes. **(A)** A 15 gauge needle electrode with eight expandable tines (RITA Medical Systems Inc., Mountain View, California). **(B)** A 14 gauge needle electrode with 10 expandable tines (Boston Scientific, Natick, Massachusetts). **(C)** A 17 gauge internally cooled needle in a three-needle cluster (Valleylab, Boulder, Colorado).

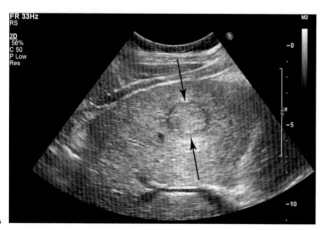

A

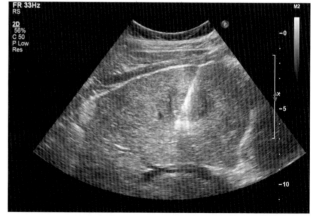

B

Figure 13–11 Sonograms obtained before and during radiofrequency ablation show a single hepatic tumor and the formation of a typical transient hyperechoic zone at the tip of the ablation needle.

(A) A 3 cm hepatocellular carcinoma (arrows) in the posterior right lobe of the liver. **(B)** Ablation needle tip positioned across the tumor. (*Continued*)

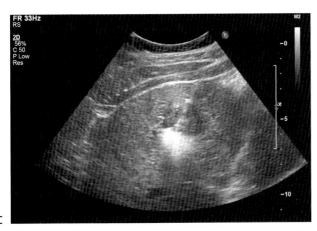

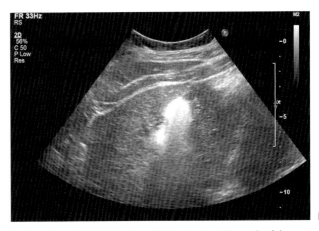

C

D

Figure 13–11 (*Continued*) **(C)** Transient hyperechoic zone formed from production of microbubbles by the ablation starts at the ends of the active electrode tip. **(D)** Hyperechoic zone has expanded to involve the entire active tip. Note resultant shadowing that obscures deeper structures.

tumors larger than 3 cm in greatest dimension necessitate multiple overlapping ablations to be completely destroyed.[12,13] Even large tumors (those with a diameter > 5 cm) may be treated with RFA, but they require many more ablations or require adjuvant techniques to increase the size of the ablation zone. The major factor that limits the size of the ablation zone with all of these devices is hepatic perfusion.

When performing multiple RFAs using sonographic guidance, it is important to plan the order of ablations so that the deepest ablations are performed before the superficial ones. This strategy minimizes the possibility that microbubbles might obscure visualization of the deeper por-

tions of the tumor and thus prevent completion of the ablation session. This feature does highlight one of the deficiencies of tumor ablation under sonographic guidance; that is, the fact that monitoring of the procedure, and especially visualization of the deep margin of the ablation zone, is increasingly limited as more and more microbubbles are formed by the ablation (**Fig. 13–11D**). The long-term follow-up posttreatment is best performed with CT (**Fig. 13–12**).

At our facility, we perform sonographically guided percutaneous tumor ablation as an outpatient procedure. Either general anesthesia or local anesthesia plus IV sedation

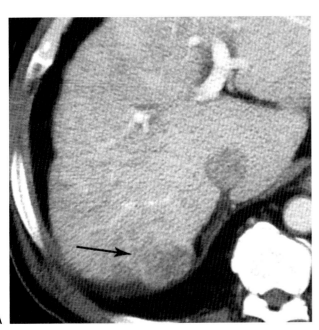

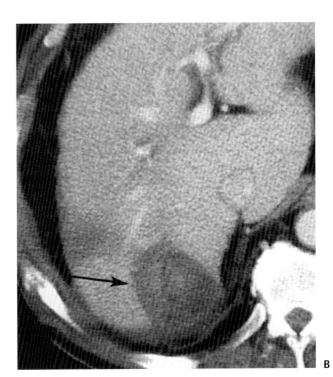

A

B

Figure 13–12 A 53-year-old man with a 3.4 cm hepatocellular carcinoma. **(A)** Computed tomographic (CT) scan before radiofrequency ablation (RFA) shows a tumor (arrow) in liver segment VIII. **(B)** CT scan after solitary RFA shows a low-attenuation ablation zone (arrow). The ablation zone is larger than the index tumor. The CT appearance of the ablations produced by all of the thermal ablation techniques is very similar.

with short-acting agents such as remifentanil or propofol can be used. Only in rare cases is general anesthesia needed. With current energy-deposition algorithms, a single ablation takes from 8 to 25 minutes and increases the temperature of the ablated tissue to between 50°C and 100°C. Total procedure time varies with the size and number of tumors to be ablated. Cases where several large tumors are ablated may be more than 1 or 2 hours in duration.

The greatest success for ablation has been shown with tumors less than 3 cm in maximum dimension. The ideal location is deep in the liver parenchyma because nodules adjacent to the major bile ducts, and especially bowel structures, should be approached with caution. In the latter case, bowel perforation can result, and therefore special interventional techniques may be needed to separate bowel from liver. Tumors adjacent to the gallbladder and diaphragm also require caution, but can be treated percutaneously with careful technique and proper choice of equipment.[14,15] Contraindications to RFA include excessive tumor burden and evidence of extrahepatic tumor. Treatment is also contraindicated in most patients with Child class C cirrhosis (i.e., hyperbilirubinemia, hypoalbuminemia, poorly controlled ascites, and severe encephalopathy). Finally, coagulation parameters, including platelet count, international normalized ratio, and partial thromboplastin times, should be corrected before ablation.

Sonography has similar utility in guiding ablation by other techniques. The most established of these is ethanol ablation, used worldwide for more than a decade.[16] Also, the up-and-coming techniques of percutaneous microwave ablation and percutaneous cryoablation are well suited for operation under sonographic guidance.

Summary

The request for a biopsy or drainage of a mass, or ablation of a tumor, should always be approached with the patient's best interest in mind. If the procedure is indicated, the guidance technique of choice should be the one with which the radiologist is most comfortable. However, radiologists who are capable of using all guidance techniques will be best equipped to handle any situation. In particular, the radiologist who is skilled in the use of sonography as a guidance technique will have a distinct advantage over those who are not.

References

1. Reading CC, Charboneau JW, James EM, Hurt MR. Sonographically guided percutaneous biopsy of small (3 cm or less) masses. AJR Am J Roentgenol 1988;151:189–192
2. vanSonnenberg E, D'Agostino HB, Casola G, Halasz NA, Sanchez RB, Goodacre BW. Percutaneous abscess drainage: current concepts. Radiology 1991;181:617–626
3. McGahan JP, Lindfors KK. Percutaneous cholecystostomy: an alternative to surgical cholecystostomy for acute cholecystitis? Radiology 1989;173:481–485
4. Yu CJ, Yang PC, Chang DB, et al. Evaluation of ultrasonically guided biopsies of mediastinal masses. Chest 1991;100:399–405
5. Nagano T, Nakai Y, Taniguchi F, et al. Diagnosis of paraaortic and pelvic lymph node metastasis of gynecologic malignant tumors by ultrasound-guided percutaneous fine-needle aspiration biopsy. Cancer 1991;68:2571–2574
6. Bret PM, Guibaud L, Atri M, Gillett P, Seymour RJ, Senterman MK. Transvaginal US-guided aspiration of ovarian cysts and solid pelvic masses. Radiology 1992;185:377–380
7. Dodd GD III, Soulen MC, Kane RA, et al. Minimally invasive treatment of malignant hepatic tumors: at the threshold of a major breakthrough. Radiographics 2000;20:9–27
8. Goldberg SN, Gazelle GS, Mueller PR. Thermal ablation therapy for focal malignancy: a unified approach to underlying principles, techniques, and diagnostic imaging guidance. AJR Am J Roentgenol 2000;174:323–331
9. Head HW, Dodd GD III. Thermal ablation for hepatocellular carcinoma. Gastroenterology 2004;127:S167–S78
10. McGahan JP, Dodd GD III. Radiofrequency ablation of the liver: current status. AJR Am J Roentgenol 2001;176:3–16
11. Leyendecker JR, Dodd GD III, Halff GA, et al. Sonographically observed echogenic response during intraoperative radiofrequency ablation of cirrhotic livers: pathologic correlation. AJR Am J Roentgenol 2002;178:1147–1151
12. Montgomery RS, Rahal A, Dodd GD III, Leyendecker JR, Hubbard LG. Radiofrequency ablation of hepatic tumors: variability of lesion size using a single ablation device. AJR Am J Roentgenol 2004;182:657–661
13. Dodd GD III, Frank MS, Aribandi M, Chopra S, Chintapalli KN. Radiofrequency thermal ablation: computer analysis of the size of the thermal injury created by overlapping ablations. AJR Am J Roentgenol 2001;177:777–782
14. Chopra S, Dodd GD III, Chanin MP, Chintapalli KN. Radiofrequency ablation of hepatic tumors adjacent to the gallbladder: feasibility and safety. AJR Am J Roentgenol 2003;180:697–701
15. Head HW, Dodd GD III, Dalrymple NC, Prasad SR, EI-Merhi FM, Freckleton MW, Hubbard LG. Percutaneous radiofrequency ablation of hepatic tumors against the diaphragm frequency of diaphragmatic injury, Radiology, in press.
16. Livraghi T, Giorgio A, Marin G, et al. Hepatocellular carcinoma and cirrhosis in 746 patients: long-term results of percutaneous ethanol injection. Radiology 1995;197:101–108

Index

Note: Page numbers followed by *f* and *t* represent figures and tables respectively.

A

Abdominal aortic aneurysm, ruptured, flank pain and, 2–3
Abdominal bruit
  celiac axis stenosis and, 106, 106*f*
  midaortic syndrome and, 106–107
  renal arteriovenous fistulas and, 106, 107*f*
  renovascular hypertension and, 97, 98*t*, 100–101, 101*f*
Abdominal pain, in right lower quadrant, 90–95. *See also* Appendicitis
Abdominal trauma
  differential diagnosis of, 29–30
  nonimaging evaluation of, 30
    in hemodynamically stable patient, 30–31
    in hemodynamically unstable patient, 30
  sonographic evaluation of, 31, 31*f*–35*f*, 33–35
    in hemodynamically stable patient, 30–31
Ablation, of tumors, 161, 162*f*–163*f*, 163–164
Abortive appendicitis, 94, 94*f*
Abscess
  drainage of, ultrasound-guided percutaneous
    hepatic abscess, 158, 158*f*
    pelvic abscess, 160, 161*f*
    periappendiceal abscess, 158, 158*f*
  epididymal tail, 47, 47*f*
  frontal lobe, intraoperative ultrasound and, 125–126, 126*f*
  as pediatric acute pyelonephritis complication
    perinephric, 82, 83*f*
    renal, 80–82, 82*f*
  retroperitoneal, flank pain and, 3
  testicular, 48, 48*f*
Accessory vessels, in renovascular hypertension evaluation, 104
Acquired immunodeficiency syndrome, deep vein thrombosis differential diagnosis in, 141, 142*f*
ACR (American College of Radiology), deep vein thrombosis imaging methods and, 142, 143*f*
Acute focal pyelonephritis, 80, 81*f*
Acute lobar nephroma, 80, 81*f*
Acute pyelonephritis
  flank pain and, 3
  focal, 80, 81*f*
  in pediatric patient, 80, 80*f*–81*f*
    complications, 80–82, 82*f*–83*f*
Acute scrotal pain
  diagnostic evaluation in, 37–38
  diagnostic imaging in. *See* Color duplex sonography
  differential diagnosis of, 37, 37*t*
Adenocarcinoma, pancreatic
  ductal, 136, 136*f*
  mucinous cystadenocarcinoma, 136–137, 137*f*
Adenoma, pancreatic microcystic, 136, 136*f*
Adrenergic blocking agents, erectile dysfunction and, 67
AIDS (acquired immunodeficiency syndrome), deep vein thrombosis differential diagnosis in, 141, 142*f*

Alcohol consumption, erectile dysfunction and, 67

Alpha-adrenergic blocking agents, erectile dysfunction and, 67

American College of Radiology, deep vein thrombosis imaging methods and, 142, 143t

Aneurysm
  abdominal aortic, ruptured, 2–3
  popliteal venous, in deep venous thrombosis differential diagnosis, 141, 141f

α 1-Antichymotrypsin, PSA bound with, 112

Antidepressants, erectile dysfunction and, 67

Anuria, in renal failure evaluation, 13, 18f

Aortic aneurysm, ruptured abdominal, 2–3

Aortography, in renal failure evaluation, 14

Appendectomy, incidence of, 89

Appendicitis
  abortive, 94, 94f
  acute nonperforated, 92, 92f
  classic presentation of, 90, 90f
  differential diagnosis of, 89–90
  disorders mimicking, 89–90, 89f–90f
  early, 91, 91f
    hyperemia in, 92, 92f
  gangrenous, appendicolith within, 92, 93f
  misdiagnosis of, 89
  perforated, 94, 94f
  RLQ pain and, 89
  sonographic diagnosis of, 91, 91f–92f
    benefits in, 94, 94f
    criteria for, 92–93, 92f–93f
    limitations in, 93–94, 94f
    vs. computed tomography, 94–95, 95f
  surgery for, incidence of, 89

Appendicolith, within gangrenous appendicitis, 92, 93f

Appendix
  normal, 91, 91f
  pelvic, 90, 90f
  retrocecal, 90

Appendix testis torsion
  Doppler findings in, 52, 52f
  imaging findings in, 51–52, 51f–52f

Arteriogenic erectile dysfunction, 66

Arteriography, in erectile dysfunction evaluation, 72

Arteriovenous fistula, renal. See Renal arteriovenous fistula

Arteriovenous malformations, intraoperative ultrasound and, 126

Astrocytoma, intraoperative ultrasound and, 126, 126f

Attached-guide technique, in ultrasound-guided percutaneous treatment of masses, 156

Autonomic nervous system evaluation, in erectile dysfunction, 70

AVMs (arteriovenous malformations), intraoperative ultrasound of, 126

B

Bacterial virulence, in pediatric urinary tract infection, 76–77

Baker's cyst, in deep venous thrombosis differential diagnosis, 140f, 141

BCR (bulbocavernosus reflex), 69

"Bell-clapper sign," scrotal pain and, 37–38

Benign prostate hyperplasia, in prostate cancer differential diagnosis, 111

Beta-adrenergic blocking agents, erectile dysfunction and, 67

Bile duct disorders, intraoperative ultrasound and, 128–130, 129f–130f

Biopsy

prostate, TRUS-guided, 113*f*–114*f,* 114–116
renal, in renal failure evaluation, 13
ultrasound-guided percutaneous, of masses, 157
    in liver, 157–158, 158*f*
    in lung, 158–159, 159*f*–160*f*
    retroperitoneal lymph nodes, 160, 160*f*
Biothesiometry, in erectile dysfunction evaluation, 69
Bladder. *See* Urinary bladder
Blunt abdominal trauma, sonographic imaging in, 34–35
Bowel, trauma to, 30
BPH (benign prostate hyperplasia), in prostate cancer differential diagnosis, 111
Brain
    intraoperative ultrasound of, 124–127, 124*f*–127*f*
    metastases to, intraoperative ultrasound and, 125, 125*f*
Bruit, abdominal. *See* Abdominal bruit
Bulbocavernosus reflex, 69
Bursitis, in lower extremity joints. *See* Baker's cyst

C
Calcifications, pancreatic, intraoperative ultrasound of, 137, 137*f*
Calculi, renal, in pediatric acute pyelonephritis, 80, 81*f*
Calculus disease
    flank pain and, 2–3
    ureteral, obstructing distal, 24–25, 24*f*–25*f*
Calf veins, in deep vein thrombosis imaging, 145–146, 146*f*
    limitations, 150–152, 151*f*–152*f*
    scanning technique, 147
Cancer. *See* Carcinoma
Candida albicans, in pediatric urinary tract infections, 85, 85*f*
Carcinoma
    cholangiocarcinoma, Klatskin-type, 130, 130*f*
    gallbladder, intraoperative ultrasound and, 129, 129*f*
    hepatocellular. *See* Hepatocellular carcinoma
    of prostate. *See* Prostate cancer
    renal cell, in hematuria evaluation, 22–23
Cardiothoracic diseases, flank pain and, 3
Cardiovascular disease, erectile dysfunction and, 68
Catheter drainage, ultrasound-guided percutaneous, 157
    of hepatic abscess, 158, 158*f*
    of pelvic abscess, 160, 161*f*
    of periappendiceal abscess, 158, 158*f*
Cavernosography, in erectile dysfunction evaluation, 72
Cavernosometry, in erectile dysfunction evaluation, 71–72
CDS. *See* Color Doppler sonography
Celiac axis stenosis, abdominal bruit and, 106, 106*f*
Cellulitis, scrotal, 48–49, 49*f*
Cervical hemangioblastoma, intraoperative ultrasound and, 127–128, 128*f*
Cervical spinal cord, intraoperative ultrasound and, 127, 128*f*
CFDI. *See* Color flow Doppler imaging
Children, urinary tract infections in. *See* Pediatric urinary tract infections
Cholangiocarcinoma, Klatskin-type, 130, 130*f*
Cholecystostomy, ultrasound-guided percutaneous, 158, 159*f*
Chronic venous insufficiency syndrome
    diagnosis of, 153, 153*f*
    ultrasound-guided treatment for, 153
Chronic venous thrombosis, diagnosis of, 152, 152*f*–153*f*

Cidex, for probe sterilization, 123–124
Cigarette smoking, erectile dysfunction and, 67
Cimetidine, erectile dysfunction and, 67
Colitis, pseudomembranous, of right colon, 92, 93*f*
Color Doppler sonography. *See also* Color duplex sonography
   in deep vein thrombosis evaluation, 141
   in intrarenal artery evaluation, 103–104*f*, 103*f*–104*f*
   in renal failure
      acute form, 16*f*
      ureteral jet and, 17–18, 18*f*
   in renovascular hypertension, 100–102, 100*f*–101*f*
Color duplex sonography
   in appendix testis torsion, 52, 52*f*
   in epididymitis, 49–51, 50*f*–51*f*
   in epididymo-orchitis, 49–51, 50*f*–51*f*
   in erectile dysfunction evaluation, 59*f*–65*f*, 72–73
      benefits, 74
      new techniques, 74
      percent arterial dilatation, 73–74
      pitfalls, 74
      technique, 59*f*–65*f*, 73
   in orchitis, 49–51, 50*f*–51*f*
   in scrotal pain evaluation, 38
      equipment and machine setup, 38–39
      rationale for using, 39
      technique, 39–41, 39*f*–40*f*
   in testicular evaluation
      torsion, 45–46, 45*f*–46*f*
      trauma, 54
      tumors, 53, 53*f*
Color flow Doppler imaging
   in chronic venous thrombosis, 152, 152*f*–153*f*
   in deep vein thrombosis evaluation, 141, 141*f*, 142
      accuracy, 148*f*, 149–150
      classic findings in, 148–149, 148*f*–150*f*
      examination protocol, 146
      limitations, 150–152, 151*f*–152*f*
      normal findings, 143–144, 144*f*
   of pancreatic islet cell tumor, 136*f*
Colorectal metastases, intraoperative ultrasound and, 132, 132*f*–133*f*
Common femoral vein
   in chronic venous thrombosis evaluation, 152, 153*f*
   in deep vein thrombosis evaluation, 144, 145*f*
      classic findings, 148*f*, 149
      limited compression examination, 146–147
Compression, ultrasound-guided, of common femoral artery, 146–147
Computed tomography
   in abdominal trauma evaluation, 29
   in deep vein thrombosis evaluation, 142
   in flank pain evaluation, 6–8
   guiding percutaneous treatment of masses, 156, 159–160
      in lung, 159*f*–160*f*
      for tumor ablation, 161
   in hematuria evaluation, 22–23, 22*f*–23*f*
   multidetector. *See* Multidetector row computed tomography
   noncontrast helical, in flank pain evaluation, 6

in prostate cancer diagnosis, 114
in renal failure evaluation, 14
single photon emission, in pediatric urinary tract infection diagnosis, 79
ultrasound *vs.*
   in abdominal trauma evaluation, 35
   in appendicitis diagnosis, 94–95, 95*f*
unenhanced multidetector, in flank pain evaluation, 3, 6
Computed tomography angiography
in deep vein thrombosis evaluation, 143
in renovascular hypertension evaluation, 99–100, 100*f*
Computed tomography arterial portography, liver lesion detection by, 131–132, 132*f*
Contrast venography, in deep vein thrombosis evaluation, 142
Corpus cavernosum
electromyography, in erectile dysfunction evaluation, 70
in penile anatomy, 61–62
Corpus spongiosum, in penile anatomy, 61–62
Creatinine, in renal failure evaluation, 13
Crohn's disease, 92, 93*f*
CT. *See* Computed tomography
CTA. *See* Computed tomography angiography
Cystadenocarcinoma, pancreatic mucinous, intraoperative ultrasound of, 136–137, 137*f*
Cystitis
hemorrhagic, in hematuria evaluation, 25
in pediatric patient, 79–80, 80*f*
Cyst(s)
Baker's, 140*f*, 141
   hepatic, 132, 132*f*–133*f*
   renal, 3

D
D-dimer test, in deep vein thrombosis diagnosis, 141
Deep dorsal vein, in penile anatomy, 59*f*, 62
Deep vein thrombosis
chronic venous thrombosis and, 152, 152*f*–153*f*
diagnosis of
   accuracy of presentation in, 140–141
   D-dimer test in, 141
   imaging evaluation in, 142–143, 143*t*
   implications for, 140
differential diagnosis of, 140*f*, 141, 141*f*–142*f*
ultrasound imaging in, 143
   accuracy of, 148*f*, 149–150
   classic findings with, 148–149, 148*f*–150*f*
   complications of, 150
   examination protocol for, 146
   limitations of, 150–152, 151*f*–152*f*
   limited compression examination and, 146–147
   normal findings in, 143–144, 144*f*–145*f*
   technique for, 144–148, 145*f*–146*f*
   unilateral *vs.* bilateral scanning in, 147–148
Degenerating myoma in pregnancy, appendicitis *vs.*, 90, 90*f*
Diabetes, erectile dysfunction and, 67
Diaphragm, abdominal trauma and, 33–34, 33*f*
Digital rectal examination, 111
   in prostate cancer screening, 113–114, 113*f*–114*f*, 119
   and TRUS-guided prostate biopsy, 111

Doppler flow imaging. *See also* Color flow Doppler imaging
   in deep vein thrombosis evaluation, 141, 150*f*
     intrarenal, 105–106
     renal response to revascularization and, 105
Doppler spectral analysis, in deep vein thrombosis evaluation, 142
     limitations of, 150–152, 151*f*–152*f*
     normal findings, 143–144, 144*f*–145*f*
Dorsal nerve conduction velocity studies, in erectile dysfunction evaluation, 69–70
Drainage, of masses. *See* Catheter drainage
DRASTIC (Dutch Renal Stenosis Intervention Cooperative) study, 98
DRE. *See* Digital rectal examination
Drug-induced erectile dysfunction, 66–67
Duodenal ulcer, flank pain and, 3
Duplex ultrasound. *See* Color duplex sonography
Duplication, of calf veins, in deep vein thrombosis evaluation, 146, 152
Dutch Renal Stenosis Intervention Cooperative study, 98
DVT. *See* Deep vein thrombosis

E
Early systolic compliance peak, 103, 103*f*, 104
Echogenicity
   of chronic thrombus, 152, 152*f*
   in liver tumor ablation, 161, 162*f*–163*f*, 163
   renal cortical, in renal failure, 16–17
ED. *See* Erectile dysfunction
Edema, with pain, in lower extremity. *See* Deep vein thrombosis
Emissary veins, in penile anatomy, 61–62
Endocrinologic erectile dysfunction, 66
Enterobacteriaceae, and pediatric urinary tract infection, 76
Enterococcus, and pediatric urinary tract infection, 76
Epididymis
   scrotal pain and. *See* Acute scrotal pain; Epididymitis
   sonographic evaluation of, 39–41, 39*f*, 40*f*. *See also* Color duplex sonography
     Doppler findings, 43*f*, 44
     normal findings, 41
     in testicular torsion, 44–46, 44*f*–46*f*
Epididymitis, imaging findings in, 46–48, 47*f*
   Doppler findings, 49–51, 50*f*–51*f*
Epididymo-orchitis, imaging findings in, 48, 48*f*
   Doppler findings in, 49–51, 50*f*–51*f*
Erectile dysfunction
   classification of, 66–67
   clinical scenarios in, 58, 59*f*–65*f*
   diagnostic evaluation, objectives of, 68
   differential diagnosis of, 58
   erection physiology and, 62–64, 66
   imaging evaluation in, 72
     sonographic, 72–75
   nonimaging tests in, 68–72
   penile anatomy and, 61–62
   prevalence of, 58
   systemic disease and, 67–68
   vascular evaluation in, 70–72
Erection
   nocturnal, 66

physiology of, 62–63
psychogenic, 63
reflexogenic, 63, 66
Escherichia coli
    pediatric renal abscess and, 81
    and pediatric urinary tract infection, 76, 77
    xanthogranulomatous pyelonephritis and, 3
ESP (early systolic compliance peak), 103, 103*f*, 104
Essential hypertension, clinical characteristics of, 98*t*
Excretory urography, in renal failure evaluation, 14, 14*f*, 15*f*
Extraperitoneal organs, trauma to, 30
Extremities, lower. *See* Lower extremities

F
False-negatives
    in deep vein thrombosis imaging, 151
    pyonephrosis, in pediatric patient, 82
False-positives
    in liver lesion detection, 131–132, 132*f*
    pyonephrosis, in pediatric patients, 82
Femoral veins, in deep vein thrombosis imaging, 146
Fibrosis, retroperitoneal, flank pain and, 3
Fibrositis, flank pain and, 3
Fistula, arteriovenous. *See* Renal arteriovenous fistula
Flank pain
    in appendicitis evaluation, 90
    causes of
        intraabdominal, 3
        renal and nonrenal, 1*t*
    differential diagnosis of, 1–3
    imaging evaluation in, 3–8, 4*f*–8*f*
    incidence of, 1*t*
Fluid collections, ultrasound-guided percutaneous aspiration of, 157
Fluoroscopy, guiding percutaneous treatment of masses, 156
Fournier's gangrene, scrotal cellulitis and, 49, 49*f*
Freehand technique, in ultrasound-guided percutaneous treatment of masses, 156
Frontal lobe abscess, intraoperative ultrasound and, 125–126, 126*f*
Fungal infection, of pediatric urinary tract, 85, 85*f*
Fungus balls, in pediatric urinary tract, 85, 85*f*

G
Gallbladder, intraoperative ultrasound and, 128–130, 129*f*–130*f*
    in gallbladder cancer, 129, 129*f*
    gallstones, 129, 129*f*
Gangrenous appendicitis, appendicolith within, 92, 93*f*
Gastrinoma, intraoperative ultrasound of, 135, 135*f*
Gene therapy, TRUS-guided, for prostate cancer, 115, 117*f*
Genital system, male
    acute scrotal pain and, 37–57
    erectile dysfunction and, 58–75
    prostate cancer and, 111–120
Genitocerebral-evoked potential studies, in erectile dysfunction evaluation, 70
Gleason scores, in prostate cancer evaluation, 116, 117*f*, 118, 118*f*
Glioblastoma, intraoperative ultrasound and, 125, 126*f*
Glioma, hyperechoic, intraoperative ultrasound and, 124, 125*f*

Glucagonomas, intraoperative ultrasound of, 135
Granuloma, sperm, postvasectomy pain and, 55–56, 55*f*–56*f*
Greater saphenous vein, ultrasound guided ablation of, 153

H
Heart rate variability, in erectile dysfunction evaluation, 70
Hemangioblastoma of cervical cord, intraoperative ultrasound and, 127–128, 128*f*
Hematoma, in deep venous thrombosis differential diagnosis, 141
Hematuria
    asymptomatic, occurrence of, 20
    causes of, 20*t*
    differential diagnosis of, 20, 21*f*
    imaging evaluation of, 22–24, 22*f*–23*f*
        cost considerations, 25, 27
        recommendations for, 27
        by ultrasound, 24–25, 24*f*–26*f*, 27
    nonimaging evaluation, 21–22
Hemodynamic stability, in abdominal trauma patient
    assessment of, 30
    sonography as screening tool in, 35
Hemoperitoneum
    in hepatorenal space, 31, 31*f*
    in posterior deep pelvis, 34, 34*f*
Hemorrhagic cystitis, in hematuria evaluation, 25
Hepatic abscess, ultrasound-guided percutaneous drainage of, 158, 158*f*
Hepatic artery, accessory or replaced, intraoperative ultrasound and, 131–132, 132*f*
Hepatic cysts, intraoperative ultrasound and, 132, 132*f*–133*f*
Hepatic metastases, intraoperative ultrasound and, 131, 131*f*
Hepatocellular carcinoma
    intraoperative ultrasound and, 133–134, 134*f*
    tumor ablation in, 163, 163*f*
Hernia, inguinal, with scrotal extension, 56, 56*f*
Host factors, in pediatric urinary tract infection, 77
Hyperlipidemia, erectile dysfunction and, 67–68
Hypertension
    erectile dysfunction and, 68
    essential, characteristics of, 98*t*
    renovascular. *See* Renovascular hypertension

I
Iliac veins, in deep venous thrombosis evaluation, 149, 150*f*
    imaging limitations, 150*f*, 151
Impedance plethysmography, in deep vein thrombosis evaluation, 142
Infection
    epididymal. *See* Epididymitis; Epididymo-orchitis
    of pediatric urinary tract. *See* Pediatric urinary tract infections
    testicular torsion *vs.*, in acute scrotal pain differentiation, 37–38
Inguinal hernia, with scrotal extension, 56, 56*f*
Insulinoma, intraoperative ultrasound of, 135, 135*f*
Intraoperative ultrasound
    abdominal applications of, 128–138
        gallbladder and bile ducts, 128–130, 129*f*–130*f*
        liver, 130–134, 131*f*–134*f*
        pancreas, 134–138, 135*f*–137*f*
    background in, 123
    efficient, technique for, 123–124

neurosurgical application of, 124–128
  brain, 124–127, 124*f*–127*f*
  spine, 127–128, 127*f*–128*f*
  probe sterilization for, 123–124
Intraperitoneal fluid, abdominal trauma and, 29
  in paracolic gutter, 34, 35*f*
Intrarenal artery evaluation, in renovascular hypertension diagnosis, 102–105, 103*f*–104*f*
Intratesticular vessels, sonographic evaluation of, 41
  Doppler findings, 42–44, 42*f*–43*f*
Intravenous pyelogram, in hematuria evaluation, 22
Intravenous urogram, in flank pain evaluation, 3
Islet cell tumors, intraoperative ultrasound of, 135, 136*f*
IVP (intravenous pyelogram), in hematuria evaluation, 22
IVU (intravenous urogram), in flank pain evaluation, 3

K
Kidneys, trauma to, 33. *See also* Renal *entries*
Klatskin-type cholangiocarcinoma, 130, 130*f*

L
Laparoscopic ultrasound, 124
  of pancreas, 135–136
Laser ablation, for chronic venous insufficiency, 153
Legs. *See* Lower extremities
Liquefactive necrosis, epididymal tail, 47, 47*f*
Liver. *See also* Hepatic *and* Hepato- *entries*
  intraoperative ultrasound of, 130–134, 131*f*–134*f*
  trauma to, 32*f*–33*f*, 33
  tumor ablation in, 161, 162*f*–163*f*, 163
  ultrasound-guided percutaneous biopsy in, 157–158, 158*f*
Liver metastases, intraoperative ultrasound and, 131, 131*f*
Lobar nephroma, acute, 80, 81*f*
Lower extremities, in deep vein thrombosis evaluation, 143–144, 144*f*–145*f*
  vessels commonly visualized, 145, 145*f*
Lung, ultrasound-guided percutaneous biopsy of, 158–159, 159*f*–160*f*
LUS. *See* Laparoscopic ultrasound
Lymph nodes, retroperitoneal, ultrasound-guided percutaneous biopsy of, 160, 160*f*
Lymphadenopathy, metastatic, intraoperative ultrasound and, 133, 133*f*
Lymphoma, non-Hodgkin's, 141, 142*f*

M
α 2-Macroglobulin, PSA bound with, 112
Magnetic resonance angiography
  in erectile dysfunction evaluation, 72
  in flank pain evaluation, 3–8
  in hematuria evaluation, 23
  in renal failure evaluation, 14
  in renovascular hypertension evaluation, 99, 99*f*
Magnetic resonance imaging
  in erectile dysfunction evaluation, 72
  guiding percutaneous treatment of masses, for tumor ablation, 161
  in hematuria evaluation, 22
  in pediatric urinary tract infection diagnosis, 79
  in prostate cancer diagnosis, 114
  in renal failure evaluation, 14–15, 15*f*
Magnetic resonance urography

in flank pain evaluation, 6
in renal failure evaluation, 14, 15*f*
Magnetic resonance venography, in deep vein thrombosis evaluation, 143
Male genital system
acute scrotal pain and, 37–57
erectile dysfunction and, 58–75
prostate cancer and, 111–120
Massachusetts Male Aging Study, erectile dysfunction and, 58
Masses, percutaneous treatment of
image guidance modalities for, 156
ultrasound-guided, 156–164. *See also* Ultrasound-guided percutaneous treatment
McBurney point, in appendicitis evaluation, 90
MDC. *See* Multidetector row computed tomography
Mesenteric adenitis, appendicitis *vs.*, 89, 89*f*
Mesenteric injury, 30
Metastases
brain, intraoperative ultrasound and, 125, 125*f*
colorectal, intraoperative ultrasound and, 132, 132*f*–133*f*
hepatic, intraoperative ultrasound and, 131, 131*f*
lymph node, intraoperative ultrasound and, 133, 133*f*
spinal, flank pain and, 3
Microbubble ultrasound contrast agents, in calf vein scanning, 147–148
Midaortic syndrome, abdominal bruit and, 106–107
Midepigastric pain, flank pain and, 3
MMAS (Massachusetts Male Aging Study), erectile dysfunction and, 58
MRA. *See* Magnetic resonance angiography
MRI. *See* Magnetic resonance imaging
MRU. *See* Magnetic resonance urography
Mucinous tumors, pancreatic, intraoperative ultrasound of, 136–137, 137*f*
Multidetector row computed tomography
in deep vein thrombosis evaluation, 142–143
in liver lesion detection, 131–132
Musculoskeletal pain, flank pain and, 3
Mycelial clumps, in pediatric urinary tract infections, 85, 85*f*
Myoma, degenerating, appendicitis *vs.*, 90, 90*f*

N
NECT (noncontrast helical computed tomography), in flank pain evaluation, 6
Nephrolithiasis, in hematuria evaluation, 24–25, 25*f*
Nephroma, acute lobar, 80, 81*f*
Nephrostomy, ultrasound-guided percutaneous, 158, 159*f*
Neurogenic erectile dysfunction, 66
Neurological testing, in erectile dysfunction evaluation, 69–70
Nocturnal erection, 66
Nocturnal penile tumescence and rigidity testing, 69
Non-Hodgkin's lymphoma, in differential diagnosis of deep vein thrombosis, 141, 142*f*
Noncontrast helical computed tomography, in flank pain evaluation, 6
Nonperforated appendicitis, acute, 92, 92*f*
NPTR (nocturnal penile tumescence and rigidity testing), 69
Nuclear medicine scan, in acute renal failure, 16*f*

O
Orchitis, imaging findings in, 48, 48*f*
Doppler findings, 49–51, 50*f*–51*f*
Osmolality, urine, in renal failure evaluation, 13
Osteomyelitis, flank pain and, 3

P

Pain
  abdominal, in right lower quadrant, 90–95. *See also* Appendicitis
  flank. *See* Flank pain
  postvasectomy, 55–56, 55*f*–56*f*
Pancreas, intraoperative ultrasound of, 134–138, 135*f*–137*f*
  pancreatic adenocarcinoma, 136, 136*f*
Pancreatitis
  calcific, intraoperative ultrasound of, 137, 137*f*
  flank pain and, 3
Paracentesis, ultrasound-guided percutaneous, 157
Paracolic gutter, intraperitoneal fluid in, 34, 35*f*
Patient history, in renal failure evaluation, 13
PBI (penile brachial pressure index), 70–71
PCR (polymerase chain reaction), PSA testing and, 113
Peak systolic velocity, in renovascular hypertension diagnosis, 102
Pediatric urinary tract infections
  bacterial, 76–77. *See also individual infections and pathogens*
  clinical outcome of, 78
  epidemiology of, 76
  fungal, 85, 85*f*
  imaging tests in, 78–79
  nonimaging tests in, 78
  pathogenesis of, 76–78
  ultrasound imaging in, 79
    acute pyelonephritis, 80–82, 80*f*–83*f*
    chronic pyelonephritis, 84*f*, 85
    cystitis, 79–80, 80*f*
    fungal infection, 85, 85*f*
    vesicoureteral reflux, 82–83
Pelvic abscess, ultrasound-guided percutaneous drainage of, 160, 161*f*
Pelvic inflammatory disease, appendicitis *vs.*, 89*f*, 90
Penile blood flow studies, in erectile dysfunction evaluation, 72–74. *See also* Color duplex sonography
Penile brachial pressure index, 70–71
Penile plethysmography, in erectile dysfunction evaluation, 71
Penile pulse volume recording, in erectile dysfunction evaluation, 71
Penis
  anatomy of, 61–62
  and erection physiology, 62–64, 66
  innervation of, 62
Perforated appendicitis, 94, 94*f*
Periappendiceal abscess, ultrasound-guided percutaneous drainage of, 158, 158*f*
Peroneal veins, in deep vein thrombosis imaging, 145, 146*f*
  classic findings in, 149*f*
PET (positron emission tomography), in prostate cancer diagnosis, 114
Pharmacological testing, in erectile dysfunction evaluation, 71
Physical examination
  in erectile dysfunction, 68
  in renal failure evaluation, 13
  in scrotal pain evaluation, 38
PI (pulsatility index), in renovascular hypertension evaluation, 104–105
Planar scintigraphy, in pediatric urinary tract infection diagnosis, 79
Pleural space fluid, abdominal trauma and, 33–34, 33*f*
Polymerase chain reaction, PSA testing and, 113
Popliteal vein, in deep vein thrombosis evaluation, 151, 151*f*
  aneurysm diagnosis and, 141, 141*f*
  classic findings in, 148*f*, 149

Positron emission tomography, in prostate cancer diagnosis, 114
Power Doppler imaging. *See also* Color duplex sonography
  in hematuria evaluation, 23, 23*f*
  in prostate cancer evaluation, 117, 117*f*
Pregnancy, degenerating myoma in, appendicitis *vs.*, 90, 90*f*
Prostate acid phosphatase, in prostate cancer diagnosis, 113
Prostate biopsy, TRUS-guided, 113*f*–114*f*, 114–116
Prostate brachytherapy, TRUS-guided, 115
Prostate cancer
  deaths from, 111
  differential diagnosis of, 111
  imaging evaluation in, 114
    by ultrasound, 114–119, 115*f*–119*f*. *See also* Transrectal ultrasound
  incidence of, 111
  nonimaging tests for, 111–114, 113*f*–114*f*
Prostate-specific antigen
  age-specific, 112
  in benign prostate hyperplasia, 112
  density of, 112
  molecular forms of, 112–113
  in prostate cancer screening, 111–113, 119
  sensitivity limitations of, 112
  synthesis of, 112
  velocity of, 112
Prostate-specific antigen density, 111
  TRUS-guided prostate biopsy and, 116
Proteus mirabilis, xanthogranulomatous pyelonephritis and, 3
PSA. *See* Prostate-specific antigen
PSAD. *See* Prostate-specific antigen density
Pseudoaneurysm, right common femoral artery, in differential diagnosis of deep vein thrombosis, 141, 142*f*
Pseudomembranous colitis, of right colon, 92, 93*f*
Pseudomonas, and pediatric urinary tract infection, 76
PSV (peak systolic velocity), in renovascular hypertension diagnosis, 102
Psychogenic erection, 63
  dysfunctional, 66
Psychological interview, in erectile dysfunction evaluation, 69
Psychometric testing, in erectile dysfunction evaluation, 69
Psychosexual history, in erectile dysfunction, 68
Pulmonary disease, erectile dysfunction and, 68
Pulsatility index, in renovascular hypertension evaluation, 104–105
Pulsus tardus, intrarenal artery and, 103, 103*f*–104*f*
Pyelonephritis
  bilateral focal, in hematuria evaluation, 23, 23*f*
  flank pain and, 3, 7–8, 7*f*–8*f*
  in pediatric patient, 77–78
    acute form, 80–82, 80*f*–83*f*
    chronic form, 84*f*, 85
Pyonephrosis
  flank pain and, 7, 7*f*
  as pediatric acute pyelonephritis complication, 82, 83*f*

R
Radiofrequency ablation
  for chronic venous insufficiency, 153
  of tumors, 161, 162*f*–163*f*, 163–164
Radiography
  abdominal

in flank pain evaluation, 3
in renal failure evaluation, 13–14, 13*f*
in pediatric urinary tract infection diagnosis, 78
Radioisotopic penography, in erectile dysfunction evaluation, 72
Radionuclide venography, in deep vein thrombosis evaluation, 142
RAR (renal:aortic ratio), in renovascular hypertension diagnosis, 102
Reflexogenic erection, 63, 66
Reflux nephropathy, 77
Renal abscess, as pediatric acute pyelonephritis complication, 80–82, 82*f*
Renal arteries
  color Doppler imaging of, 100–102, 100*f*–101*f*
  Doppler analysis and, 105–106
Renal arteriography, in hematuria evaluation, 23
Renal arteriovenous fistula
  abdominal bruit and, 106, 107*f*
  in hematuria evaluation, 23, 23*f*
Renal biopsy, in renal failure evaluation, 13
Renal calculi, in pediatric acute pyelonephritis, 80, 81*f*
Renal cell carcinoma, in hematuria evaluation, 22–23, 22*f*
Renal cortex
  echogenicity of, 16–17
  thickness of, 15–16, 17*f*
Renal cysts, flank pain and, 3
Renal failure
  acute
    neonatal, 16*f*
    postrenal, 17
  chronic, 15, 15*f*
    erectile dysfunction and, 68
  differential diagnosis of, 12–13
  imaging evaluation in, 13–15, 13*f*–15*f*
    by ultrasound, 15–18, 15*f*–18*f*
  nonimaging evaluation in, 13
  prevalence of, 12
  types of, 12*f*
Renal neoplasms, flank pain and, 3
Renal parenchymal disease, ultrasound evaluation of, 25, 26*f*
Renal scintigraphy, in renal failure evaluation, 14
Renal vascular compromise, flank pain and, 3
Renal vein thrombosis, flank pain and, 8, 8*f*
Renal:aortic ratio, in renovascular hypertension diagnosis, 102
Renovascular hypertension
  cause of, 97
  clinical characteristics of, 98*t*
  differential diagnosis of, 97–98
  imaging evaluation in, 99–100, 99*f*–100*f*
    sonographic, 100–106, 100*f*–101*f*, 103*f*–104*f*
  nonimaging evaluation in, 98–99
  prevalence of, 97
  workup for at-risk patients, 97–98
Resistive index
  in renal failure, 17
  in renal obstruction, 4–5, 4*f*, 6
  in renovascular hypertension evaluation, 104–105
Respiratory phasicity, in deep vein thrombosis evaluation, 143–144, 144*f*–145*f*, 151, 151*f*
Retrograde pyelography, in renal failure evaluation, 14
Retroperitoneal abscess, flank pain and, 3

Retroperitoneal fibrosis, flank pain and, 3
Revascularization, for renovascular hypertension, 105
Reverse transcriptase, PSA testing and, 113
RFA (radiofrequency ablation), of tumors, 161, 162f–163f, 163–164
RI. *See* Resistive index
Right colon, pseudomembranous colitis of, 92, 93f
Right lower quadrant pain. *See also* Appendicitis
   diagnostic evaluation of, 90–91
     sonographic, 91–95
RLQ pain. *See* Right lower quadrant pain
mRNA (messenger ribonucleic acid), PSA testing and, 113
RT (reverse transcriptase), PSA testing and, 113
RVH. *See* Renovascular hypertension

S
Scintigraphy
   in pediatric urinary tract infection diagnosis, 79
   in renovascular hypertension evaluation, 99
Screening
   in abdominal trauma patient, 35
   prostate-specific antigen, for prostate cancer, 111–113, 119
Scrotal cellulitis, 48–49, 49f
Scrotal pain, acute. *See* Acute scrotal pain
Scrotum
   acute pain in. *See* Acute scrotal pain
   Doppler evaluation of, 39. *See also* Color duplex sonography
   inguinal hernia and, 56, 56f
Sensory perception threshold, in erectile dysfunction evaluation, 69
Sexual stimulation, vibrotactile or visual, in erectile dysfunction evaluation, 69
SFVs (superficial femoral veins), in deep vein thrombosis imaging, 145, 146
Single photon emission computed tomography, in pediatric urinary tract infection diagnosis, 79
Somatostatinomas, intraoperative ultrasound of, 135
SPECT (single photon emission computed tomography), in pediatric urinary tract infection diagnosis, 79
Sperm granuloma, postvasectomy pain and, 55–56, 55f–56f
Spermatic cord thrombosis, imaging findings in, 54–55, 54f
   Doppler findings, 55
Spermatic cords
   scrotal pain and. *See* Acute scrotal pain
   sonographic evaluation of, 39–41, 40f. *See also* Color duplex sonography
     Doppler findings, 43–44, 43f
     normal, 41
     in testicular torsion, 44–46, 44f–46f
Spinal cord, intraoperative ultrasound of, 127–128, 127f–128f
Spinal dysraphism, intraoperative ultrasound of, 127–128, 127f–128f
Spine
   intraoperative ultrasound of, 127–128, 127f–128f
   metastases to, flank pain and, 3
Spleen, trauma to, 30, 31, 31f–32f, 33
SSR (sympathetic skin response), in erectile dysfunction evaluation, 70
Staghorn calculus, in pediatric acute pyelonephritis, 80, 81f
Staphylococcus aureus, pediatric renal abscess and, 81
Stenosis, celiac axis, abdominal bruit and, 106, 106f
Sterilization, of intraoperative ultrasound probes, 123–124
Sterrad sterilization system, 124
Superficial femoral veins, in deep vein thrombosis imaging, 145, 146
Superior mesenteric artery and vein, intraoperative ultrasound of, 136, 136f

Swelling, in leg, with pain or edema. *See* Deep vein thrombosis
Sympathetic skin response, in erectile dysfunction evaluation, 70
Sympatholytics, centrally-acting, erectile dysfunction and, 67

T
Tc-99m-DMSA scintigraphy, in pediatric urinary tract infection diagnosis, 79
Testes, scrotal pain and, sonographic evaluation of, 39–41, 40*f*. *See also* Color duplex sonography
   acute pain, 37–38, 37*t*
   in appendix testis torsion, 51–52, 51*f*–52*f*
   Doppler findings in, 42–43, 42*f*–44*f*
   in infection. *See* Epididymitis; Epididymo-orchitis
   normal findings in, 41
   in testicular torsion, 44–46, 44*f*–46*f*
   trauma and, 53–54, 53*f*–54*f*
   tumors and, 52–53, 53*f*
Testicular torsion
   imaging findings in, 44–45, 44*f*–45*f*
     Doppler findings, 45–46, 45*f*–46*f*
   infection *vs.*, in acute scrotal pain differentiation, 37–38
Testicular trauma, imaging findings in, 53, 53*f*–54*f*
   Doppler findings, 54
Testicular tumors, imaging findings in, 52–53, 53*f*
   Doppler findings, 53, 53*f*
Thoracentesis, ultrasound-guided percutaneous, 157
Thoracic spinal cord, intraoperative ultrasound and, 127, 127*f*
3-D volume acquisition ultrasound, in prostate cancer evaluation, 116, 117*f*
Thrombosis
   deep vein. *See* Deep vein thrombosis
   ovarian vein, mimicking appendicitis, 92, 93*f*
   renal vein, flank pain and, 8, 8*f*
   spermatic cord, 54–55, 54*f*
   of variocele, 56, 56*f*
Tibial veins, in deep vein thrombosis imaging, 145, 146*f*
   classic findings, 149*f*
Tissue sampling. *See* Biopsy
Torsion
   appendix testis, 51–52, 51*f*–52*f*
   testicular. *See* Testicular torsion
Transrectal ultrasound, 111
   accuracy of, 115*f*–119*f*, 116–118
   limitations of, 118–119
   prostate biopsy and, 113*f*–114*f*, 114–116
Trauma
   to abdomen. *See* Abdominal trauma
   to testes, 53–54, 53*f*–54*f*
TRUS. *See* Transrectal ultrasound
Tumor ablation, ultrasound-guided percutaneous, 160–164, 162*f*–163*f*
Tumors. *See also individually named tumors*
   islet cell, intraoperative ultrasound of, 135, 136*f*
   mucinous, pancreatic, 136–137, 137*f*
   testicular, 52–53, 53*f*
Tunica albuginea, in penile anatomy, 61–62

U
UECT (unenhanced multidetector computed tomography), in flank pain evaluation, 3, 6
Ultrasound-guided compression, of common femoral artery, deep vein thrombosis and, 146–147

Ultrasound-guided percutaneous treatment, of masses
    general applications for, 157–160, 158*f*–161*f*
    methods of, 156
    techniques for, 157
    for tumor ablation, 160–164, 162*f*–163*f*
Unenhanced multidetector computed tomography, in flank pain evaluation, 3, 6
Urea levels, in renal failure evaluation, 13
Ureteral calculus, obstructing distal, in hematuria evaluation, 24–25, 24*f*–25*f*
Ureteral jet, in renal failure
    color Doppler imaging of, 17–18, 18*f*
    obstruction of, 17–18, 18*f*
Ureteral obstruction, in flank pain evaluation, 4, 4*f*
Ureterolithiasis, diagnosis of, imaging modalities for, 3–4
Urinary bladder
    dysfunctional voiding of, in pediatric urinary tract infection, 77
    ultrasound evaluation of, 25, 26*f*
Urinary tract
    infections in children. *See* Pediatric urinary tract infections
    obstruction of, in flank pain evaluation, 3, 4*f*, 5
Urine culture, in pediatric urinary tract infection diagnosis, 78
Urine flow
    impeded, pediatric urinary tract infections and, 77
    and volume in renal failure evaluation, 13
UTI. *See* Pediatric urinary tract infections

V
Valsalva maneuver, in deep vein thrombosis evaluation, 143, 144*f*
Variocele, thrombosis of, 56, 56*f*
Vas deferens, postvasectomy pain and, 55, 55*f*
Vascular compromise, renal, flank pain and, 3
Vasculogenic erectile dysfunction, 66–67
Vasectomy, pain following, 55–56, 55*f*–56*f*
VCUG (voiding cystourethrogram), in pediatric urinary tract infection diagnosis, 78–79
Venogenic erectile dysfunction, 66
Venous enhanced subtracted peak arterial technique, in MR venography, 143, 152
Vesicoureteral reflux
    and pediatric urinary tract infection association, 77–78
    ultrasound evaluation of, 82–83
VESPA (venous enhanced subtracted peak arterial) technique, in MR venography, 143
Vibrotactile sexual stimulation, in erectile dysfunction evaluation, 69
Visual sexual stimulation, in erectile dysfunction evaluation, 69
Voiding cystourethrogram, in pediatric urinary tract infection diagnosis, 78–79
Voiding dysfunction, pediatric urinary tract infection and, 77, 78
VUR. *See* Vesicoureteral reflux

W
Weight changes, in renal failure evaluation, 13
Women, appendicitis diagnosis in, 90, 90*f*

X
Xanthogranulomatous pyelonephritis, flank pain and, 3